HQsolutions

Resource for the Healthcare Quality Professional

FOURTH EDITION

EDITORS

Luc R. Pelletier, MSN, APRN, PMHCNS-BC, CPHQ, FNAHQ, FAAN

Christy L. Beaudin, PhD, LCSW, CPHQ, FNAHQ

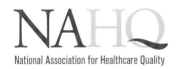

National Association for Healthcare Quality

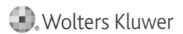 Wolters Kluwer

Philadelphia • Baltimore • New York • London
Buenos Aires • Hong Kong • Sydney • Tokyo

Acquisitions Editor: Nicole Dernoski
Development Editor: Tom Conville
Editorial Coordinator: Tim Rinehart
Editorial Assistant: Kaitlin Campbell
Marketing Manager: Linda Wetmore
Production Project Manager: Marian Bellus
Design Coordinator: Stephen Druding
Manufacturing Coordinator: Kathy Brown
Prepress Vendor: S4Carlisle Publishing Services

Fourth Edition

9 8 7 6 5 4 3 2

Printed in China

Library of Congress Cataloging-in-Publication Data

Names: Pelletier, Luc Reginald, editor. | Beaudin, Christy L., editor. |
   National Association for Healthcare Quality (U.S.)
Title: HQ solutions : resource for the healthcare quality professional /
   [edited by] Luc R. Pelletier, MSN, PMHCNS-BC, CPHQ, FNAHQ, FAAN, Christy
   L. Beaudin, PhD, LCSW, CPHQ, FNAHQ.
Other titles: Q solutions. | Resource for the healthcare quality professional
Description: Fourth edition. | Philadelphia: Wolters Kluwer Health, [2018] |
   Revised edition of: Q solutions : essential resources for the healthcare
   quality professional / editors, Luc R. Pelletier. 5 volumes. 3rd edition.
   2012. | Includes bibliographical references.
Identifiers: LCCN 2017038027 | ISBN 9781496389770 (paperback)
Subjects: LCSH: Medical care—Quality control. | Total quality management. |
   BISAC: MEDICAL / Nursing / Management & Leadership.
Classification: LCC RA399.A3 Q25 2018 | DDC 362.1—dc23
LC record available at https://lccn.loc.gov/2017038027

LWW.com

About the Editors

Luc R. Pelletier, MSN, APRN, PMHCNS-BC, CPHQ, FNAHQ, FAAN, is a healthcare consultant; senior specialist, nursing at Sharp Mesa Vista Hospital; adjunct professor at the University of San Diego Hahn School of Nursing and Health Science/Betty and Bob Beyster Institute for Nursing Research, Advanced Practice, and Simulation (BINR); and core adjunct faculty at National University, San Diego, CA. He is a graduate of Yale University (MSN) and Fairfield University (BSN). His current research focuses on recruitment and retention strategies of new graduate nurses into the psychiatric-mental health nursing profession and the measurement of patient engagement in healthcare. He is a technical writer and editor. In addition, he publishes widely in the areas of nursing administration, quality and safety, and patient engagement, including several books, numerous book chapters, and peer-reviewed articles. Mr. Pelletier participates in local and national initiatives focusing on safe and equitable care for persons with enduring behavioral health challenges. His other efforts help inform and shape systems of care and national standards of policy and performance such as a nurse expert with the U.S. Department of Justice and a scientific consultant to the National Institutes of Health. Mr. Pelletier is a Fellow of the American Academy of Nursing and NAHQ. For 9 years, he served as editor in chief for the *Journal for Healthcare Quality*.

Christy L. Beaudin, PhD, LCSW, CPHQ, FNAHQ, has more than 20 years of exceptional leadership in healthcare quality, working with health plans, acute care hospitals, primary care clinics, and behavioral healthcare facilities and supporting their achievement of mission, vision, and strategic goals for quality and patient safety. At the executive level, she delivers positive results for quality, safety, and performance improvement efforts, meeting stakeholder expectations, such as those of the Centers for Medicare & Medicaid Services, National Committee for Quality Assurance, The Joint Commission, and CARF International. Dr. Beaudin holds degrees from the University of California, Los Angeles School of Public Health (PhD), San Diego State University (MSW), and California State University San Bernardino (BA). She is a Fellow of the National Association for Healthcare Quality and the California HealthCare Foundation Health Care Leadership Program. With a strong commitment to the community, she volunteers for state and national quality initiatives, including the California Office of Statewide Health Planning and Development and National Association for Healthcare Quality (NAHQ), and is adjunct faculty at the University of Redlands. Widely published, she works with several peer-reviewed journals as an editorial board/review panel member and is an associate editor for the *Journal for Healthcare Quality*.

About the Authors

Cathy E. Duquette, PhD, RN, NEA-BC, CPHQ, FNAHQ, is executive vice president for nursing affairs for Lifespan. In this role, she is responsible for co-leading the system strategy for quality, safety, and patient experience with her physician colleague, the executive vice president for physician affairs, as well as leading nursing and the organization's efforts to implement lean and six sigma across the health system. Since 2006, Dr. Duquette has served as an appraiser for the Magnet Recognition Program. Her more than 30 years in healthcare include roles as senior vice president and chief quality officer of Rhode Island Hospital; vice president of nursing and patient care services and chief nursing officer at Newport Hospital; senior vice president at the Hospital Association of Rhode Island; and staff roles in hospital quality improvement and clinical nursing in the critical care setting. She received a Bachelor of Science and a Master of Science in Nursing from the University of Rhode Island and a PhD in Nursing from the University of Massachusetts Amherst and Worcester. In addition, she holds certifications as a Certified Professional in Healthcare Quality, Nursing Executive-Advanced, and Six Sigma Black Belt. Dr. Duquette is an active member of NAHQ and was inducted as a NAHQ Fellow (2013) for her outstanding contributions to the healthcare quality profession. Since 2010, she has served on the Editorial Board of the *Journal for Healthcare Quality* and is currently an associate editor. Other accomplishments include her involvement on a number of state and national task forces relating to leadership development, hospital performance measurement, quality improvement, public reporting, and nursing workforce.

Robert J. Rosati, PhD, is chair of the Connected Health Institute and vice president of data, research, and quality at the Visiting Nurse Association Health Group (VNAHG) in Red Bank, NJ. Dr. Rosati is responsible for implementing and evaluating new technology initiatives at VNAHG. He is also responsible for quality improvement, analysis, reporting of clinical outcomes, and conducting research related to home- and community-based care. Prior to VNAHG, Dr. Rosati was at CenterLight Healthcare, a provider and managed long-term care plan in New York, which runs one of the largest PACE programs in the country. For more than a decade, he directed the internally funded research program at the Visiting Nurse Service of New York. Dr. Rosati has varied healthcare experience in research, quality management, education, and administrative roles. He received his doctorate from Hofstra University in Applied Research and Evaluation in Psychology. Dr. Rosati has extensive experience in long-term care policy, health information technology, building data warehouses, measurement, analytics, and reporting. His research interests have included factors that contribute to adverse events in home health care, case mix adjustment, improving patient outcomes, OASIS reliability, and the Medicare home health prospective payment system. His accomplishments also include the publication of more than 40 healthcare quality-related articles and numerous presentations at national meetings. He is an associate editor for the *Journal for Healthcare Quality*.

Susan V. White, PhD, RN, CPHQ, FNAHQ, NEA-BC, is the chief of quality management at the Orlando VA Medical Center in Orlando, FL. Her areas of responsibility include quality management, performance improvement, patient safety, risk management, accreditation and continuous survey readiness, peer review, infection control, and credentialing and privileging. Dr. White received a MSN as well as a PhD from the University of Florida. She has held executive positions as the associate chief nurse, quality improvement, and Magnet coordinator for the James A. Haley Veterans' Hospital in Tampa and vice president for quality at the Florida Hospital Association. She is a member of multiple professional organizations including the Florida Association for Healthcare Quality (FAHQ), NAHQ, Florida Nurses Association, American Nurses Association, Florida Organization of Nurse Executives, American Organization of Nurse Executives, and Sigma Theta Tau. She has received numerous awards including NAHQ Fellow, the Claire Glover Quality Award (2004), the FAHQ Quality Award (2004), and the FAHQ Author Award (2007). Dr. White served as vice chair on the board of directors for the Florida Center for Nursing from its inception in 2001 until 2009 and was an initial member on the Florida Patient Safety Corporation, serving as vice chair. Published widely, she co-edited *Patient Safety: Principles and Practices* and is an editorial board member and was formerly Interviews editor for the *Journal for Healthcare Quality*.

Advisory Panel

Diane Storer Brown, PhD, RN, CPHQ, FNAHQ, FAAN
Executive Director, Medicare Strategy and Operations
Kaiser Permanente Northern California Region
Oakland, California

Robert Bunting, PhD, CPHQ, CPHRM, DFASHRM, MT(ASCP)
Health Information Manager
Anthem, Inc.
Midland, Georgia

Kathy Clinefelter, MSN, MBA, CPHQ, FNAHQ
Senior Partner
Partners in Healthcare Quality
The Villages, Florida

Jodi Eisenberg, MHA, CPMSM, CSHA
Senior Director, Accreditation Education Programs
Vizient, Inc.
Chicago, Illinois

Tricia Elliott, MBA, CPHQ
Director of Quality Measurement
The Joint Commission
Oakbrook Terrace, Illinois

Shawna Forst, BA, CPHQ
Service Excellence Manager
Pella Regional Health Center
Pella, Iowa

Jason E. Gillikin, CPHQ
Manager, Advanced Analytics
Priority Health
Grand Rapids, Michigan

Dale Harvey, MS, RN
Fellow of Patient Safety
Director, Performance Improvement, Quality & Safety
    Programs
Virginia Commonwealth University Health System
Richmond, Virginia

Stephen J. Horner, RN, BSN, MBA
Vice President, Clinical Analytics
HCA
Nashville, Tennessee

Barbara G. Rebold, RN, MS, CPHQ
Director, Engagement and Improvement
Patient Safety, Risk and Quality
ECRI Institute
Philadelphia, Pennsylvania

Jake T. Redden, DHSc, CPHQ, CPPS, FACHE
Assistant Professor
University of Maryland University College
Upper Marlboro, Maryland

Patricia Schroeder, RN, MSN, MBA, FAAN
Clinical Professor
Marquette University
Milwaukee, Wisconsin

Preface

HQ Solutions: Resource for the Healthcare Quality Professional, Fourth Edition, targets audiences across the care continuum and provides critical information to develop and strengthen essential healthcare quality skills and knowlege. Healthcare is complex, difficult to navigate, and confusing. Patients, families, and staff experience different levels of engagement in the healthcare system. This engagement includes the knowledge, skills, ability, and willingness of patients (or decision-maker) to manage their own healthcare. Engaged care means there is a culture to support the practices of active collaboration between patients and providers. Healthcare quality professionals are at the forefront to safeguard practices for patient and family-centered healthcare delivery. As leaders, healthcare quality professionals mitigate barriers to engagement and work with others to achieve the Triple Aim—*better care, smarter spending*, and *healthier people*.

Better Care

Quality professionals ensure healthy infrastructures to support effective and responsive healthcare enterprises. Efforts align care, treatment, and services with evidence-based, experience-informed structures and processes yielding care that is safe, timely, effective, efficient, equitable, ethical, and person-centered. This requires developing and deploying sustainable performance and process improvement strategies.

HQ Solutions talks to the breadth and depth of critical areas for professional development and leadership: frameworks for quality management, the linking of science with practice, and the translation of data into practical information to use and share with stakeholders, whether practitioner, third-party payer, or consumer. A learning organization is sustained by fostering creativity and encouraging the spread of person-centric, evidence-based innovations.

Smarter Spending

Quality professionals recognize that affordable healthcare happens when costs are managed side by side with quality and patient safety programs. Accountability and value result from high-reliability processes and standardized work. Comprehensive care ensures continuity and reduces the chance for error, unnecessary treatment, or rework. Techniques to identify and eradicate waste are an important part of the healthcare quality professional's toolkit. In this world of teeming technology, rapid innovation, and continuously expanding science, we rely on hope day in and day out—hope that political agendas will reflect the needs of patients, families, and other stakeholders; that resources will be available for the work to be done; and that fear will not create barriers to uncovering mistakes, flaws, and failures. Armed with analytical skills and practical tools, we are a boundless force that can wildly succeed in a universe with

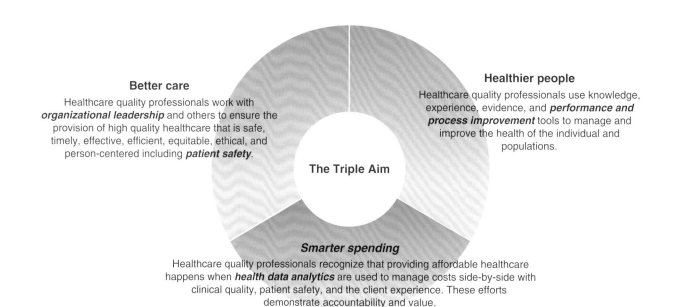

Better care
Healthcare quality professionals work with *organizational leadership* and others to ensure the provision of high quality healthcare that is safe, timely, effective, efficient, equitable, ethical, and person-centered including *patient safety*.

Healthier people
Healthcare quality professionals use knowledge, experience, evidence, and *performance and process improvement* tools to manage and improve the health of the individual and populations.

The Triple Aim

Smarter spending
Healthcare quality professionals recognize that providing affordable healthcare happens when *health data analytics* are used to manage costs side-by-side with clinical quality, patient safety, and the client experience. These efforts demonstrate accountability and value.

finite resources. *HQ Solutions* talks about how data analytics are essential to understanding where things are working and where to focus efforts for improvement. Selecting the right design tool improves quality and limits costs making healthcare efficiencies possible. Prioritization conserves resources.

Healthier People

Quality professionals use knowledge, experience, evidence, and tools to improve individual and population health. Effective care and positive outcomes result from care partnerships such as an empowered and engaged workforce or activated patients and families. Whereas prevention is an important contributor to healthier populations, monitoring care, recording variance, and exploring root causes play a role in harm reduction. An enduring and just (nonpunitive) culture supports a safe workplace. *HQ Solutions* talks about how patients can be kept safe and what leaders can do to create a strong, enduring safety culture. In addition to emerging technologies and techniques, a strong quality foundation is made possible by the collaborative relationships among stakeholders. After all, our work is relationship based. People are our business. Mutual respect and accord lead to a shared mission, alignment with core values, and a sense of camaraderie as we face complex healthcare quality challenges.

What's new with the fourth edition of *HQ Solutions*? It is innovative and timely. It is reliable and useful. It anticipates what healthcare quality professionals will face in the future. It offers setting-agnostic quality and safety tools and techniques adaptable to your organization and daily practices. It reflects recent changes in national healthcare quality and safety imperatives and initiatives, as well as the transformation of healthcare. It is the primary source for education about quality principles and practices. And, it serves as a comprehensive and contemporary review guide to prepare for the Certified Professional in Healthcare Quality (CPHQ) exam.

HQ Solutions content is informed by the Healthcare Quality Certification Commission's (HQCC) practice analysis and feedback from learners attending the CPHQ review course. The practice analysis assesses the current functions and competencies for healthcare quality professionals. Organized under the HQCC detailed content outline, this edition addresses these core competencies (Organizational Leadership, Patient Safety, Performance and Process Improvement, Health Data Analytics). *HQ Solutions* features critical information about the art and science of quality management, and environmental considerations such as legislation and healthcare reform. It delivers on the promise to be "the go-to resource" for healthcare quality and patient safety professionals. It appeals to other audiences as well: NAHQ members, academicians, researchers, consultants, administrators in healthcare organizations and systems (health plans, ACOs and HMOs), clinicians (solo,

group, facility-based practices), home health, hospice, skilled nursing facilities, rehabilitation facilities, ambulatory care, board members, students, and government agencies.

When we embarked on writing the fourth edition, there was no question about the right people to "make it happen." Esteemed authors and quality leaders, namely, Cathy E. Duquette, Robert J. Rosati, and Susie V. White, once again offer readers fresh, new perspectives on leadership, performance improvement, and data analytics. We also recognize those who contributed to previous editions—Drs. Diane Storer Brown, Jacqueline Fowler Byers, and Jean A. Grube. In addition, a thorough content examination was conducted and constructive feedback received from our expert Advisory Panel. Their efforts are greatly appreciated. We recognize the continuous support of the NAHQ Board of Directors. The Board allocated the necessary resources for *HQ Solutions*, which will contribute to the advancement of the healthcare quality profession in the 21st century. Finally, Elizabeth Kaskie from NAHQ was extraordinary in shepherding all aspects of the publication project (A-Z) to ensure a successful product launch.

The work and calling of healthcare quality professionals is noble, indeed. Nobility comes from our truth-seeking heritage. We want to share quality stories that are cogent, accurate depictions of healthcare circumstances, easily understood, and warmly received. For truth and justice in healthcare, we call on every organization and leader to

- provide resources necessary to conduct investigations and to maintain reporting systems that use state-of-the-art information technologies;
- allow and support a solid infrastructure for continuous readiness, including health information technology that supports the continuous quality improvement paradigm (and is sustained after an accreditation survey or regulatory audit);
- ensure that all organizations from the top down and bottom up are educated on the science of discovery (data, methods, analytics, and application); and
- contribute to the growing body of healthcare quality science by sharing evidence-based, outcomes-oriented quality techniques, making a difference in the safety, care, and service embraced by forward-thinking, highly reliable organizations.

May you find blessings in every day and enduring strength to lead.

Luc R. Pelletier
San Diego, CA

Christy L. Beaudin
Los Angeles, CA

Contents

Section 1: Organizational Leadership

Cathy E. Duquette

Section 2: Patient Safety

Christy L. Beaudin and Luc R. Pelletier

Section 3: Performance and Process Improvement

Susan V. White

Section 4: Health Data Analytics

Robert J. Rosati

Section 1

Organizational Leadership

Cathy E. Duquette

SECTION CONTENTS

Abstract

Organizational leadership and management of quality and safety are critical to effective continuous quality and performance improvement programs. This section provides relevant context for healthcare quality professionals regarding organizational leadership structure and integration; regulatory, accreditation, and external recognition; and education, training, and communication. Information regarding healthcare organizations as complex systems, leadership fundamentals, organizational infrastructure required to support quality and safety, strategic planning, organizational culture, and key concepts related to change and change management is provided as context to enhance the healthcare quality professional's ability to facilitate the assessment and development of the organization's culture to support organization-wide strategic planning and linking of quality, safety, and performance improvement activities to strategic goals. Regulatory, accreditation, and external recognition programs that impact healthcare quality and safety are also presented. Finally, an overview of education, training, and communication within the context of learning organizations is provided. This supports the promotion of staff knowledge and competency so the strategic goals of healthcare organizations related to quality, safety, and continuous readiness can be achieved and sustained.

Learning Objectives

1. Facilitate the assessment and development of the organization's culture to support organization-wide strategic planning and linking of quality and performance improvement activities with strategic goals.
2. Integrate the results of the quality and performance improvement process into the organization's strategic planning, and explain the value proposition for quality and safety.
3. Facilitate program and project development and evaluation, including the use of performance measures, key performance and quality indicators, and performance improvement models.
4. Discuss the functions and types of regulatory agencies (federal, state, and local) and recognize the impact of regulations on healthcare quality and safety; understand the different types of accreditation and processes associated with different accreditation procedures.
5. Identify the benefits and outcomes of continuous readiness and promote staff knowledge and competency to achieve the healthcare organization's goal of continuous readiness.

Healthcare Organizations as Complex Systems

Healthcare quality professionals often take on a leadership role in creating a culture of quality and safety, and making operational the strategies to attain performance excellence. They are typically members of the senior leadership team and provide coaching and teaching related to principles and practices of quality, safety, and performance improvement. For the leadership team to be informed and agile in their pursuit of excellence, they must understand the concepts of organization as complex systems, leadership, culture, strategic planning, change, innovation, and creativity.

The Institute of Medicine (IOM; now the Health and Medicine Division of the National Academies of Science, Engineering, and Medicine) defines *healthcare quality* as "the degree to which health services for individuals and populations increase the likelihood of desired health outcomes and are consistent with current professional knowledge."[1(pp128–129)] Care should be based on evidence-based practice and provided in a technically and culturally competent manner with good communication and shared decision making.[2] *Quality management*, derived from *total quality management*, is "a strategic, integrated management system, which involves all managers and employees and uses quantitative methods to continuously improve an organization's processes to meet and exceed customer needs, wants, and expectations."[3(p58)] For the last several years, consumers increasingly scrutinized the U.S. healthcare delivery system, and the results of their examination are not favorable. In response to the public's concern and outcry, the IOM identified six aims for healthcare improvement:

1. *Safety*—avoiding injuries to patients from care that is intended to help them;
2. *Effectiveness*—providing services based on scientific knowledge to all who could benefit and refraining from providing services to those who are not likely to benefit (avoiding overuse and underuse);
3. *Patient-centeredness*—providing care that is respectful of and responsive to individual patient preferences, needs, and values and ensuring that patient values guide all clinical decisions;
4. *Timeliness*—reducing waits and sometimes harmful delays for both those who receive care and those who give care;
5. *Efficiency*—avoiding waste, particularly waste of equipment, supplies, ideas, and energy; and
6. *Equity*—providing care that does not vary in quality with respect to personal characteristics, ethnicity, geographic location, or socioeconomic status.[2(p6)]

Healthcare quality professionals can use these aims when developing quality and safety strategies with senior leadership.

Leaders in healthcare organizations continuously search for ways to improve the quality and safety of the care and service provided in their organizations. The current healthcare environment, however, is complex and constantly changing, making continuous quality improvement a challenge. In 2001, the IOM report *Crossing the Quality Chasm* highlighted the gap between the current and ideal state of the healthcare industry regarding the quality of patient care and framed the need to provide care to patients that focuses on six specific aims as described earlier. This seminal work triggered a call to action for healthcare providers to develop strategies for closing the chasm in quality and safety in alignment with the IOM aims. Nearly two decades later, "There's no doubt we've made progress—but it's also clear that making any headway has been agonizingly slow"[4(p554)] and many opportunities remain to improve the healthcare delivery system.

Healthcare organizations are among the most complex entities, with ever-changing technology, new environmental pressures presenting almost daily, and complicated relationships among professionals, disciplines, departments, stakeholders, and organizations. Healthcare leaders and quality professionals must consider the science of complex systems to be effective in the management and continuous improvement of their organizations.

The primary dictionary definition of system is "a regularly interacting or interdependent group of items forming a unified whole."[5] The value of having a systems perspective is that systems thinking is a discipline for seeing wholes. It is a framework for seeing interrelationships rather than things; for seeing patterns of change rather than static snapshots.[6] "Today, systems thinking is needed more than ever because we are becoming overwhelmed by complexity."[6(p69)] Benefits of systems thinking include

1. aiding in solving complex problems by identifying and understanding the "big picture";
2. facilitating the identification of major components in early-stage product conception and design;
3. addressing recurring problems;
4. identifying important relationships and providing proper stakeholder perspectives;
5. avoiding excessive attention to a single part;
6. allowing for a broad-scope solution;
7. fostering integration, including who to partner with to address capability or core competency challenges; and
8. providing a basis for architecture, design, development, and redesign.[7,8]

Complexity science, or the study of complex adaptive systems (CASs), is a field applied to healthcare to understand complex human organizations. *Complex* implies the inclusion of a significant number of elements. *Adaptive* refers to the capacity to change and the ability to learn from experience.

A *system* is a set of interdependent or connected items that are referred to in CAS as independent agents.[9] CAS theory provides a useful alternative to the machine metaphor, which was first used by Newton to make sense of the world.[10] A Newtonian model of a machine suggests that the parts can explain the whole, whereas complexity science suggests that organizations are living systems in which the whole is not the sum of the parts. Rather than attempting to understand organizations by examination of the parts in a linear model, CAS theory is an acknowledgment that groups of people create outcomes and effects that are far greater than prediction by summing up the resources and skills available within the group. Three concepts—independent agents, distributed control, and nonlinearity—create conditions for perpetual innovation as the CASs develop and implement new strategies from experience. History shapes the future.

Viewing organizations as complex systems is consistent with the principles held by quality pioneers like Deming[11] and Juran[12] because quality, safety, and performance improvement practices influence all processes, functions, and departments within an organization. Making changes in one process or department naturally requires changes in other processes, functions, and departments because of their interdependencies. All the potential consequences of change need to be considered when making strategic decisions. Thus, effectiveness depends on alignment of the parts of the system. These concepts may resonate with healthcare quality professionals when reflecting on current and previous organizational experiences.

Although it is long recognized that organizations are complicated, further differentiation is necessary if one is to understand complexity and its effect on healthcare quality and safety programs. Healthcare organizations are CASs. Because they are systems of interdependent parts or agents, such as people or departments, a significant number of connections exist between their numerous elements. Those involved could have the opportunity to learn from the experiences of others in the system.[10]

The various agents of the system can respond in different and unpredictable ways, which can manifest as innovation, creative behavior, and errors,[13] or more recently as disruptive innovation.[14] Each person or department acts based on local knowledge and conditions, and a central body does not control their actions; control is distributed throughout the CAS rather than centralized. Centralized control slows down the capacity to react and adapt. Consider that in many healthcare delivery systems organizational executives typically work Monday through Friday predominantly during daytime business hours, although operations may be extensive as 24 hours a day, 7 days a week, 365 days a year. CASs may also be agents of other, larger CASs. For example, a physician is a CAS but also an agent in the department; the department is a CAS and an agent in the

hospital; the hospital is a CAS and an agent in a multisystem organization; and the organization is a CAS and an agent in the healthcare system. The entire system emerges from a pattern of interactions.

Relationships between individuals are a critical component of the CAS model. Using team sports as an analogy, a team with the best individual players can lose to a team of poorer players when the second team focuses on creating outcomes that are beyond the talents or capabilities of an individual. Team members on healthcare improvement projects who use diverse thinking styles are more likely to produce the information to solve problems or improve care.

The outcomes of a CAS emerge from a process of self-organization, which emerges from interrelationships.[10] How the system will evolve is therefore unpredictable. The coevolution of a CAS and its environment is difficult to map because it is not linear. The size of the outcome may not be correlated to the size of the input. One can relate to experiences in which a small effort resulted in huge change and, conversely, situations in which a huge effort resulted in little, if any, demonstrable or sustainable change. For example, a big push after a retreat or strategic planning session may not result in change. In contrast, one small push to the system, such as a piece of gossip or bad press, may create radical or rapid change in an organization.

CASs are drawn to attractors, which are patterns or areas that draw the energy of the system to it.[10] Using this concept flips change management perspectives from overcoming resistance to change or fighting against it to using the natural energy of the system. Studying CASs in nature and applying this knowledge to organizations provides insight into how change occurs in human systems.[15] A key finding is that change occurs naturally within the existing system. Reflection on how healthcare changed over the years demonstrates the natural adoption of many new procedures, medications, systems, and information and medical technologies. Change is not so much about overcoming resistance as it is about creating attraction. What was labeled "resistance" is an attraction to factors in the current system that might not be fully understood or appreciated. Resistance is a natural, but potentially changeable, reaction of a system attracted to something else. If organizations can change the attractors or tap into existing ones that are better, the system may do the rest of the work of change on its own. The challenge for leaders is to look for and leverage the subtle attractors that may not always be obvious.

Consistent with this understanding of organizations as CAS, Zimmerman and colleagues[10] propose practical principles of management for the real world that are ways of thinking about roles healthcare quality professionals play as quality leaders in organizations. **TABLE 1-1** compares key characteristics of leaders in traditional (bureaucratic) systems and CAS.

Table 1-1 Characteristics of Leaders in Traditional and Complex Adaptive Systems

Traditional Systems	Complex Adaptive Systems
• Value positions	• Value persons and relationships
• Use tight structuring	• Use loose coupling
• Simplify	• Complicate or link
• Socialize	• Diversify
• Make decisions	• Make sense
• Do planning based on forecasting	• Think about the future
• Are controlling, in charge	• Are collaborative
• Know	• Listen and learn
• Are self-preserving	• Are adaptable
• Repeat the past	• Offer alternatives

Adapted from Anderson RA, McDaniel RR. Managing health care organizations: where professionalism meets designing organizations. *Healthcare Manag Rev*. 2000;25(1): 83–92; Center for the Study of Healthcare Management. *Applying Complexity Science to Health and Health Care*. Minneapolis, MN: Plexus Institute; 2003.

Constraints management, a management philosophy developed by Goldratt, offers another systematic approach to managing complex organizations by identifying and controlling key leverage points in a system or process to yield faster system throughput. A system constraint is anything that limits the system from attaining higher performance.[16] Put simply, the strength of any process or system is dependent upon its weakest link. Improvements to the system under constraints management aim to identify (1) what to change, (2) what to change to, and (3) how to cause the change.[16] Improvement proceeds in five general steps, namely,

1. identification of the system constraint,
2. determination of how to exploit the identified constraint,
3. subordination and synchronization of the other processes in the system to maximize the capacity of the system,
4. elevation of the system constraint by investing more resources, and
5. repetition of the cycle to ensure ongoing improvement.

Leadership Frameworks and Models

Leadership and management are distinct functions. Kotter[17] notes that leadership involves coping with change by developing a vision and aligning the subsystems of the organization. In contrast, management involves coping with complexity through planning and budgeting; setting goals; organizing, staffing, and creating a structure to foster goal attainment; setting up mechanisms for monitoring; and controlling results. *Leadership* is the ability to influence an individual or group toward achievement of goals[18] and includes determining the correct direction or path. *Management* involves doing the correct things to stay on that path. Both strong leadership and skilled management are necessary for high-reliability performance. Some individuals are great leaders but poor managers, whereas others are great managers but poor leaders. In some cases, an individual may be successful in both roles.

Healthcare quality professionals possess an awareness of different frameworks for driving organizational performance when working with organizational leadership. Frameworks can assist in guiding and organizing leadership activities to achieve improvement. Many systems models exist. "The model that the manager selects is less important than how [the person] uses it to begin recognizing, understanding, and anticipating how the parts of the systems interact as a whole."[19(p73)] The healthcare quality professional assists the organizational leaders, employees, and physicians in understanding the principles and common frameworks for healthcare quality and safety strategies. Recent and classic literature point the healthcare quality professional to a wealth of evidence-based frameworks. Descriptions of some popular models and frameworks follow.

Donabedian. Avedis Donabedian is credited as being the founder of the quality assurance field. As a researcher and physician at the University of Michigan, he developed a theoretical framework, with focus on structures, processes, and outcomes, for patient care evaluation.[20] Donabedian's framework describes the importance of relating healthcare structures and processes to how clients fared because of their care. *Structure* represents the resources available for care delivery and system design, whereas *processes* involve the "set of activities that go on within and between practitioners and patients."[20(p79)] *Outcomes* include the results of that care (e.g., increased engagement, decreased morbidity, improved quality of life or well-being) or the "change in a patient's current and future health status that can be attributed to antecedent health care."[20(p83)]

Donabedian was the first to describe an approach to assessing quality through a systems framework. However, the model is very basic and does not describe interrelationships. This gap led to the development of other models to illuminate the interrelationships necessary for quality performance. However, Donabedian's triad is lauded as a "lasting framework" for healthcare quality.[21] This evidence-based theoretical work became personal after experiencing the healthcare system firsthand. Donabedian shared in an interview published in *Health Affairs* that

> Health care is a sacred mission. . .a moral enterprise and a scientific enterprise but not fundamentally a commercial one. We are not selling a product. We don't have a consumer who understands everything and makes rational choices—and I include myself here. Doctors and nurses are stewards of something precious. ... Ultimately the secret of quality is love. ... If you have love, you can then work backward to monitor and improve the system.[22(p140)]

As a leader and pioneer in healthcare quality, Donabedian was always cognizant of the social, emotional, and ethical factors related to quality and safety.

The Baldrige Performance Excellence Framework. A second framework used to understand quality, safety, and performance improvement in complex systems is Baldrige's framework for the 2017–2018 Baldrige Excellence Framework Overview in Health Care,[23] depicted in FIGURE 1-1. The Malcolm Baldrige National Quality Award, named for former U.S. Secretary of Commerce Malcolm Baldrige in tribute to his managerial ability, is given to organizations demonstrating a commitment to excellence. This framework displays core values and concepts that support principles of quality, safety, and performance improvement. The organizational profile at the top of the figure reflects the specific circumstances within which the organization functions. This element highlights the need to consider the organization's operating environment (e.g., service offerings, vision and mission, workforce profile, assets, regulatory requirements), relationships (e.g., customers and stakeholders, suppliers and partners, structure and relationship between senior leaders and the governing body), and specific strategic situation when developing a performance management system.

Three components of the framework—leadership, strategy, and customers—constitute the leadership triad and highlight the value of leadership focus on strategy and customers. The results triad includes workforce, operations, and results—these emphasize the impact of workforce-focused and operational process—leading to results. The six elements of the leadership and results triads constitute the performance management system. The central arrows represent the important integration between leadership and results where integration is defined as the "harmonization of plans, processes, information, resource decisions, workforce capability and capacity, actions, results, and analyses to support key organization-wide goals."[23(p50)] Integration is different from alignment. Alignment is a state of consistency among the above-mentioned elements of the performance management system. Integration is attained when the elements not only are consistent but also operate as a fully interconnected unit.

At the base of the framework are the critical elements that represent the foundation of the performance management system—measurement, analysis, and knowledge management, which also serve as the foundation for effective organizational management.[23]

Health and Medicine Division, National Academies of Sciences, Engineering, and Medicine. In 2001, the IOM's report *Crossing the Quality Chasm: A New Health System for the 21st Century*[2] offered new rules for the healthcare system. Contrasted with the then-current healthcare

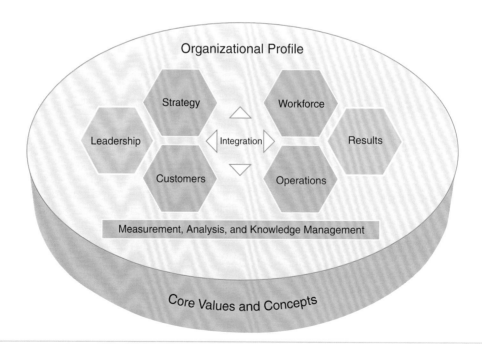

Figure 1-1 **2017–2018 Baldrige Excellence Framework Overview (Health Care).** (Reprinted from Baldrige Performance Excellence Program at the National Institute of Standards and Technology, with permission. https://www.nist.gov/baldrige/publications/baldrige-excellence-framework/health-care.)

Table 1-2 Rules for the 21st-Century Healthcare System

Current Approach	New Rule
Care is based primarily on visits.	Preference is given to professional roles over the system.
Professional autonomy drives variability.	Care is customized based on patient needs and values.
Professionals control care.	The patient is the source of control.
Information is a record.	Knowledge is shared, and information flows freely.
Decision making is based on training and experience.	Decision making is evidence based.
"Do no harm" is an individual responsibility.	Safety is a system priority.
Confidentiality is necessary.	Transparency is necessary.
The system reacts to needs.	The system anticipates needs.
Cost reduction is sought.	Waste is continuously decreased.
Preference is given to professional roles over the system.	Cooperation among clinicians is a priority.

Reprinted from Institute of Medicine, Committee on Quality of Health Care in America. *Crossing the Quality Chasm: A New Health System for the 21st Century*. Washington, DC: National Academies Press; 2001. Copyright 2011 by National Academies Press, with permission.

system approach (**TABLE 1-2**), the new rules were characterized as simple. Today's healthcare system continues to struggle with adopting these rules, with multiple sectors of the healthcare system experiencing varying degrees of success on each rule. Leaders and healthcare quality professionals consider these rules in the development and implementation of improved care delivery systems and other improvement strategies across their organizations.

Institute for Healthcare Improvement. The Institute for Healthcare Improvement's Framework for Leadership Improvement[24] outlines five specific core leadership activities to drive improvement. The activities are described below (see FIG. 1-2):

- *Establish the mission, vision, and strategy* to set the direction of the organization. Organizational incentives are aligned with the purpose, and the purpose should be communicated to all stakeholders.
- *Establish the foundation* for an effective leadership system by choosing a leadership team with the right balance of skills to build relationships and improvement capability.
- *Build will* through a plan for improvement that sets aims, allocates resources, measures performance, provides encouragement, and makes financial linkages to the impact of quality on cost when customer expectations are not met.
- *Generate ideas* about clinical and organizational best practices through benchmarking and listening to patients. Invest in research and development, manage knowledge, and understand the organization as a system.

- *Execute change* through a standardized approach that is used for improvement daily. Assess the effectiveness of execution efforts, spread ideas, and communicate results to sustain higher levels of performance.

High-Impact Leadership

High-impact leadership[25] provides a roadmap for individuals at every level of leadership in healthcare organizations to drive organization-level results from improvement efforts to achieve the Triple Aim. The term "Triple Aim" refers to the simultaneous pursuit of improving the patient experience of care, improving the health of populations, and reducing the per capita cost of healthcare. The Triple Aim, a single aim with three dimensions, is a framework that was developed by the Institute for Healthcare Improvement (IHI) in Cambridge, MA, and is widely referenced as a statement of purpose for healthcare system transformation to better meet the needs of people and patients. Its successful implementation will result in fundamentally new systems contributing to the overall health of populations while reducing the overall cost of care.[26] Three interdependent dimensions of high-impact leadership in healthcare—new mental models, high-impact leadership behaviors, and the IHI High-Impact Leadership Framework—are depicted in FIGURE 1-3 and will be described next.

High-impact leadership is critical to success for leaders shepherding the transition from volume-based to value-based care delivery systems. Success requires leaders to think differently about the world around them, to change their mental

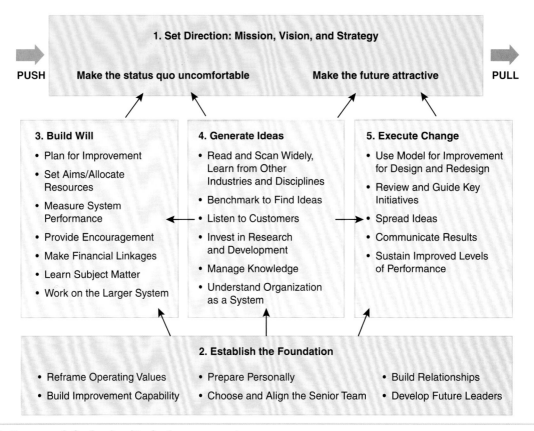

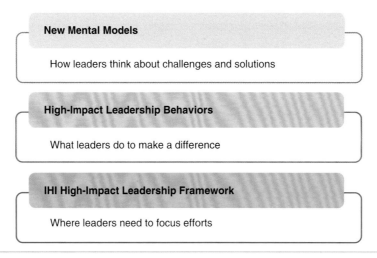

models and focus on value (FIG. 1-4). Four new ways of thinking provide the context necessary for considering approaches to promote innovation and achieve the Triple Aim:

1. Recognize that individuals and families are partners in their care;

2. Compete on value, with continuous reduction in operating cost;

3. Reorganize services to align with new payment systems; and

4. Operate from the perspective that everyone is an improver.[25(p4)]

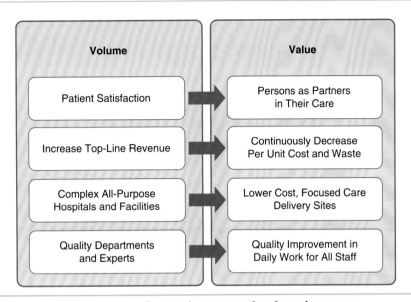

Figure 1-4 **New mental models: transitioning from volume- to value-based systems.** (Reprinted from IHI High-Impact Leadership Framework. *Outlines New Mental Models; High-Impact Leadership Behaviors.* Cambridge, MA: Institute for Healthcare Improvement; 2013. http://www.ihi.org/. Copyright 2013, with permission.)

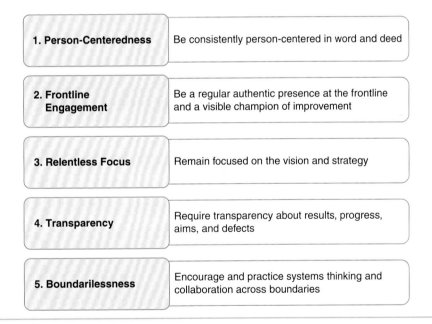

Figure 1-5 **High-impact leadership behaviors.** (From IHI High-Impact Leadership Framework. *Outlines New Mental Models; High-Impact Leadership Behaviors.* Cambridge, MA: Institute for Healthcare Improvement; 2013. http://www.ihi.org/. Copyright 2013. Reprinted with permission.)

Certain high-impact leadership behaviors are closely aligned with new ways of thinking and the High-Impact Leadership Framework. The IHI[25] offers five behaviors to be used as a starting point for leaders who are examining their own practices as they develop efforts and strategies to achieve Triple Aim results (FIG. 1-5): Person-Centeredness,

Frontline engagement, Relentless focus, Transparency, and Boundarilessness.

The IHI High-Impact Leadership Framework consists of six domains and provides a method of organizing and focusing leadership efforts for leading improvement and innovation. The following six domains are critical for leaders at all levels in

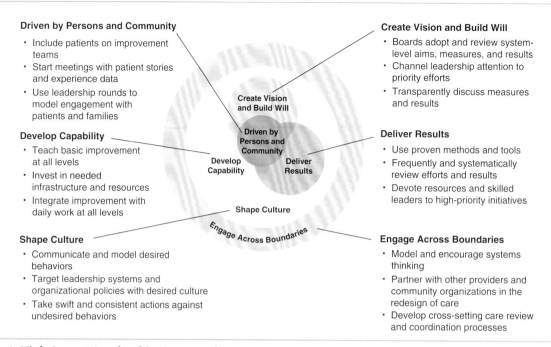

Driven by Persons and Community

- Include patients on improvement teams
- Start meetings with patient stories and experience data
- Use leadership rounds to model engagement with patients and families

Develop Capability

- Teach basic improvement at all levels
- Invest in needed infrastructure and resources
- Integrate improvement with daily work at all levels

Shape Culture

- Communicate and model desired behaviors
- Target leadership systems and organizational policies with desired culture
- Take swift and consistent actions against undesired behaviors

Create Vision and Build Will

- Boards adopt and review system-level aims, measures, and results
- Channel leadership attention to priority efforts
- Transparently discuss measures and results

Deliver Results

- Use proven methods and tools
- Frequently and systematically review efforts and results
- Devote resources and skilled leaders to high-priority initiatives

Engage Across Boundaries

- Model and encourage systems thinking
- Partner with other providers and community organizations in the redesign of care
- Develop cross-setting care review and coordination processes

Figure 1-6 High-Impact Leadership Framework. (Reprinted from IHI High-Impact Leadership Framework. *Outlines New Mental Models; High-Impact Leadership Behaviors*. Cambridge, MA: Institute for Healthcare Improvement. http://www.ihi.org/. Copyright 2013, with permission.)

healthcare to consider to drive improvement and innovation to achieve the Triple Aim:

1. Driven by Persons and Community
2. Create Vision and Build Will
3. Develop Capability
4. Deliver Results
5. Shape Culture
6. Engage Across Boundaries

FIGURE 1-6 displays the High-Impact Leadership Framework with some examples of leadership actions for each of the six domains.

Leadership Styles

Leadership styles are often presented within the context of the approaches to decision making and problem solving as well as the specific approaches used to influence change. Leaders, through their own management style, also can influence the degree to which employees share information, knowledge, rewards, and power in the organization. Several different styles of leadership are as follows:

- *Autocratic*—leader is directive and controlling; employees have little discretionary power in their work.
- *Participative*—leader allows employees some degree of autonomy in completing their work while maintaining some control of the group and the decision-making

process; leader seeks input from employees and serves as facilitator.

- *Empowering*—leader shares power and decision making with employees, enabling others by providing the necessary resources and support.
- *Transactional*—leader views the leader–follower relationship as a process of exchange where compliance or performance is achieved through the process of giving rewards and punishment.
- *Transformational*—leader can inspire others to change expectations and motivations to work toward common goals.[28]

Contemporary leaders tend to adapt their style to the situation, ideally resulting in a style best suited to the needs of the organization. Goleman[29] defines six styles within situational leadership, namely,

1. coaching,
2. pacesetting,
3. democratic,
4. affiliative,
5. authoritative, and
6. coercive.

The coaching style is most effective when employees understand their weaknesses and want to improve their performance and is least effective when employees are resistant to learning how to change.[29] The pacesetting style involves the leader setting high standards and then demonstrating them at times causing many employees to feel overwhelmed. The democratic style involves taking time to get employees' input and works best when the leader is not certain about the solution and wants fresh ideas. A key tenet of the affiliative style is a desire of the leader to keep employees satisfied and engaged. With this style, leaders place employees first. The authoritative style is where leaders demonstrate self-confidence and empathy. Leaders take charge and work to mobilize employees toward a vision. Finally, with coercive leadership style, leaders just tell employees what to do and how to do it. This style works best in crisis situations. One key to a situational leadership style is to understand and select the most effective leadership style for the situation.

Leadership Practices

An organization's leadership must be aware of the impact of both leadership styles and leadership practices on organizational performance. Several leadership practices are noted to produce a positive impact on organizational outcomes. Kouzes and Posner[30] explored practices of exemplary leaders and identified five important general practices that apply to any type of organization. A listing of the five practices and brief overview of each follows.

1. *Model the way.* Much behavior is learned through role modeling. This practice involves setting example by aligning actions and values. Leaders who expect employees to make changes to support quality, safety, and performance improvement must model those desired behaviors each day; actions speak louder than words.

2. *Inspire a shared vision.* If a change is to be successful, leaders must provide a vision for quality, safety, and performance improvement and influence others to share that vision. This means getting people to accept the core values underlying healthcare quality by developing a strong culture for quality and performance improvement. This effort requires more than just telling others what needs to be done; leaders need to communicate the vision in a manner that causes others to embrace it.

3. *Challenge the process.* Challenging the process means questioning the status quo and leading the way as an early adopter of innovation. It also means recognizing good ideas and demonstrating a willingness to experiment and take risks to improve the quality of care. Adoption of core values as a learning organization is key to success. Leaders ask what *should be* instead of accepting what *is*.

4. *Enable others to act.* This practice involves enabling others to act by sharing decision making and power in a way that enables others to move toward the direction of the vision. Along with sharing power, enabling involves having an appropriate structural design and the appropriate resources to support quality, safety, and performance improvement initiatives.

5. *Encourage the heart.* Change is difficult, even if it is done for the right reasons, and many employees need much more encouragement and feedback than many leaders realize. Encouraging the heart means recognizing the contributions that employees make and celebrating the core values and victories. The most important point of any reward system is to reward the desired behaviors.

Leaders use these five practices to keep subsystems aligned. However, leaders must first get people to support a vision of quality. One way this occurs is through the development of a strong culture of quality, safety, and performance improvement. Healthcare quality professionals typically take on a central role in defining and fostering the organization's culture of quality and safety.

Leadership and Organizational Culture

Culture is defined as the set of shared attitudes, values, goals, and practices that characterize an institution or organization[31] and the social glue that holds people together.[32] At the heart of culture is the notion of shared values, what is important, and behavioral norms, how things are done.[33] Perrin defines organizational culture as "the sum of values and rituals which serve as 'glue' to integrate the members of the organization."[34(¶10)] Cultures are described as strong when the core values are intensely held and widely shared. Strong culture

- provides a sense of identity for employees and a commitment to something larger than themselves;
- enhances cooperation;
- creates a system of informal rules spelling out how people are expected to behave; and
- creates distinctions between organizations, allowing a definitive competitive advantage to develop.

Elements of Culture

Culture has both invisible and visible elements. Invisible elements include values and norms, whereas visible elements include symbols; language, slogans, and brands; rituals and ceremonies; stories, legends, and myths; and heroes.

- **Values and Norms.** The core values described in the Baldrige Performance Excellence Program criteria are one example. The role of leaders is to inspire commitment to these underlying quality values. Norms are usually locally established such as how customers are greeted.

- **Symbols.** Symbols are things that represent an idea. The purpose of symbols is to reflect the culture, trigger values and norms, and help people make sense of their organization. For example, one hospital wanted to strengthen the value for reporting adverse events. To do this, staff wore buttons that said, "We care, We report, We learn." Another uses a "Stop the Line" approach to indicate staff are empowered to ensure the correct actions are taken (see Red Rules in the *Patient Safety* section).
- **Language, Slogans, and Brands.** Language and slogans are intended to convey cultural meaning to employees and stakeholders. They should be easy to learn, remember, and repeat (e.g., "Quality is Job 1," "Thrive"). Brands help build loyalty to a product or service.
- **Rituals and Ceremonies.** Rituals and ceremonies reinforce an organization's core values and goals, thereby strengthening culture. For example, healthcare quality week with annual quality forums and celebration of improvement projects conveys the importance of these activities.
- **Stories, Legends, and Myths.** Stories, legends, and myths are narrative examples repeated by employees to inform (often new) employees about culture. Stories are based on fact; legends are based on facts but embellished; myths are consistent with the culture but are not based on fact. For example, stories about an extraordinary event and the organization's response may illustrate a new patient safety program.
- **Heroes.** Heroes are company role models whose ideals, character, and support of the organizational culture highlight the values and norms a company wants to reinforce. Heroes provide a role model for success. For example, an employee or leader who is remembered for a transformative event may be considered an organizational hero.

By design or default, an organization develops a culture. It is better to actively direct the evolution of that culture than to try to change a strong culture that is not aligned with the organization's quality and safety goals.

Assessing Organizational Culture

Organizations must measure their culture, provide feedback to the leadership and staff, and undertake interventions to change the culture in a way that will promote quality and reduce patient safety risk.[35] How can it be determined whether quality and safety are core values in the culture of an organization? Experts in the field of culture suggest posing the following questions[36,37]:

- Do leaders regularly pay attention to, measure, and control quality and safety?

- Are adequate resources allocated to quality, safety, and performance improvement?
- Are behaviors supporting quality, safety, and performance improvement rewarded?
- Do staff knowledge, skills, and behaviors important for quality, safety, and performance improvement figure into decisions regarding recruitment, selection, and promotion?
- Is active involvement in quality, safety, and performance improvement activities one measure of status in the organization?
- Are people spending time or being supported for spending time on quality, safety, and performance improvement?
- Does staff frequently discuss quality, safety, and performance improvement and its related activities?
- Is the prevailing attitude toward quality, safety, performance improvement, and organizational quality outdated or progressive?

Several tools exist to measure an organization's culture from the perspective of quality and safety. Healthcare quality professionals may be asked to coordinate survey processes related to a culture of safety with an outside vendor or to lead organizational efforts to measure the patient safety culture across the organization using one or more currently available survey instruments. For example, Agency for Healthcare Research and Quality (AHRQ) currently offers five surveys on patient safety culture appropriate for hospital, medical office, nursing home, community pharmacy, and ambulatory surgery settings.[35,38] The University of Texas has developed the Safety Attitudes Questionnaire to measure healthcare provider attitudes important to patient safety.[39] Additional information on culture of safety is discussed in the *Patient Safety* section. Healthcare quality professionals typically take the lead in coordinating the survey efforts and working with leaders across the organization to address identified improvement opportunities through specific actions to drive culture alignment and improvement.

Leadership and Culture Change

Many actions for establishing and strengthening a quality culture flow from the above questions. First, leaders must show visible support through such actions by embracing quality, safety, and performance improvement as an important part of the strategic planning process. Quality, safety, and performance improvement are everyone's responsibility. Adequate resources are allocated in the annual budget for quality, safety, and performance improvement activities and behaviors that support quality and safety are rewarded. Second, leaders need to be evaluating and providing attention to the visible elements of culture. For example, accomplish the following:

- Replace old, negative stories about quality that are acting as barriers to cultural change with new, positive ones.

- Reinforce values by using symbols and creating rituals critical to quality.
- Celebrate successes when quality, safety, and performance are achieved.

Finally, leaders invest persistent effort, knowing that culture takes a long time to change.

Although inspiring people with a vision is critical, leaders must also enable others to achieve goals and objectives. One way to enable others is to design the organization in a way that supports quality, safety, and performance improvement. Leaders must integrate healthcare safety practices into the plan for the organization's strategic direction, and goals must be developed to ensure adoption and measurement of safety practices. The organization's quality and patient safety programs are aligned with the mission, vision, core values, and goals of the organization. High-performing organizations embrace approaches that serve as a solid foundation for promoting quality and patient safety. Two examples are provided here, and more examples and details are provided in *Patient Safety*.

Just Culture. Many organizations incorporate the principles of a *just culture* to promote shared accountability and a learning environment as part of the organizational response to error. In a fair and just culture, everyone throughout the organization is aware that medical errors are inevitable, and all errors and unintended events are reported—even when the events may not cause patient injury. This culture can make the system safer. A just culture recognizes that competent professionals make mistakes and acknowledges that even competent professionals develop unhealthy norms such as shortcuts or routine rule violations, but a just culture has zero tolerance for reckless behavior or willful disregard for established policy and procedure. Key principles of a just culture can be summarized as follows:

- A just culture is not an effort to reduce personal accountability or discipline. It is a way to emphasize the importance of learning from mistakes and near misses to reduce errors in the future.
- In a just culture, an individual is accountable to the system, and the greatest error is to not report a mistake and thereby prevent the system and others from learning. Policies that encourage or require any healthcare provider to self-report errors are in alignment with a fair and just culture.
- A culture of patient safety is successfully created when all employees serve as safety advocates regardless of their positions within an organization. Providers and consumers will feel safe and supported when they report medical errors or near misses and voice concerns about patient safety.

Healthcare organizations committed to a fair and just culture identify and correct the systems or processes of care that contributed to the medical error or near miss; they do not assign blame but ensure that individuals are held accountable when circumstances warrant individual action, such as events that occur because of willful disregard of policy or procedure. Feeling protected by a nonpunitive culture of medical error reporting, more healthcare professionals will report more errors and near misses, which will further improve patient safety through opportunities for improvement and lessons learned.

Focus on Patient Safety. In the current environment, reducing and eliminating medical errors is a major aim for most of the healthcare industry. Healthcare organizations are very complex and variability in processes can lead to patient harm. In some organizations, leaders set the tone for patient safety as a priority through clearly articulated goals such as the aim for zero harm or in committing to the journey toward high reliability. These and other concepts will be discussed in more detail in *Patient Safety*. Whether the focus is on procedure booking processes, medications, or surgery, the goals are the same—to assure patients that they are being treated in a safe environment.

Through ongoing scans of the healthcare quality scientific literature and new and evolving regulation, healthcare quality professionals can keep the leadership team up to date and facilitate the adoption and integration of key leadership practices that support the quality and safety function within the organization. See *Patient Safety* for more discussion of safety culture, harm reduction, and mitigating risk.

Strategic Planning and Performance Excellence

The environment surrounding healthcare organizations is both dynamic and complex because it changes frequently and has many constituents. With continued emphasis on improving the patient experience of care, improving the health of populations, and reducing the per capita cost of healthcare, external forces in healthcare continue to be important. Strategic planning for healthcare quality is even more important as the impact of the shift from volume-based to value-based reimbursement is felt. Other considerations are the expanded focus on accountable care organizations (ACOs) and alternative payment models (APMs). And, there is a significant shift from higher cost acute care settings as a focus for delivery of care to lower cost subacute, ambulatory, and primary care settings.

Strategy is defined as "the plans and activities developed by an organization in pursuit of its goals and objectives, particularly in regard to positioning itself to meet external demands relative to its competition."[40(p220)] Strategic planning is one way of coping with a dynamic and complex environment. The goals of strategic management[7] are to

- provide a framework for thinking about the "business";
- create a fit between the organization and its external environment;
- provide a process for coping with change and organizational renewal;
- foster anticipation, innovation, and excellence;
- facilitate consistent decision making; and
- create organizational focus.

Quality, safety, and performance improvement received increased attention in recent years because organizations realize that if they are to be successful, quality and safety must be an integral part of the strategic plan. The healthcare quality professional plays a key role in strategic planning for quality and safety.

Strategic Planning Process

The strategic planning process includes all the decisions and actions required to meet the strategic goals. Several steps are offered by various sources. FIGURE 1-7 shows some of the common steps in the strategic planning process. Before a strategy is formulated, leaders consider what they want to do, what they should do, and what they can do.[41] Consideration

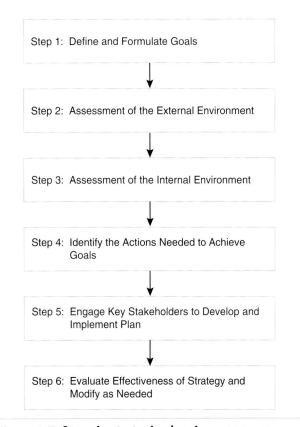

of these three issues leads to the development of a strategic plan. Per the Baldrige Framework,[23] strategy planning and development refer to the organization's approach to preparing for the future. In developing the strategy, the level of acceptable enterprise risk is determined. Various types of forecasts, projections, options, scenarios, knowledge, analyses, or other approaches might be used to envision the future. This aids in decision making and resource allocation.

Strategy is defined broadly and might be built around new healthcare services; differentiation of the organization's brand; new core competencies; new partnerships, alliances, or acquisitions to improve access, grow revenue, or reduce costs; and new staff or volunteer relationships.[23] The strategic planning process must include a focus on long-term organizational sustainability and consideration of the environment from competitive and collaborative perspectives.[42]

Step 1: What the Organization Wants to Do (Define and Formulate Goals)

Mission and Vision. Organizations must define what they want to accomplish in the future, in part, by evaluating the current state against the desired future state. Ideally, what the organization wants to accomplish will be in alignment with the organization's mission and vision. *Mission* refers to the organization's purpose or reason for existing. It answers questions such as "Why are we here?" "Whom do we serve?" and "What do we do." For example, the mission of SSM Health Care, the first healthcare Malcolm Baldrige National Quality Award recipient, is "Through our exceptional healthcare services, we reveal the healing presence of God." Its core values are compassion, respect, excellence, stewardship, and community.[43] This provides a long-term direction for the organization. In contrast, the 2015 Baldrige recipient's (Charleston Area Medical Center) mission is "Striving to provide the best health care to every patient every day" with core values of quality, service with compassion, respect, integrity, stewardship, and safety.[44] *Vision* is an organization's statement of its goals for the future, described in measurable terms that clarify the direction for everyone in the organization. An organization's direction is built upon its mission and guided by its vision.

References to quality and safety are often included in organizational mission and vision statements to show that these values are priorities in what the organization wants to do. The healthcare quality professional may be expected to work with senior leaders and the governing body to evaluate and refine the mission and vision of the organization through participation in strategic planning processes. They may also be asked to assist leadership in developing the goals, objectives, and metrics for measuring the effectiveness of their mission and vision.

Guiding Principles and Core Values. *Guiding principles* and *core values* facilitate development of leadership values and

Step 1: Define and Formulate Goals

↓

Step 2: Assessment of the External Environment

↓

Step 3: Assessment of the Internal Environment

↓

Step 4: Identify the Actions Needed to Achieve Goals

↓

Step 5: Engage Key Stakeholders to Develop and Implement Plan

↓

Step 6: Evaluate Effectiveness of Strategy and Modify as Needed

Figure 1-7 Steps in strategic planning processes.

commitment to quality. They define the organization's attitudes and policies for employees and thereby help to direct the vision. The following list displays the core values and concepts identified in the Baldrige Performance Excellence Program as a set of beliefs and behaviors embraced by some organizations as a foundation for performance excellence:

- systems perspective,
- visionary leadership,
- patient-focused excellence,
- valuing people,
- organizational learning and agility,
- focus on success,
- managing for innovation,
- management by fact,
- societal responsibility and community health,
- ethics and transparency, and
- delivering value and results.[23(piii)]

The organization's plans integrate the perspectives of the customer. The organization must first identify its customers. The needs of various customers, such as patients, clients, families, and other stakeholders, help the organization to refine its mission, vision, guiding principles, and core values.

Goals and Objectives. Goals and objectives are essential components of any planning process; they guide actions and serve as a yardstick for measuring the organization's progress and performance. Confusion sometimes arises about the terms *goal* and *objective*; they differ with respect to scope and specificity. In general, goals are broad, general statements specifying a purpose or desired outcome and may be more abstract than objectives. One goal can have several objectives.

Establishing goals is the initial step in the strategic planning process and sets the direction for the activities to follow. A goal is a general statement about a desired outcome and is accompanied by one or more specific objectives that specify in precise terms exactly what is to be accomplished. Goals describe accomplishments, not tasks or activities. As a guide, goals need to be SMART:

- Specific,
- Measurable,
- Achievable,
- Relevant, and
- Time-bound.[45]

Objectives are specific statements that detail how the goals will be achieved through specific and measurable action; they therefore are relatively narrow and concrete. They clearly identify who is going to do what, by when, and to what extent. Objectives representing the organization's commitment to achieving specific outcomes are written as action-oriented statements. Specific activities are implemented to yield measurable and observable qualitative or quantitative performance outcomes. An example of a mission statement, vision statement, values statement, strategic goals, and strategic objectives can be found in **TABLE 1-3**.

After strategic goals and objectives are developed at the executive level, corresponding goals and objectives must be established for other levels in the organization, for example, the business level and functional level (e.g., human resources/ talent management, research and development) or the unit or departmental level (e.g., nursing, diagnostic imaging, pharmacy). Both long-term and short-term goals and corresponding objectives are established for all levels. Goal congruence is the integration of multiple goals, either within an organization or between multiple groups. Congruence is a result of the alignment of goals to achieve an overarching mission.[46]

Step 2: What the Organization Should Do (Assessment of the External Environment).
Once the goals and objectives are established or revised, the organization must look at the external environment. On the roadmap, the environment is shown to influence what the organization wants to do: all organizations must adapt to the forces of the external environment to survive, stretch, and grow. In other words, the organization is one system among a variety of systems in the external environment. Adaptation includes maintaining good relationships with key constituents who can influence the organization's ability to meet the stated objectives. FIGURE 1-8 depicts some of the key categories of various environmental influences on quality and safety by multiple constituents whose needs must be met and balanced with the needs of other stakeholders. The outer ring pertains to the overall environment in which the organization exists. A variety of factors—sociocultural, political and legal, economic, technologic, global, and demographic—indirectly influence the organization. For example, economic forces can influence the amount of resources (e.g., labor, capital) available to organizations. For this reason, organizations must scan the general external environment looking for threats to, or opportunities for, meeting strategic goals and objectives. The second ring represents the immediate environment in which the organization operates. With respect to quality and safety in healthcare organizations, the key constituent is the customer as the consumer of care or service. However, other constituents also are important. For example, payers, regulatory agencies, and entities through which the patient acquires healthcare insurance are also key stakeholders.

Public Reporting. Public reporting of quality information may be considered as one of the key external drivers for transparency and accountability.[47] Releases of public data began in the late 1980s when the Health Care Financing Administration (now Centers for Medicare & Medicaid Services [CMS]) released case-mix-adjusted mortality rates for hospitals throughout

Table 1-3 Example of Mission, Vision, Values Statement, and Strategy

Mission Statement	We provide hope, care, and cures to help every child live the healthiest and most fulfilling life possible.
Vision Statement	Seattle Children's will be an innovative leader in pediatric health and wellness through our unsurpassed quality, clinical care, relentless spirit of inquiry, and compassion for children and their families. Our founding promise to the community is as valid today as it was over a century ago. We will care for all children in our region, regardless of their family's ability to pay. We will: • Practice the safest, most ethical, and effective medical care possible. • Discover new treatments and cures through breakthrough research. • Promote healthy communities while reducing health disparities. • Empower our team members to reach their highest potential in a respectful work environment. • Educate and inspire the next generation of faculty, staff, and leaders. • Build on a culture of philanthropy for patient care and research.
Values Statement	*Compassion.* Empathy for patients, their families, and staff is ingrained in our history and inspires our future. We do more than treat the child; we practice family-centered care as the cornerstone of compassion. *Excellence.* Our promise to treat, prevent, and cure pediatric disease is an enormous responsibility. We follow the highest standards of quality and safety and expect accountability from each other. *Integrity.* At all times, we approach our work with openness, transparency, decency, and humility. It is our responsibility to use resources wisely to sustain Seattle Children's for generations to come. *Collaboration.* We work in partnership with patients, their families, staff, providers, volunteers, and donors. This spirit of respectful cooperation extends beyond our walls to our business partners and the community. *Equity.* We embrace and find strength in the diversity of our patients, their families, staff, and community. We believe all children deserve exceptional care, the best outcomes, respect, and a safe environment. *Innovation.* We aspire to be an innovative leader in pediatric healthcare, research, and philanthropy. We continually seek new and better solutions. Because innovation springs from knowledge, we foster learning in all disciplines.
Strategic Goal	Provide the safest, most effective care possible.
Strategic Objectives Related to Goal	Eliminate medical errors by focusing on systems, people, and technology. *Systems* • Accelerate the implementation of Clinical Standard Work. • Establish systems to prevent and respond rapidly to medical errors and hospital-acquired infections. *People* • Improve our management systems to support safe practice. • Improve medication safety through enhanced oversight and pharmacy staffing. • Support a family-centered model of care. *Technology* • Utilize technology to improve medication safety. • Complete the transition to an electronic medical record system. *Measure and Report Our Progress* • Develop an integrated safety index to track our progress toward eliminating preventable harm.
Measures of Success	• Develop an integrated safety index to track our progress toward eliminating preventable harm. • The hospital will reduce its hospital-acquired infections by 25% to eliminate preventable harm in surgical services and chase zero by December 31, 2013.

Table created for general educational use by Christy L. Beaudin, PhD, LCSW, CPHQ, from information available on the Seattle Children's Hospital website. http://www.seattlechildrens.org/about/strategic-plan/. Accessed August 4, 2014.

the country. Eventually, these reports were no longer issued because of hospitals' criticisms of case-mix-adjusted methodology. In the early 1990s, New York State began releasing mortality data on patients who underwent open-heart surgery by hospital and ranked hospitals according to how much they deviated from case-mix-adjusted values. Hospitals were then labeled as providing either "good" or "poor" care. Hospitals that had poor outcomes were encouraged to improve their care

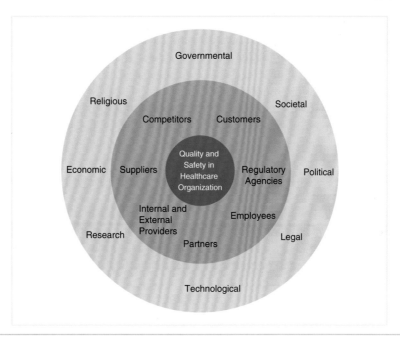

Figure 1-8 **Environmental influences on quality and safety.**

processes. Eventually, New York released data on individual surgeons and other procedures such as angioplasty.

The broad implementation of mandatory public reporting was intended to guide hospitals and physicians, through incentives, toward improving the quality of care and service delivered to patients. The 2003 Hospital Inpatient Quality Reporting program aimed to provide consumers with quality information to support efforts to make informed decisions about healthcare.

The current emphasis for public reporting is on reporting structural, process, and outcome measures, and the focus of reporting is highly variable. Examples of government-sponsored reporting include CMS efforts related to nursing homes (Nursing Home Compare), home healthcare agencies (Home Health Compare), dialysis facilities (Dialysis Facility Compare), and hospitals (Hospital Compare). Many private organizations emerged with varying missions around healthcare quality and safety, several of which publish different types of reports that include information about the quality and safety. These reporting entities use similar, yet differing and proprietary approaches, comparing healthcare providers to national benchmarks and providing a rating as to whether care meets specific standards. The Leapfrog Group is a not-for-profit organization founded by employers and private healthcare experts that aims to make giant "leaps" forward in the safety, quality, and affordability of healthcare in the United States by promoting transparency through their data collection and public reporting initiatives.[48] Healthgrades is an online resource for information about physicians and hospitals. Per their website, more than one million people a day use the

Healthgrades website to search, compare, and connect with hospitals and physicians based on the most important factors when selecting a healthcare provider: experience, hospital quality, and patient satisfaction.[49]

Early evidence indicated that public reporting of performance data stimulates quality, safety, and performance improvement activities at the hospital level.[50] More recent review of the available evidence indicates that public reporting programs at different levels of the healthcare sector are a challenging but rewarding public health strategy and stimulate providers to improve healthcare quality.[47]

Incentives and Penalties. As national pressures continue to increase, new expectations emerge for leaders, including those of government agencies (e.g., CMS), public reporting groups (e.g., The Commonwealth Fund, The Leapfrog Group), accreditation agencies (e.g., The Joint Commission [TJC], DNV GL Healthcare), and third-party payers (e.g., Blue Cross Blue Shield, UnitedHealthcare, Tufts). Third-party payers implemented the practice of nonpayment for certain conditions that could have been reasonably prevented ("serious reportable events [SREs]," formerly known as "never events," e.g., pressure ulcers) and serious preventable events (e.g., leaving a sponge in the patient during surgery).

The organization's external environment relative to national and local practices that involve rewarding or penalizing organizations and providers based on specific outcomes serves as another external factor requiring consideration as part of planning for quality, safety, and performance improvement. For example, one of the key principles behind the development of the Leapfrog Group was to support value-based purchasing. Leapfrog's mission is to reward healthcare providers that provide excellent care. Further, it suggests that the rewards for superior healthcare value be based on four critical ingredients: reliable use of proven methods to ensure patient safety, improved clinical information systems, routine use of modern performance improvement methods in managing and delivering care, and routine and active engagement of consumers in healthcare decision making. Purchasers are directly encouraged to shift their resources to better providers, to educate their employees about the importance of comparing the performance of healthcare providers, and to assist them in using the measures to make informed healthcare choices.

The pay-for-performance movement is expected to expand further over the next several years to include additional levels of providers. Third-party payers continue to expand their pay-for-performance initiatives through increasingly robust programs. All the major payers (including Blue Cross, Aetna, Cigna, and UnitedHealthcare) are linking reimbursement to quality in their contracts with organizations and providers.

Customer Demands. The organization must consider what it should do from the perspective of its customers. A review of the healthcare market segments as well as an assessment of the specific needs, requirements, and expectations of various patient and stakeholder groups will help determine what the organization should do. The organization determines appropriate mechanisms for obtaining information from its customers.

Value-Based Service Delivery. As organizations plan, evaluate, and refine their strategy in response to the ever-changing healthcare market as the healthcare delivery system transforms from fee-for-service to value-based service, understanding where an organization is in the transition is critical to determining the impact of the external demands on the organization relative to planning. To meet external demands and optimize performance and align clinical outcome priorities with current quality and revenue-cycle opportunities, healthcare quality professionals need to understand and demonstrate key competencies related to population-health management and care transitions to best guide leaders in understanding the healthcare quality implications of this external force.

Step 3: What the Organization Can Do (Assessment of the Internal Environment). After the organization establishes what it *wants* to do and what it *should* do based on an assessment of the external environment, it needs to know what it *can* realistically do to ensure effective planning for success in achieving its goals. This requires an examination of the internal environment—the resources, capabilities, and core competencies of the organization. Resources can be tangible, such as human, financial, or physical, or intangible

such as reputation. For example, if an organization wants to be recognized as a leader in breast cancer detection and treatment, it must have qualified staff and equipment, as well as an engaged workforce and activated patients.

Step 4: Strategy Formulation. Based on the strategic goals, objectives, and evaluation of external and internal environments, strategic opportunities and threats are identified. Generally, organizations perform a gap analysis in which they evaluate the extent to which the present strategy needs change to meet the goals and objectives. Strategy formulation clearly stipulates actions to be taken to achieve goals. Any identified gaps between the current and needed resources, capabilities, and competencies identified in the assessment of the internal environment are appropriately planned in the strategy formulation.

Step 5: Strategy Implementation. Although various organizational departments and service lines may develop their own strategies and plans, they need to align with the overall goals and objectives of the organization. Members of senior leadership can take many approaches to integrate quality, safety, and performance improvement with strategic planning and to ensure that plans and strategies are being carried out.

Overseeing and Communicating Goals. An organization's strategic goals must be communicated to all levels of the organization. Because most strategic planning processes yield a set of strategic goals that are established for a period of more than 1 year, organizational leaders and healthcare quality professionals need to conduct an annual review of key services, customer expectations, regulatory requirements, and other aspects of organizational performance to establish annual priorities and project plans for quality and safety. Leaders in high-performing/high-reliability organizations consistently demonstrate—in both words and actions—a commitment to quality.[51] Leaders can emphasize quality and safety in forums with new employees and make connections between specific daily activities and quality priorities for the organization. Healthcare quality professionals support leadership efforts by communicating organizational values and commitment to staff in daily improvement activities and huddles, "connecting the dots" between activities and priorities wherever possible.

Hoshin Planning. Hoshin planning, a Japanese term that means policy deployment, is one approach for integration in a quality, safety, and performance improvement system used to ensure that the vision set forth by top management is being translated into planning objectives and actions that both management and employees will take to accomplish long-term organizational strategic goals (FIG. 1-9). "The primary reason to undertake Hoshin planning is to focus effort and resources on those few strategies and processes that will best

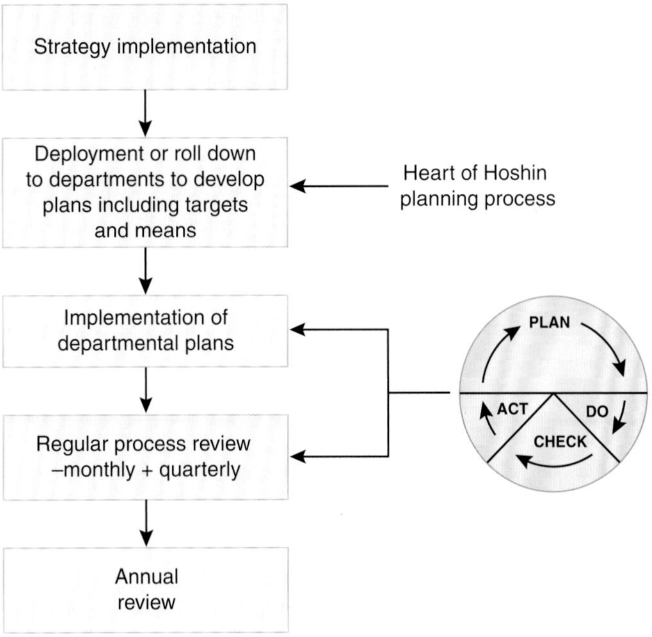

Figure 1-9 **Core Hoshin planning process.**

achieve the organization's survival and vision and to develop an effective process to align the goals and efforts of the organization."[52(p492)] The planning typically is performed at three levels: general (senior management), intermediate (middle management), and detailed (implementation teams). By using integrated and aligned cascading goals and objectives, individuals and groups across the organization can be guided to lead or contribute to the attainment of one of more specific goals identified as critical to success of the overall strategy. Furthermore, the Hoshin concept is based on the principle that high-performance organizations are those that harness the creative thinking power of all its employees. In this model, each employee is regarded as the expert at their own job and their contributions are consistently acknowledged.[53]

Step 6: Measure and Monitor Progress. In this last step of strategic planning, management seeks to evaluate the extent to which the strategy is accomplishing the goals set forth in the first step of strategic planning and ensure that improvement opportunities are identified and corrective action is implemented. Actual performance is evaluated and compared with the performance goals and objectives established as part of the strategic plan. Gaps between desired performance and actual performance require action. Many factors influence the effectiveness of strategy. Among the most important is the need for effective leadership.

As an expert facilitator, the healthcare quality professional may be expected to facilitate one or more of the planning steps outlined earlier. The healthcare quality professional can ensure a more informed strategic planning process by ensuring that the

results of quality, safety, and performance improvement processes, as relevant, are incorporated into various steps in the strategic planning process. Lessons learned from improvement efforts can inform several steps in the process. In addition, the healthcare quality professional may be expected to support or assist in strategy implementation and in measurement and control. As efforts to support the strategy are deployed throughout the organization, the expertise of the healthcare quality professional is critical to ensuring the development of appropriate metrics to monitor and evaluate success. Senior-level healthcare quality professionals are expected to use their advanced sense of organizational awareness to support the strategic planning process through seeing and communicating "the big picture" for both present and future.[54]

Identifying and Engaging Key Stakeholders

Identifying key stakeholders and ensuring their engagement is an important part of leadership's role in maintaining quality, safety, and performance improvement strategies. The healthcare quality professional can also assist leadership in engaging board members, senior leaders, physicians, staff, and patients and families.

Board Members. At the highest level, the organization's governing body is ultimately responsible for the quality of care provided in an organization. In most organizations, the governing body either assumes full responsibility for oversight of the organization's quality activities or delegates a large portion of the oversight responsibility to an oversight group (e.g., Quality Council; Steering Council; Quality, Safety, and

Performance Improvement Committee; Clinical Governance Committee) that consists of members of the governing body, medical staff leaders, and organizational senior leaders. Stakeholder representatives on these quality oversight committees might also sit on these committees (e.g., patients, families, community agency representatives).

Senior Leaders. The organization's senior leaders perform an important role in moving the organization to achieve strategic goals tied to safety and effectiveness. All senior leaders need to be fully engaged in the safety and quality journey. The healthcare quality professional can increase the engagement of the organization's senior leaders in several ways:

- Provide periodic education on senior leaders' roles and responsibilities related to responsibility for the quality of care and service provided in the organization and on targeted quality and safety topics.
- Ensure that senior management meeting agendas are structured so that quality and safety issues receive as much attention as financial and other issues.
- Communicate the status of organizational progress on key patient safety, quality, and service measures through the dissemination of quality dashboards.

Physicians. Although all members of the clinical staff are critical for patient safety and quality efforts, physicians often need focused attention to become fully engaged in quality, safety, and performance improvement efforts. Physicians are more likely to connect with quality and safety efforts that are important to them.[55] Organizations achieve success in engaging physicians in quality, safety, and performance improvement by embarking on projects that are led or co-led by physicians. A framework for engaging physicians in quality and safety can include engaged leadership, a physician compact, appropriate compensation, realignment of financial incentives, data plus enablers, and promotion.[56]

Staff. Leaders need to communicate that improving quality and safety is everyone's job and take steps to ensure that teamwork and collaboration are supported and rewarded. As this message spreads to the organization's frontline staffs, the healthcare quality professionals can further ensure staff engagement by ensuring appropriate frontline staff and physician representation on quality, safety, and performance improvement teams when teams are chartered. And, healthcare quality professionals can provide support to frontline managers by offering suggestions for quality- and safety-related staff meeting agenda items along with data, information, stories, and other evidence to support the discussion.

Patients and Families. In patient-centered environments, patients and families play a key role in advancing safety and quality.

Many organizations add patient and family representatives to relevant committees to keep the patient's perspective visible in all discussions about quality and safety. Patients and their families may need a higher level of detail when information about their medical situation is shared if they are to be effective partners in their own care.[14] The ever-present focus on quality and safety also requires that clinicians engage patients and families in their care. Patients and their families need to understand their role and responsibilities related to quality and safety. And leaders must heed the imperative to engage and activate patients.[57]

Resource Requirements

Healthcare quality professionals may be expected to work with senior leaders across the organization to identify the resources needed to implement and evaluate the quality and safety plan. As the gap between what the organization should do and what the organization is currently doing is identified, and specific goals and objectives are established, the healthcare quality professional will need to determine the staff and other resources needed to appropriately address the priority goals and objectives identified in the plan. For example, if reducing hospital-acquired conditions becomes a strategic priority as part of the quality, safety, and performance improvement plan for the organization, the healthcare quality professional will need to evaluate current performance, identify opportunities, and determine a strategy to meet the objective. The strategy will involve resources such as people, equipment, training, technology, external consultants, and other resources which need to be quantified so that appropriate resources may be allocated in the appropriate departmental budgets.

Program Development and Evaluation

The organization's strategic plan takes into consideration results of the quality, safety, and performance improvement process. These results serve as the basis for objectively evaluating the gaps between what the organization is doing and could be doing. Program evaluation considers progress on these results as well as other key metrics to determine the overall effectiveness of the program. Healthcare quality professionals are involved in collecting and analyzing specific outcome metrics tied to the quality program as part of the evaluation process. The results and analyses of findings are shared internally and action plans developed to address opportunities using one or more of the performance improvement models accepted by the organization. Various performance improvement models are discussed in detail in *Performance and Process Improvement*. Results and analyses are also shared with senior leadership and the governing body so that findings may be incorporated into key steps in the next strategic planning cycle.

Organizational Infrastructure for Quality and Safety

Organizational leadership is responsible for establishing the organizational infrastructure for quality and safety. For practical purposes, day-to-day leadership is delegated to the CEO and senior leaders, elected or appointed members of the medical staff (e.g., chairs, chiefs), and administrative and clinical staff (e.g., nurses, healthcare quality professionals). Organizational senior leadership is expected to work closely with the governing body and the organized medical staff. These groups are expected to regularly communicate with each other on issues of safety and quality. Senior leaders are expected to create and maintain a culture of safety and quality throughout the organization and use organization-wide planning processes to establish structures and processes that focus on safety and quality. Organizational senior leadership is also expected to work with other leaders to effectively manage the organization's programs, services, sites, or departments. Healthcare quality professionals can be instrumental in working with organizational leadership to ensure that the quality and safety structures are organized in the most efficient and effective manner. The quality structure of an organization is defined and organized with clear linkages and reporting structures. Donabedian[20(p82)] believed "that good structure, that is, a sufficiency of resources and proper system design, is probably the most important means of protecting and promoting the quality of care."

Governance and Leadership

The organization's governing body (e.g., board of directors, board of trustees) bears ultimate responsibility for the setting of policy, for financial and strategic direction, and for the quality of care and service provided by all its practitioners and nonclinical staff. The role and focus of the governing body evolved from a primary focus on financial health and reputation to a focus that includes direct responsibility for the hospital's mission to provide high-quality care.[58] Together with the organization's management and medical staff leaders, the board sets priorities for quality, safety, and performance improvement activities.

The development of meaningful board involvement in quality and safety requires assessment of the board's knowledge regarding healthcare quality. This is a key role of healthcare quality professionals, who are responsible for organizing and coordinating quality, safety, and performance improvement activities for the organization and its medical and professional staff. Healthcare quality professionals can promote the board's commitment to quality by providing useful information in a format easily understood by members who may lack familiarity with healthcare terminology and procedures.

Healthcare quality professionals work with the organization's leaders to maximize the effectiveness of the governing body's quality and safety committee. The Governance Institute[59] offers several insights, strategies, and practices to achieve this aim. Agendas and topics are organized to facilitate the governing body's quality and safety committee to focus on governance and not operations. Quality outcomes receive the same amount of focus and expectation of accountability in the governing body's quality committee as financial outcomes do in the governing body's finance committee. Clear messages about the expectation for transparency related to quality and safety come from the governing body through board adoption of policies to support fair and just culture and strong error disclosure and apology plans.

Organized Medical Providers

In many healthcare organizations and health systems, the physicians and other licensed independent practitioners are organized into a "medical and professional staff" and the leaders of the medical staff contribute to the leadership of the organization. In hospitals and other organizations, the medical staff functions according to a set of bylaws that are adopted by the medical staff and approved by the governing body. Bylaws establish standards for appointment, reappointment, and privileges whereby there is assurance that all members of the medical staff meet certain requirements to provide patient care. In hospitals, the organized medical staff is responsible for the quality and safety of medical care provided to patients. Medical staff departments have formal committee structures for evaluating quality of care and service provided to patients. These are critical and strengthen the organization's ability to meet its goals (e.g., clinical quality, financial).

In managed care networks, providers are organized as part of a healthcare delivery system to manage cost, utilization, and quality. The health plan manages the health benefits and additional services offered by a public or private third-party payor (e.g., Medicare, employer-sponsored plans). Healthcare is provided through contracted arrangements with individual and group providers. Providers go through an initial credentialing process prior to seeing health plan members and are recredentialed at set intervals (e.g., every 3 years). The "rules" for participating providers are typically informed by local, state, and national regulations and accreditation standards.

Other Organizational Structures and Departments

The healthcare quality professional's role is to evaluate the effectiveness of the various structures, paying close attention to alignment, coordination, and communication. Effective quality structures with clear lines of reporting ensure ongoing effective communication between and among structures and the alignment of activities with organizational priorities.

Operational Structures. Most organizations define one or more operational-level groups of senior leaders, physicians, mid-level managers, and staff members to manage the coordination of quality, safety, and other performance improvement efforts across the organization. The number, type, and focus of these operational quality structures will vary by the size, scope, and culture of an organization. Focus areas may include, but are not limited to, clinical quality, patient safety, and patient experience through Clinical Quality Councils, Patient Safety Committees, and Patient Experience/Engagement Councils.

Quality Departments. Many operational departments within healthcare organizations advance the quality and safety agenda and some have healthcare quality professional staff focused on one or more department-specific quality functions. However, most healthcare organizations establish an organized and staffed quality department responsible for most of the quality functions across the organization. How quality departments are staffed and structured impact how well the organization's quality, safety, and performance improvement processes are aligned, integrated, and effective.

Although limited evidence exists regarding best practices for quality functions and structures, the National Association for Healthcare Quality (NAHQ) and IHI cosponsored a research and development project that found the focus of quality departments changing from simple identification and reduction of defects to adding value to the organization. The quality department includes facilitators to educate and mentor staff to reduce variation, standardize workflow, and decrease defects in their everyday work. The department is viewed by the organization as experts in quality, safety, and performance improvement with adding value to efficiency in processes and decreasing operating costs.[60,61] How an organization's quality department is organized, structured, and staffed, as well as how it is regarded by key organizational stakeholders from a value perspective for quality, safety, and performance improvement, will influence an organization's overall ability to improve.

Other Elements Influencing Quality

When designing the infrastructure to influence quality, safety, and performance improvement, leaders need to consider approaches with the greatest positive impact. Evans and Dean[62] identified six basic elements with great influence on quality, namely,

- focus on processes,
- recognition of internal customers,
- reduction of hierarchy,

- creation of a team-based organization,
- use of steering committees, and
- development of an agile organization.

Focus on Processes. A focus on processes concerns the structural elements referred to as *departmentation*, that is, how jobs are grouped together. Jobs can be grouped by function, product or service, geography, and process or customer. Quality, safety, and performance improvement tend to focus on process structure rather than functional structure, supporting both Deming and Juran, who noted that quality issues more often arise from processes than from individual worker issues. Some organizations have reorganized their organizational quality structures to assign staff resources to focus on and standardize core processes.

Reduction in Hierarchy. One direct approach leaders can take to enable others to act is to modify the structure of the organization by reducing the hierarchy. Hierarchy relates to the number of managerial levels in the organization. The trend in recent years is toward a significant "flattening" (reduction in the number of levels), with more focus on employee participation through cross-functional collaboration (usually in the form of teams). Flatter organizations also tend to abolish silos—replacing a department-specific focus with interdepartmental, interprofessional, and cross-functional work.

Deming[11] maintains that improvements in quality are more likely to be realized when workers are empowered to solve problems, including changing processes and systems (most likely developed by management).

To work effectively, teams must be empowered. Empowerment enables people to take ownership of their jobs and make decisions concerning their department or area. People can take responsibility for their decisions, and add value to their jobs. Empowerment does not mean that people can be free to do whatever they want or reassign work that they do not want to do themselves. Empowerment means regarding existing policies and practices, accepting accountability for results, and giving advice.

Creating a Team-Based Organization. Another important structural element for quality, safety, and process improvement is creating a team-based organization. Because patient care involves multiple disciplines, the linchpin for improvement is frontline employees with regular communication and contact that allows them to coordinate and problem-solve to continuously improve quality of care. The organization must develop an infrastructure within which the cycle of improvement can operate. One feature of this infrastructure is teams.

Use of Steering Committees. A steering committee is usually an advisory committee consisting of key stakeholders and experts who come together to provide guidance on a specific issue or strategic objective. Steering committees are usually formed to advise and guide the development and implementation of a major program, project, or initiative.

Development of an Agile Organization.

In the current environment, organizations must be able to adapt rapidly to changes, executing strategy more quickly than previously and with more flexibility and adaptability to survive.

In addition to the elements offered by Evans and Dean, healthcare organizations require increasingly robust data management systems to manage data for quality, safety, and performance improvement. As the focus of care extends beyond the walls of the individual healthcare organization, healthcare quality professionals need more complex tools for data analytics to meet the data and information needs of organizational leaders related to the overall strategy for quality and safety. A detailed discussion of data management systems to include data warehouses, business intelligence tools, and implementing health information technology is provided in *Health Data Analytics*.

Change Management

Within the healthcare environment, change is not only inevitable, but it is also an ingredient essential for growth. Without change, systems would stagnate, and new knowledge and technology would not be adopted. Change is constant and occurs at all levels of healthcare organizations. Each level of change requires different strategies, depending on the type of change, the people involved, and the magnitude of the behavior that must be modified to make the required change. An overview of the key concepts associated with change, models describing how change occurs, strategies to manage change, and tools to help accelerate successful change is provided. Healthcare quality professionals can use this information to help leadership facilitate successful change in their organizations.

Change Models

Six change models will be presented to suggest different ways to think about change and the way various strategies, techniques, or tools can be used to effect change. This list is not exhaustive but rather provides foundational knowledge about change and common strategies. No single model will fit every type of change or organization. For this reason, healthcare quality professionals need a repertoire of principles and skills or a toolkit from which to draw for each situation.

Models explain a phenomenon and provide an approach for applying techniques at strategic points. The models have many common elements or similarities, such as description of movement from a current state to a future state. The impetus for this transition is dissatisfaction with the current state. Some common elements among models are readiness for change, communication of the change, and lead implementing the change. Using an approach in which change is planned provides the best results for a successful change.

Similarities in models also include the characteristics of the change itself and views of how these characteristics make it likely to be readily accepted by "users" (healthcare professionals, etc.). Common factors increasing the speed of change within an organizational setting are also identified in each model. The primary differences in the models are the scope and level of change. Most of the models address complex changes within complex organizations that often involve systems and processes, whereas other models focus on individual behavior changes.

Healthcare quality professionals are frequently asked to support or serve as change agents. A change agent is a person who helps members of an organization adapt to organizational change or creates organizational change.[63] Healthcare quality professionals can use various change models to guide them in their roles as change agents. The following change models will be described next:

- Lewin's Change Model.
- Palmer's Change Model.
- DeWeaver and Gillespie's Change Model.
- Galpin's Human Side of Change Model.
- Kotter's Heart of Change Model.
- Prochaska's Transtheoretical Change Model.

Lewin's Change Model.

Lewin had a strong impact on the theory and practice of social and organizational psychology. Of interest is his change model, the first premise of which is, motivation and readiness for change must occur before the change takes place. The impetus to change is based on a force field of driving and restraining forces. For change to occur, the force field must be altered so that driving forces are stronger than restraining forces. A key concept of Lewin's model is that the force field—and therefore the impetus to change—could be affected more by removing restraining forces than by adding more driving force. To create the motivation to change, some level of frustration or dissatisfaction with the current situation must exist. This dissatisfaction creates a level of anxiety or creative tension that will spur the desire to change. Effective change managers will use the dissatisfaction with the status quo to begin the movement to change.

This first step in Lewin's change process, known as "unfreezing," assumes that beliefs, expectations, and norms can be remolded into new beliefs and behaviors. Through a process of learning new information, attitudes, and processes, people can redefine their current beliefs and "refreeze" these new concepts into their behaviors. This model is useful in approaching change in behaviors and identifying strategies to accelerate change and sustain new desired behaviors.

Current State	Transition State	Future State
Unfreeze old behavior	Intervening change	Refreeze new behavior

Figure 1-10 Model for unfreezing and refreezing behavior.

Models of change typically show movement from a current state or an old system to a new or future state. This involves first unfreezing or changing the old system and moving it out of a "comfort zone" so that change can occur. This progresses to a transition state or middle ground, through which the now unfrozen process is altered. Finally, a new system or future state of equilibrium emerges. This new state must be refrozen so the new change "sticks." This model is used to integrate human system change with technology and work systems changes. It also can be used to create new systems to foster new activities needed by redesigned or reengineered work processes. The focus of the change effort is to invent a new status quo by directing all the activities and people involved in the change process.[64,65]

FIGURE 1-10 depicts the change model of moving from a current state by unfreezing behavior, through the transition state, and finally to a future state by refreezing a new behavior. The tool that can be used to analyze a situation or process to be changed, based on Lewin's work, is force-field analysis (FIG. 1-11). A diagram of two columns—"driving" and "restraining" forces—is developed to analyze opposing forces related to a specific change. Brainstorming, in a verbal format, and "brainwriting," in a written format, are tools that can be used to identify the driving and restraining forces if they are not clear. Driving forces, such as incentives and competition, tend to push change in a direction and keep it going. Restraining forces, which might include apathy or hostility, tend to restrain or decrease the driving forces. For change to be possible, the driving forces must be greater than the restraining forces. However, the force-field analysis shows not only the number of opposing forces but also the significance of each force. It is useful, for clarity, to indicate the relative "weights" of the opposing forces with the size of arrows (FIG. 1-11). For example, if a new law requires that a change be made, this mandate, together with the threat of a large fine for noncompliance, would be a more powerful driving force than would a manager's lack of interest in the change (the lack of money could also be a strongly weighted restraining force).

A key change management strategy using force-field analysis is to reduce the number of restraining forces; this approach increases the chances of success. Note, however, that adding powerful drivers does not necessarily make change happen faster.

Palmer's Change Model. Palmer, like Lewin, sees change involving movement from a current state through a transition state to an improved future state (FIG. 1-12). Palmer's change model lists seven key elements of implementing change, namely,

1. leading change,
2. creating a shared need,
3. shaping a vision,
4. mobilizing commitment,
5. monitoring progress,
6. finishing the job, and
7. anchoring the change in systems and structure.[66]

TABLE 1-4 assists with the assessment of failure points and indicates the needed change element for success using Palmer's model.

A key strategy to manage change using Palmer's model is to first assess readiness. By using the guidelines for change readiness listed in **TABLE 1-5**, one can assess an organization's readiness for change.[66,67] If a check of the elements in the guidelines does not indicate organizational readiness, then strategies are developed to achieve readiness.

DeWeaver and Gillespie's Change Model. Most change models used in healthcare follow a reductionist approach and are based on the assumptions that the change process can be broken into component parts and that healthcare quality professionals can then objectively measure the system inputs and outputs for each part. This model, described by DeWeaver and Gillespie,[37] is most useful when objective measures that can predict accurate results are in place. It depends on an orderly system in which objects behave predictably and new information can fit into existing structures. The following is a breakdown of the stages within this change model:

- *Awareness stage.* The person knows something about the change or is aware of the change and may have heard it mentioned and explained. However, the individual generally does not have a strong opinion about it and may deny that the change will affect him or her.
- *Curiosity stage.* The person expresses concern or curiosity about the change or asks questions about the effect of the change on him or her and may be defensive, resistant, or in denial about the change.
- *Visualization stage.* The person seeks to understand one's relationship to the change and the effect of the change on the person or the organization, by asking questions and seeking information.
- *Learning stage.* The person takes part in learning how to implement or use the change and may offer opinions and concerns about specifics of the change.

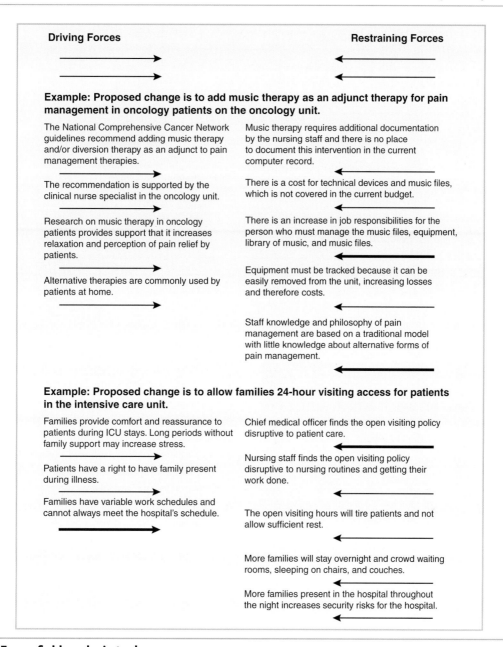

Figure 1-11 Force-field analysis tool.

- *Use stage.* The person actively uses the change and integrates the change into his or her daily work habits and can describe or explain the change to others.[68]

Individuals progress through these stages at different rates and can revert to previous stages at any time. The model is not linear: some may never make it through all the stages. The change agent cannot force people into later stages if they have not dealt with earlier stages. Whatever actions the facilitator takes to assist people through the change process will need to be repeated many times for various groups of people. Some individuals may need the same process repeated several times. Others may take a "What's in it for me?" approach; they will

need more time and more examples of benefits before they can commit to a change.[68]

Specific strategies can be used at each stage of the change model to increase the speed of the change process: awareness, curiosity, visualization, learning, and use.

- *Awareness stage.* Advertising in various media is used to inform people that the change is coming. Take the opportunity to highlight the positive effects of the change, and link the change to meeting staff needs and eliminating problems. Increasing awareness about the change early on provides an opportunity to shape perceptions positively.

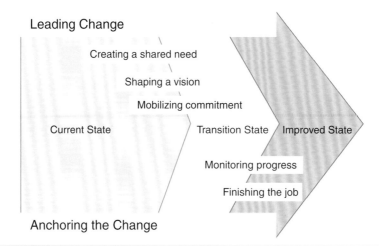

Figure 1-12 Palmer's change model. (Reprinted from Palmer B. *Making Change Work: Practical Tools for Overcoming Human Resistance to Change*. Milwaukee, WI: ASQ Quality Press; 2004, with permission from American Society for Quality, Quality Press © 2004 ASQ, www.asq.org.)

Table 1-4 Change Elements Necessary for Success	
Change Model Element	**Consequence of Missing a Model Element**
Leading change	Change is slow, lacks attention and resources.
Creating a shared need	Change has a low priority; receives no attention; and starts, then stops.
Shaping a vision	Change gets off to a fast start that fizzles; there is no clear direction.
Mobilizing commitment	Nobody "owns" the change; the project is not sustainable.
Monitoring progress	There is no chance for feedback and improvement.
Finishing the job	Cynicism, naysaying, and a "fad-of-the-month" attitude abound.
Anchoring the change	Mixed signals, anxiety, and frustration increase.

Reprinted from American Society for Quality. *Making Change Work*. Milwaukee, WI: ASQ; 2004, with permission. Copyright 2004 by the American Society for Quality. No further distribution allowed without permission.

- *Curiosity stage*. Strategies for the curiosity stage include providing frequent, clear, concise explanations and answering all questions. Taking time to elicit staff concerns and acknowledge the difficulties that the change may or will cause engenders support later in the change process. At the same time, it is important to present a viable approach to the change that acknowledges staff concerns. The curiosity stage is the time to create a level of dissatisfaction with the status quo and to generate interest in a new approach.

- *Visualization stage*. The strategy in this stage is to demonstrate the change for people and conduct user testing and reviews of the proposed changes. This gives people implementing change the opportunity to try the change before it is put into place.

- *Learning stage*. The strategy for this stage is to focus on educating staff regarding the change, conducting workshops or training sessions for as many staff members as possible, and giving them the opportunity for simulation or hands-on involvement when appropriate. An additional strategy is to provide materials that will make the change easier to use, such as quick reference guides, frequently asked questions (FAQs), troubleshooting tips, implementation teams, or help desks.

- *Use stage*. Technical assistance may be needed to make the change happen efficiently and effectively, with enough resources allocated to enable people to become experts at the change.

Users will be at different stages of accepting and implementing the change. Early in the change process, facilitators meet with all stakeholder groups to communicate the change, especially discussing the reason it is needed at that time for that stakeholder group. They take time to elicit reactions to the change and be sure to correct any misunderstandings. Also, it is important to acknowledge people's reactions to the changes and ask for suggestions that will help overcome any obstacles. In summary, key strategies include multiple approaches to garner support for the change and keep people informed of the change process.

Table 1-5 Guidelines for Assessing Change Readiness

Category	10% Readiness	50% Readiness	90% Readiness
Leading change	No one is in charge.	The leader is pretty clear; management's commitment is clear in some areas.	The change has a clear sponsor and clear commitment from management.
Creating shared need	Most people are happy with the status quo.	Many people think a change is needed.	Everybody knows a change is needed.
Shaping a vision	People ask, "What vision?"	Some consensus exists on what is needed, but also some apathy.	Everyone knows the needed outcome.
Mobilizing commitment	A staffer might help someone.	Some resources have been dedicated, but more are needed to finish the job.	All the needed resources have been dedicated and are available.
Monitoring progress	Everyone has her or his own opinion.	Some things are measured, but staff members also go by gut feeling sometimes.	Clear metrics exist for every activity being performed.
Finishing the job	The situation looks like a "dump and run."	Some plans have been made, but more remains to be done.	A pilot run, training, and recognition have occurred; everyone is ready.
Anchoring the change	People ask, "Why does anything have to be done?"	Discussion about this problem has begun but hasn't been finished.	Everyone knows exactly what needs to be adjusted to embed this change.

Instructions for Use:

1. Use to assess readiness in each of the categories listed and identify the corresponding percentage (e.g., if no one is in charge, then a rating of 10% is assigned).
2. After each category is assessed, total the percentages for the first three categories. If the sum of categories 1 + 2 + 3 <50%, then the likelihood of success for the change is low, and even starting a project is risky. Consider delaying the change project until support is garnered.
3. If any category is rated <50%, then the likelihood of success is also low (e.g., if no one is in charge, then chances of success are slim).
4. If the sum of categories 6 + 7 <50%, then proceeding to implementation of a successful change is unlikely.
5. The greater the percentage of readiness for change, the greater the likelihood of success. This approach also demonstrates the interrelatedness of each factor for change; all elements are important.
6. Plotting the percentage of readiness by category helps planners visualize the state of readiness and consider strategies for various stages of the change project and the critical elements at different points.

As the change is being implemented, it is important to continually assess the degree of its acceptance by the staff. This requires observing people's behavior and noting responses. Then, it is necessary to determine the stage of the change process in which people are operating. People will use many different methods to demonstrate resistance to change, and some may try to sabotage the change. It will be necessary to find ways to help people identify with the change and understand it and to anticipate and address their concerns. For change to succeed in an organization, a critical mass must support the new change.

People tend to fall into three groups related to change: those who are for change, those who are against the change, and those who are undecided. If efforts are focused on individuals who are already positively disposed to the change, they can in turn encourage those who are undecided, thereby allowing the facilitator to amass critical support. At this point, the focus turns to individuals who are not supportive, so that they can be influenced to accept the change.

Early in the change process, a communication plan must be developed to ensure that everyone becomes aware of the changes that will occur. This task may be easier to accomplish if the people's concerns are anticipated and proactively addressed. This can be achieved by providing a forum in which individuals can express their concerns openly and honestly. Forums (town halls, etc.) involve supportive stakeholders in an

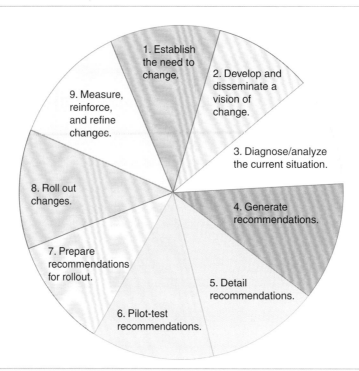

early demonstration of the change and include enough time for people to deal with their emotions regarding the change and to help them let go of the past and embrace the future.[68]

To summarize, key strategies that a change agent or project champion can use to accelerate change using this model include

1. assessing change readiness,
2. leading the change process proactively,
3. creating a shared need with stakeholders,
4. shaping a vision with clear goals,
5. mobilizing commitment with those who support the change,
6. monitoring progress toward completion,
7. completing the job, and
8. anchoring the change in systems and structures.

Galpin's Human Side of Change Model. Traditional views of change claim that most organizations focus on the technical, financial, and operational aspects, with little regard for the human aspect.[69,70] This mindset has since shifted to a strong appreciation of the human side of change. After all, people do the work, people must make the changes, and people will support or resist the changes. Galpin's approach is based on a nine-step process in which change is a deliberate, planned process. Having a well-planned, carefully thought-out process is the best approach to change management. Except in unusual

circumstances, planning for change, rather than allowing it to occur haphazardly, will ensure the greatest degree of success. Galpin's change management model involves the steps depicted in FIGURE 1-13.

Galpin correlates these stages with suggested time frames to guide the facilitator in planning and correlates the stages with either strategic change or grassroots change. Strategic change involves stages 1, 2, 3, 4, and 5, and grassroots change involves stages 6, 7, 8, and 9. Teams are basic infrastructure for the use of this model.[70]

Using his nine-step model, Galpin identifies four communication phases of a change effort. First is the "build awareness" phase (corresponding to stages 1 and 2). Next is the "project status" phase (corresponding to stages 3, 4, 5, 6, and 7). Then the communication plan is rolled out (corresponding to stage 8). Finally, follow-up with staff takes place at the end of the change process (corresponding to stage 9).

Galpin identified a practical change management tool, which he calls a "cultural screen." This tool focuses on the cultural aspect of change and identifies those factors associated with the culture of the organization assessed to achieve successful change. If, while using the screening tool, items are found that will impede the change process, a proactive approach to manage these specific items can be developed. If items are not identified prior to change efforts, then a risk exists that the change will be slow, arduous, or may even fail.

Implementation Actions

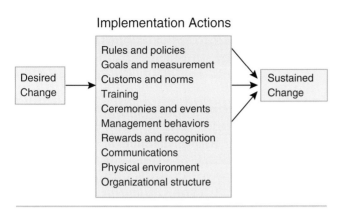

Figure 1-14 Cultural screening tool.

The cultural screening tool, which is used in implementing change,[44] includes the following 10 items (FIG. 1-14):

1. *Rules and policies.* To support positive implementation of change, identify and eliminate the rules and policies that will impede or restrain the change process. Develop new policies and procedures that will reinforce or drive the change. This effort corresponds to a recognition of the restraining and driving forces in Lewin's model.
2. *Goals and measurement.* Develop clear goals and measurements that reinforce the desired change. These will help sustain change and hold gains over time.
3. *Customs and norms.* Replace the old way of doing things by making it harder to revert, and reinforce the new change by making it easier to implement.
4. *Training.* Develop training and education that will reinforce the new change. Provide real-time, hands-on experience with the new process to support acceptance.
5. *Ceremonies and events.* Implement ceremonies that reinforce the new change and recognize both individual and team contributions to the success of the change effort.
6. *Management behaviors.* Publicly recognize and reward managers who support and implement the change. Link pay, merit, and promotion to desired behaviors.
7. *Rewards and recognition.* Make rewards specific to the change goals. Be sure that the performance system rewards the desired change. Rewards and recognition are key principles to successful management.
8. *Communications.* Communicate in ways that demonstrate commitment to the change. Use multiple methods to deliver a consistent message throughout the change process.
9. *Physical environment.* Ensure that the physical environment reflects and supports the change.
10. *Organizational structure.* Ensure that the organizational structure reinforces the change.[69]

In a humanistic approach to change, communication during all stages of the change process is critical for success.

Communication is realistic and honest, and it must be proactive, not reactive. Link messages to the purpose of the change and repeat consistently through the entire process. Multiple avenues of communication are needed, including a feedback mechanism. This includes communication up and down as well as across the organization. Most experts on change reiterate that the most important aspect of change is communication.

Because communication is an essential aspect of Galpin's humanistic approach to change, it is important to discuss some associated pitfalls. Leaders must be clear and precise about the change. If the leaders cannot succinctly and accurately describe the change, then inaccuracies and rumors will abound throughout the organization. Leaders who believe in limiting information will quickly find that the "grapevine" is a powerful force and that the desired message will not be delivered as intended. Open, honest communication is important to create credibility and trust. Leaders who are promoting significant change cannot delegate communication and ownership of the change to others. A well-written communication plan with the involvement of senior leaders will be necessary throughout the entire change process. A common pitfall is to slow down communication when the process is under way. Ensuring that the change is complete and sustained is one of the more difficult tasks and is often overlooked or neglected. Providing infrastructure to maintain the change is also critical. Leaders need to communicate with staff even after the change is made to ensure that it endures.

Management strategies based on Galpin's humanistic model focus specifically on assessing the organization's culture. This approach allows for the elimination of rules and policies that hinder the change and the development of new rules that reinforce the desired approach or behavior (like restraining and driving forces). These strategies also include the development of goals and measurements that reinforce the desired changes and provide greater leverage for advancing change.

Kotter's Heart of Change Model. Kotter writes extensively on leadership and change management. His view of change is based on ensuring that people fully accept and incorporate the change into their belief system. His work also details a humanistic approach to get to the "heart" or emotional aspects associated with change.[71] Common errors of organizational change efforts include:

- allowing too much complacency,
- failing to create a sufficiently powerful guiding coalition,
- underestimating the power of vision,
- undercommunicating the vision,
- permitting obstacles to block the new vision,
- failing to create short-term wins,
- declaring victory too soon, and
- neglecting to anchor changes firmly in the corporate culture.

Kotter[72] provides an eight-stage process of creating a major change that proactively addresses errors common to organizational change efforts. The first four steps in the process help "defrost" a hardened status quo, the next three phases introduce many new practices, and the last stage grounds the changes in the corporate culture and helps make them stick.

1. *Increase urgency.* The first and most critical step in Kotter's model is to shake up the status quo and create a feeling of urgency. At this stage, people must be shocked into action. ("We must do something!") The major challenge at this stage is to get people ready to move. Methods that will advance this stage include dramatic presentations with compelling stories and items that people can see, touch, and feel, such as seeing a visual display of performance levels, touching a new computer, or feeling the emotional fear of job reductions. This step requires evidence that change is required.

2. *Build the guiding team.* The next step is to organize a team of influential, effective leaders. It is important to get the right people in the right place with the right change process. Team members must be fully committed to the change initiative, be well-respected within the organization, and possess power and influence to drive the change effort. It is a challenge to get the right people with the best tools to be an effective trusted team. The team makeup is diverse enough to provide multiple perspectives on the change and the stakeholders' interests.

3. *Get the vision right.* As with other models presented, a clear vision is essential. Without clear direction, the team cannot focus on the change and the implementation process. Providing this direction is leadership's responsibility. It is the vision that will steer the team into the new direction. Visioning activities about possible futures will help create strategies for the change initiative.

4. *Communicate for buy-in.* It has already been said: communicate, communicate, communicate! Once a vision and strategy are developed, they must be communicated to the organization. Sending clear, credible, and heartfelt messages about the direction of change establishes genuine, gut-level buy-in, which sets the stage for getting people to act. Keep communication simple and sincere; find out what people are feeling and address their anxiety, confusion, anger, and distrust. Rid communication channels of "junk" so that the important message can be delivered. Constantly reassess this step throughout the change effort.

5. *Empower action.* The next step is to empower people to act by removing barriers. Removing obstacles will promote confidence in change, allowing more people to feel able to act.

6. *Create short-term wins.* Short-term wins provide visible immediate successes and inspire people to believe that the change can be implemented. The challenge is to create short-term wins and energize users about the change.

7. *Don't let up.* The process is not complete until the change is a reality. Leaders need to support the change over time, building on the momentum of short-term wins by keeping the sense of urgency alive. It is difficult to sustain excitement and energy over time and easy to become sidetracked by other tasks.

8. *Make change stick.* The end of the change process often is one of the most difficult stages. Once the change is implemented, it must be ingrained (hardwired) in the organization, so that gains can be sustained, and a return to the previous way of doing things is prevented.[71]

Successful change goes through all eight stages, usually in sequence, although it is also normal to go through multiple phases at once. Most major change initiatives are made up of several smaller projects, with each going through the multi-step process. So, at any one time, people might be halfway through the overall effort, finished with a few smaller pieces, and just beginning other projects. Thus, with multiple steps and multiple projects, the result is often complex, dynamic, and messy rather than the conclusion of a simple, linear, analytical process (in other words, a CAS).

Prochaska's Transtheoretical Change Model. Prochaska's approach to changing behavior is known as the transtheoretical, or "stages of change," model.[73] The concepts of this model are applicable to numerous individual behavior changes including those related to maintenance of a healthy weight, smoking cessation, and substance abuse treatment. The stages of change explain the individual's readiness to change behavior, rather than a process change. This model is useful for working with individual staff members, patients, and providers to change behaviors.

Six stages that individuals use to change behavior (based on psychotherapy) are identified:

1. *Precontemplation.* The person has no intention to act within the next 6 months;

2. *Contemplation.* The person has an intention to act within the next 6 months;

3. *Preparation.* The person has an intention to act within the next 30 days and has taken some behavioral steps in this direction;

4. *Action.* The person's behavior changed for a period of less than 6 months;

5. *Maintenance.* The person's behavior changed for a period of more than 6 months; and

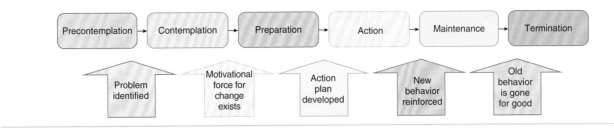

Figure 1-15 **Prochaska's stages in changing behavior.**

6. *Termination.* The person is confident the behavior will never return and complete confidence in the ability to cope without fear of relapse.[73]

FIGURE 1-15 illustrates the stages in changing behavior along a time continuum. Prochaska, director of the Cancer Prevention Research Center, led the development of measures that can be used with the transtheoretical model. Using this model requires some different strategies from those used in the other models presented. This model assumes that a person will not change his or her behavior until ready. Therefore, planned change is dependent on the readiness of the individual, not the organization. The person must move from a state of precontemplation to contemplation; only when this occurs can change take place. The application of this model may be useful with special populations (e.g., patients with congestive heart failure, renal failure, or diabetes) and certain health behavior changes (e.g., smoking cessation, adherence to medication regimen, and weight loss). It also may be effective in changing the practice patterns of individual providers, for example, influencing providers to adopt a new product or technology. It is not useful for planned system change.

Leading Change

To effect true change, one must become a compassionate leader, requiring "a paradigm shift from the present dehumanizing model of the organization as a machine to one of the organization as a living complex adaptive system."[74(p1)] Such leadership is difficult because no formula exists, and one must be willing, for starters, to change oneself.

Although management involves a set of processes that can keep a complex system of people and technology running smoothly, leadership defines what the future looks like, aligns people with that vision, and inspires them to make it happen despite the obstacles.[72] This distinction is crucial, because successful transformation is 70% to 90% leadership and only 10% to 30% management. An emphasis on management rather than leadership is often institutionalized in corporate cultures that discourage employees from learning how to lead. Managing change is important because without

competent management, the transformation process can go out of control. But for most organizations, the much bigger challenge is leading change. Leadership often begins with just one or two people, but that number needs to grow over time. Modern organizations are far too complex to be transformed by a single individual.

The ability to manage change in a planned, productive manner is a core competency of healthcare quality professionals. It is therefore necessary to understand various aspects of change, change models, and ways to use tools to successfully manage change for improvement. One of the most important change concepts to understand is that "all changes do not lead to improvement, but all improvement requires change."[75] People may make changes with no impact on improving services or products but that certainly disrupt routines. This reality must be clearly understood by healthcare quality professionals because of the turmoil and upheaval that constant change creates for daily workflow. When change improves services and products, healthcare quality professionals and other members of the change team can more easily and positively influence those who must make the change. Change merely for the sake of change usually causes frustration and dissatisfaction, not to mention additional work. Healthcare quality professionals play vital roles as change agents, improvement advisors, and facilitators and must be attuned to the personal side of change to manage the change process successfully.

Healthcare is a complex system in which demands change quickly. The intense competition among various healthcare organizations is intensified when resources are scarce. The question facing most organizations is not whether changes are needed, but rather how much and how often. Two factors are critical to assessing change in organizations: first, the limits of human performance in being able to respond to change, and second, the actual capacity of the systems to handle change. An organization's ability to handle frequent change depends largely upon the individuals within the organization, including its leaders.

In a 2014 Pew Research Center Survey, the top seven leadership qualities that matter most to the public included honest, intelligent, decisive, organized, compassionate, innovative, and ambitious. Women leaders were more compassionate and men more decisive.[76] Having evaluated over 30,000 leaders over 12 years, Olivo found that effective healthcare leaders exhibited these six characteristics:

1. *Directing*—Assertive yet collaborative with reasoned diplomacy and bluntness
2. *Engaging*—Verbal and social
3. *Challenging*—Very logical, but still supportive and tolerant
4. *Methodical*—Achieving and structured
5. *Adventurous*—Very ambitious, competitive, and willing to take risks
6. *Concrete*—Practical and experience-based.[77]

The resiliency of individuals is another critical element in an organization's ability to make changes quickly and rebound from one change to the next. "Resilience is the process of adapting well in the face of adversity, trauma, tragedy, threats, or significant sources of stress—such as family and relationship problems, serious health problems, or workplace and financial stressors. It means 'bouncing back' from difficult experiences."[78(¶1)] The American Psychological Association (APA) recommends that individuals follow these guidelines to build and sustain resilience, such as make connections (good relationships), avoid seeing crises as insurmountable problems, accept that change is a part of living, move toward goals, and look for opportunities for self-discovery. Although the APA principles were developed for individuals, they are also applicable to organizational behavior.

Although individual resiliency affects an organization's response to change, the leaders establish the culture of change, role-model flexibility, and the behaviors needed to adapt to change. If participants view the change as positive, they are more likely to value the results. However, if they are not part of the change process, they probably will not accept the

changes that result; this rejection will be evident in several ways. Commonly, unengaged or disgruntled staff will return to the old way of practice. They may devise work-around solutions or outright sabotage to avoid the change. Healthcare is in constant flux, and the success of healthcare organizations in the future will depend on their reliability, flexibility, resilience, and implementation of change in a purposeful, collaborative manner.

Although change generally is focused on moving people from an existing state through a transition state to a future state, no single model or tool will fit every situation in which change is desired. A repertoire of skills, knowledge, and abilities will help healthcare quality professionals understand different views of how change occurs and to use a variety of tools and techniques to effectively manage change. Reviewing a few change models that describe how change occurs, as well as some change management strategies based on their theoretical frameworks, will be useful.

Planning and Managing Change

Planning and managing change will be described in three major areas: the assessment of readiness for change, Plan-Do-Study-Act (PDSA; previously known as Plan-Do-Check-Act [PDCA]) cycles of change, and change concepts.

Assessment of Readiness for Change. Tools can assist with assessing an organization or unit for readiness to change. FIGURE 1-16 illustrates in a simple manner how to assess readiness for change. If the organization is ready and a plan is followed, chances for success are good. If the organization is not ready, the change agent must determine whether the person

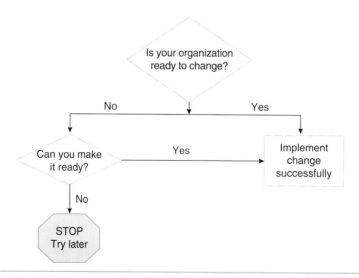

Figure 1-16 **Assessing readiness for change.** (Reprinted from Palmer B. *Making Change Work: Practical Tools for Overcoming Human Resistance to Change.* Milwaukee, WI: ASQ Quality Press; 2004, with permission from American Society for Quality, Quality Press © 2004 ASQ, www.asq.org.)

can help make the organization ready or whether the change instead be considered later. If a change effort proceeds in an organization that is not ready, the costs of failure will be high.

It is important to reiterate that "all changes do not necessarily lead to improvement, but all improvement requires change."[79] This concept is strongly voiced by IHI, which also provides several tools for performance improvement that will now be addressed.

Plan-Do-Study-Act Cycles of Change. The point of change is to make an improvement. Until this point the discussion focused on change models; it now moves to a performance improvement model to make change for improvement. Variations were made to the original PDCA model, including PDSA and others.[80]

Change Concepts. Langley and colleagues[81] introduced the idea of the *change concept* as a general approach to developing specific ideas for improvement. Nine change concepts fitting the PDSA improvement cycle are identified as ways to introduce creative or innovative approaches to change and improvement. These nine change concepts, which can be further subdivided into 70 major ideas, also align with core tenets of Lean and Six Sigma:

1. Eliminate waste,
2. Improve work flow,
3. Optimize inventory,
4. Change the work environment,
5. Enhance producer–customer interface,
6. Manage time,
7. Manage variation,
8. Design error-proof systems, and
9. Focus on the product or service.

This is described in more detail in *Performance and Process Improvement*.

Factors Supporting or Accelerating Change

Several factors are identified as accelerators for success and can be thought about in several ways. In healthcare, there is a divide and struggle with change—spearheading fiscal progress for the organization and understanding the burden that change causes on the frontline of care. Change is accelerated when the organization's culture exhibits and encourages a capacity for continuous learning and closing the divide with executives, clinical leaders, and staff.

A recent report suggests that disconnects in transforming healthcare delivery can slow change. However, the "more exposure executives and clinical leaders receive on the impact increased patient engagement and disruptors have on clinicians, the easier it will be to figure out how to alleviate system stressors. And the more clinicians see the positive impacts that patient engagement, market disruptors, and value-based care have on quality and cost outcomes, the more enthusiastic they will be about these opportunities."[82(p8)]

Having knowledge of its internal stakeholders, customers, and key business processes will allow an organization to identify driving and restraining forces quickly and move into the phases of planned change more easily. Every change requires some access to resources. The availability of resources, such as training, project materials, information systems, personnel, and financial support, will accelerate the change process. **TABLE 1-6** lists characteristics that accelerate change and innovation within four categories: leadership, culture, structure, and techniques.

In addition, the values of high-performing organizations outlined in the Baldrige Health Care Criteria (2017) are built on the following set of interrelated core values and concepts, such as the systems perspective, visionary leadership, patient-focused excellence, valuing people, organizational learning and agility, ethics and transparency, and delivering value and results. Organizations exhibiting these values have a greater capacity to adapt to change and to implement innovations than organizations that do not.

Resistance to Change

In managing resistance to change, three key areas need to be assessed: attitude, skill, and knowledge. Fear accompanies change, and fear cannot be eliminated, so the change strategy needs to actively address this emotion. Fear is usually associated with the unknown effects that the change will bring. This fear can be reduced by clearly identifying the effect of the change effort and communicating openly with those involved.

- Strategies to reduce resistance in people who are not willing to make the change include setting goals, measuring performance, providing coaching and feedback, and rewarding and recognizing positive efforts.
- Strategies to reduce resistance in people who are not able to perform the new change include educating and training staff in the new skills and the use of various management techniques.
- Strategies to reduce resistance in people without the necessary knowledge to make the change include
  ○ communicating the what, why, how, when, and who of the change process;
  ○ presenting a positive outlook on the proposed change;
  ○ having a clear focus and goal for the change and expectations of those involved;
  ○ being flexible and adaptable during the change process;
  ○ using a structured approach to manage ambiguity and confusion;

Table 1-6 High-Performing Organizations: Factors Affecting Speed of Change

Aspect of Organization	Accelerator of Change or Innovation
Leadership	• Sets expectations for organizational performance, includes a focus on creating and balancing value for patients, other customers, and other stakeholders • Focuses on creating and balancing the value of change for patients, other customers, and other stakeholders • Creates a focus on action that will improve the organization's performance and assesses readiness for the change • Identifies needed actions and makes the focus or goal of the change clear • Active, visible, and supportive of change involving all leaders with clear expectations for results • Takes a direct role in motivating the workforce toward high performance and a patient, other customer, and healthcare focus, including by participating in reward and recognition programs • Creates and promotes a culture of patient safety • Demonstrates personal accountability for the organization's actions • Communicates as marketplace, patient, other customer, or stakeholder requirements change • Encourages open, two-way communication, including use of social media, when appropriate • Communicates key decisions and needs for organizational change • Addresses any adverse societal impacts or public concerns related to changes in healthcare services and operations
Culture	• Fosters patient and other customer engagement • Values relationships • Encourages new ideas • Supports creativity, innovation, and risk-taking • Accepts failures (without blame) as well as successes • Creates an environment for the achievement of mission and organizational agility • Cultivates organizational learning, learning for people in the workforce, innovation, and intelligent risk-taking • Supports participative structure with staff-level involvement • Focuses on group learning • Values continuous learning and improvement • Supports succession planning and the development of future organizational leaders • Encourages diversity • Focuses on systems and processes • Rewards individuals and teams for performance
Structure	• Develops a strong team infrastructure and empowers team members • Makes resources available for the change • Enables mechanisms to obtain actionable items for desired change taking into consideration the voice of the customer • Creates the means to listen to, interact with, and observe patients and other customers
Linkages	• Makes connections between processes and the results achieved • How data are measured and analyzed in the strategic planning process and for improving operations • Connects workforce planning and strategic planning • Need for patient, other customer, and market knowledge in establishing strategy and action plans • Connects action plans with changes needed in work systems
Techniques	• Makes tools and technology available to teams and ensures they are used • Applies change models and concepts • Uses constraints and forcing functions • Replaces old ways of doing things with new customs or norms and reinforces the change • Makes it easy to accomplish the change • Uses training that reinforces the change • Puts procedures in place to reinforce the change • Evaluates sustainability of change • Recognizes and rewards by linking promotion and pay to desired behaviors

Adapted from Baldrige Performance Excellence Program. 2017–2018 *Baldrige Excellence Framework: A Systems Approach to Improving Your Organization's Performance*. Gaithersburg, MD: U.S. Department of Commerce, National Institute of Standards and Technology; 2017. https://www.nist.gov/baldrige. Accessed 27, June 2017; Fraser SW, Schall M. Accelerating the spread of better practice. Presented at the 14th Annual Institute for Healthcare Improvement Conference in Orlando, FL, December 2002.

- planning and coordinating the change process in a systematic way with clear expectations; and
- using a proactive rather than a reactive approach.

An area that also must be considered in relation to change management is special populations. Both individuals and patient populations often require behavioral changes in healthcare practices to facilitate compliance with discharge instructions and thus improve the likelihood of positive outcomes. Change management approaches commonly are needed for patients with chronic conditions such as congestive heart failure, renal failure, or diabetes. Patients with complex medication or treatment schedules also may require change management. Some situations in which individuals or patient groups may require change management include

- substance use (e.g., abuse of tobacco, alcohol, or illegal substances);
- conditions involving dietary and weight management (e.g., bowel disorders, obesity, eating disorders, diabetes); and
- mental health disorders (e.g., medication adherence, therapeutic behaviors).

Change management techniques also are utilized with specific providers, such as physicians, to engage them as champions of a change initiative or to enlist them in making a major change. Change strategies require special attention to these restraining forces and to the development of culture and methods to communicate the rationale for the change. Driving forces for this group often include a demonstration of the value of the change (the return on the investment), such as its relevance to practice or to pay-for-performance programs. The last change factor to consider with this group is accountability and how it can be applied in implementing and evaluating the change.

Best Practices, Creativity, and Innovation

A *best practice* is "a procedure that has been shown by research and experience to produce optimal results and that is established or proposed as a standard suitable for widespread adoption."[83] Organizational leaders need to create the environment where review, consideration, and adoption or adaptation of best practices are promoted as part of quality, safety, and performance improvement. Additional details will be provided about best practices in *Performance and Process Improvement*.

If an organization desires a reliable, creative, resilient, and regenerative culture that promotes learning, then it must look at human relationships. In this context, people are more willing to change and are more adaptable when they believe that they are not alone and that together they can manage almost anything. Maher et al.[84] identified seven dimensions that impact an organization's culture for innovation: (1) risk-taking, (2) resources, (3) knowledge, (4) goals, (5) rewards, (6) tools, and (7) relationships. The concept of creativity corresponds to individual resiliency and capacity to change and moving forward may be impacted by the culture.

To encourage creativity in an organization, leaders must be accessible and must acknowledge the value of people's contributions. They must create opportunities in which people can take risks and be allowed to fail. Creativity allows organizations to generate new ideas, remain competitive, and face the constant barrage of new challenges. Hundreds of ideas must be generated to find a true innovation that can be put into practice.[85] Common themes across models of creativity include the creative process (purposeful, imaginative idea generation and critical evaluation) and purposeful generation of new ideas that are directed and action-oriented. Several techniques can be used to create new ideas like break routine ways of thinking and conduct activities to generate ideas; inspire breakthrough performance; use brainstorming (and brainwriting, its written form); use metaphors; develop prototypes and models; and use traditional tools such as fishbone (cause and effect or Ishikawa) diagrams, flowcharts, and process maps.

Creativity must be nurtured and identified as an expectation within the organizational culture. The three principles that underpin creative thinking are attention, escape, and movement. Plsek[85] described these principles in action as focusing attention, escaping the current reality, and moving mentally toward inventing or generating new ideas. The principle of attention primarily occurs in the preparation stage of creativity in which attention is focused on an idea or item in a different or uncommon way. According to Plsek,[85] the principle of escape allows one to see familiar objects in a new light; one must escape or abandon the tendency to "oversimplify the world into neat conventional explanations."

The principle of movement involves moving away from familiar or traditional ideas toward an innovative or novel approach. Plsek[84] identifies four general phases, or steps, in directed creativity:

1. *Preparation*: pausing and noticing, seeking other points of view, refocusing a topic, looking closer and analyzing, searching for analogies, and creating new world.
2. *Imagination*: brainstorming, using analogies, provoking imaginations, "leaping," combining concepts systematically, organizing and displaying ideas, and harvesting ideas.
3. Development: final harvesting.
4. Action.

A structured approach within each of these four phases of directed creativity, depicted in FIGURE 1-17, guides creativity and the generation of tangible ideas and products.

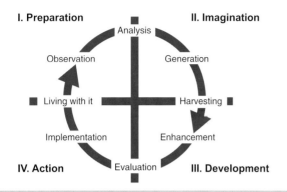

Figure 1-17 Four phases of directed creativity cycle.
(Reprinted from Plsek P. Directed creativity cycle. In: Plsek P, ed. *Creativity, Innovation and Quality*. Milwaukee, WI: ASQ Quality Press. www.DirectedCreativity.com. Copyright 1997 by P. Plsek, with permission.)

Leaders and healthcare quality professionals need to foster creativity and innovation in their employees. The Center for Creative Leadership[86(pp16–17)] identified important components of an innovation leadership mindset:

- *Curiosity*. Curiosity fuels the acquisition of new information.
- Paying Attention. Paying attention is sometimes phrased as "slowing looking down" or "slowing down to power up."
- *Customer-Centric*. With this approach, you combine paying attention with looking through the eyes of a client—creating opportunities to adapt existing products and services or to create new ones.
- *Affirmative Judgment*. Versus letting people know what you don't like, more valuable to the growth and development of the organization are leaders who take on the more difficult task of letting people know what they do like.
- *Tolerance for Ambiguity*. Balance the need to move forward with the need to hold oneself open to additional possibilities.

When creativity and innovation are fostered and nurtured in the culture, innovations can emerge, and creative endeavors can be transformed into innovations. Baldrige's *2017– 2018 Health Care Criteria for Performance Excellence* focuses on managing for *innovation*, defined as "making meaningful change to improve an organization's services, processes and organizational effectiveness and create new value for stakeholders."[23] Managing for innovation leads to new dimensions of performance. Innovation builds on the knowledge of the organization and its staff. These nine rules of innovation can be adopted by the organization as strategies:

1. Innovate or imitate best-performing innovative organizations.
2. Practice both research and development, and search and development. Do not reinvent the wheel.
3. Engage in both product innovation and process innovation. (Most healthcare organizations implement process innovations.)

4. Invest in new processes and products as well as in old ones. There is a typical life span for each product and process. The usefulness of these products and processes is maximized during this period.
5. Practice both "big-bang" (breakthrough) innovation and continuous (incremental) improvement.
6. Be both market-driven and technology-driven.
7. Be totally committed to innovation as a strategy.
8. Conduct both basic and applied research in a coordinated way, and make basic research more application-oriented.
9. Use speed strategies to bring products to market.

Creativity is necessary for innovations, and innovations depend on a creative organization with leaders who possess an innovation mindset.

Disruptive Innovation

The theory of disruptive innovation was first introduced by Christensen in his research and later popularized by his book *The Innovator's Dilemma*, published in 1997. The theory explains the phenomenon by which an innovation transforms an existing market or sector by introducing simplicity, convenience, accessibility, and affordability where complication and high cost are considered the norm. Initially, a disruptive innovation is formed in a specialized market that may appear unattractive or inconsequential to industry insiders, but eventually the new product or idea completely redefines the industry.[87] One of the most frequently cited examples of a disruptive innovation is the personal computer. Prior to its introduction, mainframes and minicomputers were the prevailing products in the computing industry. The theory of disruptive innovation helps explain how complicated, expensive products and services in healthcare are eventually converted into simpler, affordable ones.

Healthcare leaders who want to understand or even introduce disruptive innovation can explore opportunities in terms of the four Ws—who, what, when, and where. This involves asking the following questions about the service delivery model for a specific type of care:

Who is actively and substantially carrying out the process? Consider whether the patient could become a more active and substantial participant, rather than just a somewhat passive recipient, and whether clinical protocols may reduce the role of physicians in managing the process.

What happens in the process? Consider possible changes in the sequence of events, the content of the work, the use of different technologies, etc.

When are patients able to access the service? Consider shifts in thinking regarding 24/7 access, weekends versus weekdays, etc.

Where are patients able to access the service? Consider shifts that make the service accessible at home, in the community, or in a referring provider's office, rather than at a medical center.[88]

Nurse practitioners, general practitioners, and even patients can do things in less-expensive, decentralized settings that could once be performed only by expensive specialists in centralized, inconvenient locations. Examples include remote monitoring using technology for renal transplant patients and nurse-managed healthcare clinics.

Healthcare quality professionals are in a key position to influence leadership on the importance of fostering creativity and innovation in an organization. Pradhan and Pradhan[89] identified several disruptive innovations such as Google Glass, noninvasive healthcare, automation in healthcare, 3D printing, personal health devices, gene mapping, e-Patients, and digital checkup in their work describing emerging healthcare innovations.[90]

Spread of Change and Innovation

Although generating and implementing innovative ideas take effort and can be challenging, one of the most frustrating aspects of promoting creativity and innovation is the difficulty of making sure that the innovation spreads throughout the organization.[91] Rogers[92] and IHI[93,94] each offer models to facilitate the spread of innovation.

Rogers' Diffusion of Innovation Model. To be widely implemented, new ideas, products, or technology must be disseminated throughout an organization. *Diffusion* is the process by which an innovation or new idea is communicated through certain channels over time among members of a social system (*dissemination* is synonymous with *diffusion* for purposes of this work). An *innovation* is an idea, practice, or object that is perceived as new by those who adopt it. Directed creativity activities may lead to an innovation, or the innovation may be adopted from an external source. Rogers'[92] diffusion model includes innovation; communication channels about the innovation; time (the time span from the point of someone first hearing of the innovation to the point of decision to accept or reject it, the number of individuals in a social system who adopt an innovation in each period, and the innovativeness of the individual or agency to determine the time needed to achieve adoption); and the social system in which an innovation is adopted.

The decision process on innovations consists of five stages. Rogers[92] defines five stages in adopting an innovation:

1. *Knowledge*—socioeconomic characteristics, personality variables, and communication behavior (the level of the person's innovativeness determines the type of adopter);

2. *Persuasion*—attending to the perceived cha[ ] the innovation: relative advantage, compa[ ] plexity, trialability (suitability for trial), observability or visibility, reversibility, uncertainty;

3. *Decision*—adoption or rejection;

4. *Implementation*—direct application, reinvention, indirect application, or effect; and

5. *Confirmation*—evaluation of the innovation's effectiveness to determine whether it will be continued or discontinued.

Before the five stages occur, however, other factors must be considered, such as the history and culture of change in the organization, support of change given by leaders; the needs of the organization within a competitive market; the innovativeness of the organization; and the norms of the system (including the organization's culture of change, readiness for change, boundaries and relationships, channels of communication, and priorities).

The dissemination or diffusion of innovations is affected by influences in three major areas as outlined in Rogers' model[92]:

- Perceptions of the innovation
  - the perceived benefit of the change or innovation (people are more likely to adopt a change or innovation if they think it can help them);
  - the compatibility of the change or innovation with the values, beliefs, history, and current needs of individuals (people are more likely to adopt a change or innovation that is consistent with their own values);
  - the complexity of the change or innovation (generally, simple changes and innovations are adopted more quickly than complicated ones);
  - the trialability of the change or innovation by users (people are more likely to adopt a change or innovation that they can try before being required to use it); and
  - the observability of the change or innovation by people who can watch others try the change first (people are more likely to adopt a change or innovation that they can see in use before having to use it).
- Characteristics of individuals who may (or may not) adopt the change, depending on their degree of innovativeness
  - innovators (2.5%),
  - early adopters (13.5%),
  - early majority (34%),
  - late majority (34%), and
  - laggards (16%).
- Managerial and contextual factors (e.g., communication, incentives, leadership, and management) within organizations involved (the rate of adoption of innovations is greater with increased communication, positive incentives, and supportive leaders).

By using Rogers' model (which Berwick adapted to healthcare in 2003),[95] healthcare quality professionals can develop plans that incorporate these concepts, increasing the likelihood that desired changes and innovations will be successfully implemented. The rate of adoption of specific innovations can be affected using strategies that target specific groups of adopters. Targeting innovators and early adopters is usually sufficient to create the necessary support and momentum for adoption of a change or innovation, with the other groups following.[92] The individuals in specific adopter categories are shown in the bell curve in FIGURE 1-18.

Tools can assess the rate of adoption of innovations. The scorecard tool for new ideas (FIG. 1-19) can be used to assess the possibility for and rate of adoption of an innovation or new change based on specific criteria defined in Rogers' model.[96] If the assessment indicates that the adoption is not likely to be successful, additional strategies can be developed to improve the odds.

Ratings are determined independently based on a 5-point scale where a score of 1 signifies that the change is very weak relative to the attribute being scored and 5 signifies that the change is very strong. The higher the rating of each item on the scorecard, the greater the likelihood that a specific innovation or change will be successfully adopted. The items in the scorecard are defined as follows:

- *Relative advantage*—the degree to which an innovation is perceived as better than the idea it supersedes;
- *Simplicity*—the degree to which an innovation is perceived as simple to understand and use; and
- *Compatibility*—the degree to which an innovation is perceived as being consistent with the existing values, experiences, beliefs, and needs of potential adopters;

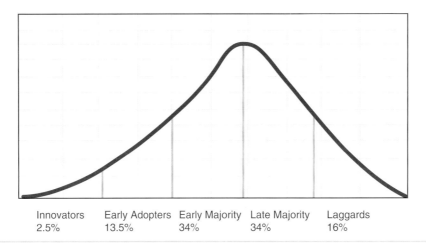

| | Innovators 2.5% | Early Adopters 13.5% | Early Majority 34% | Late Majority 34% | Laggards 16% |

Figure 1-18 **Categories of adopters of innovations.**

	Relative Advantage	Simplicity	Compatibility	Trialability or Suitability for Trial	Observability
Name of Innovation	Score	Score	Score	Score	Score

SCORING DIRECTIONS: Group exercise with individuals rating independently.
Score on 1–5 scale
1 = change is very weak relative to the attribute
5 = change is very strong relative to the attribute

Figure 1-19 **Scorecard tool for new ideas.** (Reprinted from Fraser SW and her Associates. *New Idea Scorecard*. Cambridge, MA: Institute for Healthcare Improvement. http://www.ihi.org/resources/Pages/Tools/NewIdeaScorecard.aspx, with permission.)

- *Trialability or suitability for trial*—the degree to which an innovation can be tested on a small scale;
- *Observability/visibility*—the degree to which the use of an innovation and the results it produces are observable or visible to those who should consider it;
- *Communicability*—the ability to clearly communicate to stakeholders a description of the innovation and its value;
- *Reversibility*—the ability to stop the adoption or use of the innovation and return to a normal or "safe" position if the innovation is not effective; and
- *Uncertainty*—the fear and discomfort associated with the implementation of the innovation.[96]

Institute for Healthcare Improvement Framework for Spread. This aspect of dissemination or diffusion is addressed by IHI with a model for spreading change and innovations to promote rapid dissemination of quality, safety, and performance improvement practices across an organization. This framework (FIG. 1-20) includes seven major components to be considered broadly and not in a specific order.[94]

1. *Leadership*—Leadership is required to ensure that the goal to be spread throughout the organization is aligned with strategic goals. Responsibility for day-to-day leadership must be assigned to provide guidance on the spread. Communication channels need to be established and supported by leaders as part of an ongoing process.
2. *Setup for spread (infrastructure)*—The setup for spread is a structure for coordinating the activities in which the target population is identified, the sites are selected for initiating the spread, the key partners are identified, and a plan for implementation is established.
3. *Better ideas*—Better ideas are the ideas for changes or improvement with demonstrated success and desired to be spread throughout the organization.
4. *Communication*—Communication is a key underpinning of the spread model, and communication strategies include the purpose and methods of communication for the target population.
5. *Social system*—The social system for spread includes the individuals and groups in the target population. The relationships within the social system must be understood so that problems related to communication, support, and other issues can be identified and resolved.
6. *Knowledge management*—Knowledge management is the process of collecting information about the spread with the aid of the measurement and feedback component so that the spread process can be modified as necessary. It is critical to the systems foundation that effective management be fact-based and knowledge-driven, permitting the system agility for improving performance and competitiveness.[23] This enables the "focus on the quality and availability of data and information and on organizational knowledge, including the sharing of best practices."[23(p46)] Not all information is valuable, so individual organizations need to determine what information qualifies as a knowledge-based asset. The challenge of accumulating knowledge is figuring out how to recognize, generate, share, and manage it to foster innovations.

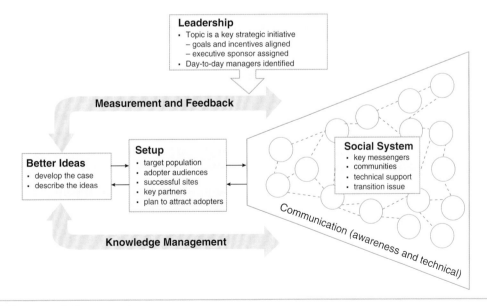

Figure 1-20 A framework for spread. (Reprinted from Massoud MR, Nielsen GA, Nola K, Schall MW, Sevin C. *A Framework for Spread: From Local Improvements to System-Wide Change.* Cambridge, MA: IHI; 2006. Copyright 2006 by the Institute for Healthcare Improvement, with permission.)

7. *Measurement and feedback*—A system for measurement and feedback is needed to ensure that the spread of the change proceeds as planned. This system provides data about the process and outcomes, and, in combination with knowledge management, allows adjustments to the spread strategy.

To maximize results, a strategy is needed to spread change and improvements. These strategies include assessing readiness for spread, developing a plan for the spread, leveraging pilot sites, developing a communication plan, and developing a measurement and feedback system. These are helpful in making the business case for quality and determining investments that should be made by the organization. Employers, patients, providers, and insurers are all financial beneficiaries of quality improvement.[27] Overuse, defective, inefficient, and underuse care is not patient-centered but is most often reimbursed. The business case for reducing overuse and underuse of care lies not with the healthcare organization, but with self-insured employee populations and capitated plans. The business case for reducing inefficient care is derived from the benefit of reducing variation, defect, and waste and associated financial savings. However, reducing defects of care almost always improves business bottom lines, even if the defective care is reimbursed.

> A business case for a healthcare improvement intervention exists if the entity that invests in the intervention realizes a financial return on its investment in a reasonable time frame, using a reasonable rate of discounting. This may be realized as 'bankable dollars' (profit), a reduction in losses for a given program or population, or avoided costs. In addition, a business case may exist if the investing entity believes that a positive indirect effect on organizational function and sustainability will accrue within a reasonable time frame.[97(p18)]

Healthcare quality professionals may be the ones in the organization who build and defend a business case for quality. The framework for establishing a business case for quality is set forth by Bailit and Dyer.[98] The framework rests on three broad categories for which a business case can be established:

1. Return on investment (ROI), the amount of financial return that an investment provides in a year, reduced expenditures or cost avoidance, and costs.
2. Investments in quality and safety initiatives may be undertaken by a healthcare facility because of regulatory or contractual requirements or because of performance incentives (or disincentives) offered to the organization by groups such as purchasers or providers, their alignment with explicit performance incentives (e.g., pay-for-performance initiatives).
3. The desire to gain a strategic advantage over competition by bolstering image and reputation or by marketing a product (development of brand identity).

Although strategic considerations typically focus staff members' efforts on the external world, organizations also must consider the nature of the internal environment when deciding whether to fund quality and safety initiatives.

External Consultants

Healthcare quality professionals interact with external consultants on a wide range of quality and safety-related topics. Whether one is entering an agreement with an external consultant as part of efforts toward regulatory or accreditation preparedness or working with a consultant on a focused improvement project, an external consultant is typically needed when internal resources and talent in the organization are not sufficient to address the specific need.

When the determination is made that a consultant is needed, the healthcare quality professional checks with relevant trade groups and industry partners for available options. After options are identified, the healthcare quality professional reviews available background information to help narrow the selection. The nature of the specific need may necessitate a meeting to discuss the specific expectations and deliverables of the project—what needs to be done, on what timeline, and with what resources. The healthcare quality professional will need to involve relevant key organizational representatives and ensure that the consultant fully understands the expectations, work with organizational points of contact for the specific project and the consultant to establish a series of milestones and deadlines, and address as early as possible any questions or issues that arise.

As the work progresses and the consultant offers recommendations, the healthcare quality professional needs to evaluate the advice offered and translate the recommendations to colleagues. These questions are considered during the evaluation process: Has the consultant delivered what was promised? Have the core issues been addressed? Do the recommendations make sense for the organization? Finally, the healthcare quality professional needs to be clear about what the next steps are and how the consultant will be involved as recommendations are implemented.

The business case for quality often justifies the need for the investment in the use of external consultants and additional resources. The quality professional is key to ensuring the effective utilization of consultants.

Regulation and Leadership

Healthcare regulations and accreditation standards are dynamic and ever-changing. This requires organizations to commit resources to sustain performance and ensure compliance, which is important for maintaining an organization's public reputation for providing safe, effective, reliable, and high-quality care. Healthcare is not a unique industry in this regard; other industries are also highly regulated. Like these other industries, there is an opportunity for staff to have specialized knowledge and skill sets focusing on regulatory and accreditation compliance. Titles of these professionals may vary, but large organizations often have personnel titles or department names, such as compliance, regulatory affairs, accreditation and regulatory readiness, or licensing. Other organizations might use an integrated approach in which the quality or administration departments and operational leaders assume these responsibilities. Alternatively, organizations may outsource or purchase consultation services in this area.

Healthcare quality professionals are responsible for supporting the organization in ensuring ongoing compliance with many of the laws and regulations pertaining to their business operations. This includes working with federal, state, and/or local regulatory agencies on specific requirements for their business lines. For example, the requirements for an outpatient medical practice are different from those for an outpatient ambulatory surgery center (ASC), a critical access hospital (CAH), comprehensive medical rehabilitation hospital, or acute freestanding psychiatric hospital. General acute care hospitals have different requirements than medical homes, disease management programs, or ACOs. Advising organizations on myriad requirements and helping these organizations sustain compliance is a vital role of the healthcare quality professional. This includes ensuring the infrastructure for safety, quality, and performance improvement programs supports continuous readiness and understanding the nuances of implications of regulations or standards applicable to the healthcare setting.

Federal Regulations

The healthcare industry is regulated by all levels of government—federal, state, and local—presenting challenges for healthcare organizations and quality professionals, such as being confident that they possess an understanding of regulatory requirements. A simple early 2017 Internet search on "healthcare regulation" yields about 151,000,000 citations—an overwhelming place to start. Healthcare regulations create circumstances in which healthcare quality professionals spend inordinate amounts of time responding to changing rules concurrently with demonstrating compliance with complex existing rules. In a dynamic marketplace, organizations are driven to expand and refine the services offered to meet the needs of the community. This creates an ongoing need for healthcare quality professionals to research and interpret regulations that are applicable to the organization's new or unique situation.

Although there are federal laws and regulations significantly impacting healthcare organizations, healthcare quality professionals will want to become familiar with the following five federal laws and regulations, four of which are among the many that CMS oversees:

- *Emergency Medical Treatment and Active Labor Act (EMTALA)*: Any hospital participating in Medicare

and offering emergency services must provide a medical screening examination when a request is made for examination or treatment for an emergency medical condition (EMC), including active labor, regardless of an individual's ability to pay. The hospital is then required to provide stabilizing treatment for patients with EMCs. If a hospital is unable to stabilize a patient within its capability, or if the patient requests, an appropriate transfer should be implemented.[99]

- *Health Insurance Portability and Accountability Act (HIPAA):* HIPAA provides federal protections for personal health information and provides patients with rights.[100]

- *Clinical Laboratory Improvement Amendments (CLIA):* In 1988, the CLIA established quality standards for all laboratories (regardless of where the test was performed) to ensure the accuracy, reliability, and timeliness of patient test results. CLIA regulations are stratified based on the complexity of the test method: waived complexity; moderate complexity, including the subcategory of provider-performed microscopy; and high complexity. The regulations specify quality standards for laboratories performing moderate- and/or high-complexity tests and require waived laboratories to enroll in CLIA and follow manufacturers' instructions.[101]

- *Patient Protection and Affordable Care Act (PPACA)* was signed into law in 2010, putting in place comprehensive U.S. health insurance reforms that will greatly impact accountability (Public Law, 111–148, PPACA). The intent of the Affordable Care Act (ACA) was to transform and modernize the American healthcare system. The ACA created new programs and payment models with goals of rewarding value and quality. These models include ACO models, medical home models focused on primary care, and new models of bundling payments for episodes of care. In these APMs, healthcare providers are accountable for the quality and cost of the care they deliver to patients and have a financial incentive to coordinate care for their patients—who are therefore more likely to receive high-quality, team-based care. The start of 2017 saw a strong push, under a new President and federal administration, to repeal the PPACA. Healthcare quality professionals are encouraged to monitor the impact of federal governmental action on the PPACA and the resultant impact on their respective healthcare organization.

- *Medicare Access and CHIP Reauthorization Act (MACRA) Quality Payment Program (QPP)* was signed into law in 2015 and final rule issued in late 2016. This act impacts the way providers are reimbursed through Merit-Based Incentive Payment System and APMs, collectively referred to as the QPP. Healthcare quality professionals are encouraged to refer to the most up-to-date CMS information as elements of this law go into effect.

Detailed information about these and additional federal laws and regulations is readily available on the Internet.

Federal Regulatory Agencies

There are federal agencies with which healthcare regulatory and healthcare quality professionals interface. A few are described briefly.

Occupational Safety and Health Administration. The U.S. Department of Labor's Occupational Safety and Health Administration (OSHA) is an agency that most healthcare professionals will be familiar with no matter where in the healthcare continuum services are provided. OSHA was created by Congress with the Occupational Safety and Health (OSH) Act of 1970 to ensure safe working conditions. The OSH Act covers most private sector employers and their workers, in addition to some public sector employers and workers in the 50 states and certain territories and jurisdictions under federal authority. This agency is visible within government structures, because OSHA's administrator answers to the Secretary of Labor, who is a member of the Cabinet of the President of the United States.

U.S. Department of Health & Human Services. The U.S. Department of Health & Human Services (HHS) describes its role as being the principal agency for protecting the health of all Americans, providing essential human services, and promoting economic and social well-being for individuals, families, and communities, including seniors and individuals with disabilities. A huge government agency with more than 300 services, HHS has 11 operating divisions, including eight agencies in the U.S. Public Health Service and three human services agencies which administer a wide variety of health and human services. HHS works closely with state and local governments, and because many HHS-funded services are provided by state or county agencies, or through private sector grantees, it may be difficult for healthcare professionals to distinguish between the federal role in regulation versus the role as an insurer, and the state role acting on behalf of the federal programs. Several of the HHS agencies and offices are described below.

- Administration for Children and Families (ACF). Established in 1991 and promotes the economic and social well-being of families, children, individuals, and communities through a range of educational and supportive programs in partnership with states, tribes, and community organizations.
- Administration for Community Living (ACL). Established in 2012, bringing the Administration on Aging, the Administration of Developmental Disabilities, and Office on Disabilities together. Increases access to community support and resources for the unique needs of older Americans and people with disabilities.
- Agency for Healthcare Research and Quality (AHRQ). Established in 1989 with the mission to produce evidence to make healthcare safer, higher quality, more accessible, equitable, and affordable, and to work within HHS and with other partners to make sure that the evidence is understood and used.
- Agency for Toxic Substances and Disease Registry (ATSDR). Established in 1980 and prevents exposure to toxic substances and the adverse health effects and diminished quality of life associated with exposure to hazardous substances from waste sites, unplanned releases, and other sources of environmental pollution.
- Centers for Disease Control and Prevention (CDC). Established in 1946, part of the Public Health Service, protects the public health of the nation by providing leadership and direction in the prevention and control of diseases and other preventable conditions, and responding to public health emergencies.
- Centers for Medicare & Medicaid Services (CMS).[102] Established in 1977 as the Health Care Financing Administration. CMS combines the oversight of the Medicare program, the federal portion of the Medicaid program and State Children's Health Insurance Program, the Health Insurance Marketplace, and related quality assurance activities.
- Food & Drug Administration (FDA). Established in 1906 as part of the Public Health Service, ensures that food is safe, pure, and wholesome; human and animal drugs, biologic products, and medical devices are safe and effective; and electronic products that emit radiation are safe.
- Health Resources & Services Administration (HRSA). Established in 1982, improves health and health equity through access to quality services, a skilled health workforce, and innovative programs.
- Indian Health Service (IHS). Established in 1921, part of the Public Health Service, provides American Indians and Alaska Natives with comprehensive health services by developing and managing programs to meet their health needs.
- National Institutes of Health (NIH). Established in 1887, part of the Public Health Service, supports biomedical and behavioral research with the United States and abroad, conducts research in its own laboratories and clinics, trains promising young researchers, and promotes collecting and sharing medical knowledge.
- Substance Abuse and Mental Health Services Administration (SAMHSA). Established in 1992, part of the Public Health Service, improves access and reduces barriers to high-quality, effective programs and services for individuals who suffer from or are at risk for addictive and mental disorders, as well as for their families and communities.

Leadership for the HHS operating divisions is divided into geographic regional offices; these are the offices with which healthcare quality professionals work directly. Healthcare quality professionals may need to be familiar with the names and contact information for staff in their geographic offices (**TABLE 1-7**).[103] Healthcare quality professionals may be involved with one or more operating divisions depending on the segment of healthcare where they are employed. However, most will become familiar with several key divisions, including CMS, CDC, FDA, and AHRQ. Additional, up-to-date information is available on each agency's respective websites.

Federal Role in Quality and Safety

The Social Security Act mandates the establishment of minimum health and safety standards that must be met by providers and suppliers participating in the Medicare and Medicaid programs.[104] In 1935, the Social Security Act was signed by President Franklin D. Roosevelt to provide benefits for retirees and the unemployed. This was amended in 1965, signed by President Lyndon B. Johnson, to create the Medicare and Medicaid programs.

As a federal insurance program, Medicare provides a wide range of benefits for most people 65 years and older, Social Security beneficiaries younger than 65 years who are entitled to disability benefits, and individuals needing renal dialysis or renal transplantation. The care is provided through "providers and suppliers" that participate in the Medicare program by providing care and receiving reimbursement from Medicare. In Medicare terminology, *providers* include patient care institutions, such as hospitals, CAHs, hospices, nursing homes, and home health agencies (HHAs). *Suppliers* are agencies for diagnosis and therapy rather than sustained patient care, such as laboratories, clinics, and ASCs. The providers and suppliers are subject to federal healthcare quality standards; thus, the federal government plays a large role in setting quality standards and oversight of compliance to these standards for Medicare beneficiaries.

CMS developed Conditions of Participation (CoP) and Conditions for Coverage (CfC) that healthcare organizations must meet to participate in the Medicare and Medicaid programs and receive reimbursement for services. These standards are the foundation for improving quality and protecting the health and safety of beneficiaries. CoP and CfC apply to all types of healthcare organizations like Comprehensive Outpatient Rehabilitation Facilities, federally qualified health centers, HHAs, Intermediate Care Facilities for Persons with Mental Retardation, and Programs of All-Inclusive Care for the Elderly organizations.

Table 1-7 U.S. Department of Health & Human Services Regional Offices

Region	Geographic Area
Region 1 Boston	Connecticut, Maine, Massachusetts, New Hampshire, Rhode Island, Vermont
Region 2 New York	New Jersey, New York, Puerto Rico, the Virgin Islands
Region 3 Philadelphia	Delaware, District of Columbia, Maryland, Pennsylvania, Virginia, West Virginia
Region 4 Atlanta	Alabama, Florida, Georgia, Kentucky, Mississippi, North Carolina, South Carolina, Tennessee
Region 5 Chicago	Illinois, Indiana, Michigan, Minnesota, Ohio, Wisconsin
Region 6 Dallas	Arkansas, Louisiana, New Mexico, Oklahoma, Texas
Region 7 Kansas City	Iowa, Kansas, Missouri, Nebraska
Region 8 Denver	Colorado, Montana, North Dakota, South Dakota, Utah, Wyoming
Region 9 San Francisco	Arizona, California, Hawaii, Nevada, American Samoa, Commonwealth of the Northern Mariana Islands, Federated States of Micronesia, Guam, Marshall Islands, Republic of Palau
Region 10 Seattle	Alaska, Idaho, Oregon, Washington

Although each program's CoP or CfC will be different, the table of contents from the hospital program (**TABLE 1-8**; U.S. Government Publishing Office)[105] provides an example to gain insight into the kinds of regulations found in the CoP and how they are organized (*Code of Federal Regulations*, Title 42, Volume 3, Part 482).[106] These federal quality standards are organized in *State Operations Manuals* (*SOMs*) as conditions, with subsidiary standards under each condition.[107] There are individual sets of conditions or requirements for each type of provider or supplier subject to certification. The condition or requirement in the *SOMs* is expressed in a summary paragraph, which describes the quality or result of operations to which all the subsidiary standards are directed.

The HHS Secretary delegates to CMS regional offices the authority for ensuring healthcare providers and suppliers participating in the Medicare, Medicaid, and CLIA programs meet applicable federal requirements. CMS regional offices use state health agencies to determine whether healthcare entities meet federal standards. This process is called certification.

State and local agencies with agreements under section 1864(a) of the Act perform the following functions:

- Survey and make recommendations regarding the organization or providers' ability to meet the Medicare CoP or requirements;
- Conduct validation surveys of deemed status facilities, providers, and suppliers;
- Perform other surveys and carry out other appropriate activities and certify their findings to CMS;
- Make recommendations regarding the effective dates of provider agreements and supplier approvals in accordance with §489.13 of this chapter.[108]

Table 1-8 Hospital Conditions of Participation

Subpart A: General Provisions	
§482.1	Basis and scope.
§482.2	Provision of emergency services by nonparticipating hospitals.
Subpart B: Administration	
§482.11	Condition of participation: Compliance with federal, state, and local laws.
§482.12	Condition of participation: Governing body.
§482.13	Condition of participation: Patient's rights.
Subpart C: Basic Hospital Functions	
§482.21	Condition of participation: Quality assessment and performance improvement program.
§482.22	Condition of participation: Medical staff.
§482.23	Condition of participation: Nursing services.
§482.24	Condition of participation: Medical record services.
§482.25	Condition of participation: Pharmaceutical services.
§482.26	Condition of participation: Radiologic services.
§482.27	Condition of participation: Laboratory services.
§482.28	Condition of participation: Food and dietetic services.
§482.30	Condition of participation: Utilization review.
§482.41	Condition of participation: Physical environment.
§482.42	Condition of participation: Infection control.
§482.43	Condition of participation: Discharge planning.
§482.45	Condition of participation: Organ, tissue, and eye procurement.

Table 1-8 **Hospital Conditions of Participation** (*continued*)	
Subpart D: Optional Hospital Services	
§482.51	Condition of participation: Surgical services.
§482.52	Condition of participation: Anesthesia services.
§482.53	Condition of participation: Nuclear medicine services.
§482.54	Condition of participation: Outpatient services.
§482.55	Condition of participation: Emergency services.
§482.56	Condition of participation: Rehabilitation services.
§482.57	Condition of participation: Respiratory care services.
§482.58	Special requirements for hospital providers of long-term care services ("swing-beds").
Subpart E: Requirements for Specialty Hospitals	
§482.60	Special provisions applying to psychiatric hospitals.
§482.61	Condition of participation: Special medical record requirements for psychiatric hospitals.
§482.62	Condition of participation: Special staff requirements for psychiatric hospitals.
§482.68	Special requirements for transplant centers.

From Code of Federal Regulations: Title 42, Public Health: Chapter IV—Centers for Medicare & Medicaid Services, Department of Health & Human Services: Subchapter G—Standards and Certification: Part 482—Conditions of Participation for Hospitals. 2015. https://www.gpo.gov/fdsys/pkg/CFR-2015-title42-vol5/xml/CFR-2015-title42-vol5-part482.xml.

The state agencies used to evaluate healthcare entities against federal regulations are usually the same agencies responsible for state licensing; however, they are reimbursed with federal funds for this work. There are also provisions for CMS-approved accreditation bodies to determine if healthcare entities meet the Medicare CoP. These providers are referred to as deemed status providers for participation, also known as the deeming process. Therefore, CMS-certified healthcare entities can receive a visit from federal, state, or accreditation agencies to evaluate federal standards for certification or recertification, for compliance investigations, or as part of random validation programs to confirm accreditation or state survey findings as valid and reliable.

To ensure evaluations are done in a consistent manner by these agencies, the *SOMs* are published and available publicly on the Internet. Healthcare quality professionals are encouraged to search for the relevant *SOMs* and review them for further guidance in preparing an organization for on-site survey. The *SOMs* include very explicit survey methods and processes as well as specific interpretive guidance for determining if an organization meets a standard.

The survey process varies depending on the services under review and may vary slightly depending on individual state resources, such as the staff or disciplines available to conduct surveys. During a survey, healthcare professional surveyors determine if each standard is met by conducting document reviews, interviewing staff and leaders, and observing routine procedures and patient care. After a CMS survey, the state agency (acting as CMS surveyor) prepares a certification report for the CMS regional office and sends the healthcare organization a statement of deficiencies. The healthcare organization needs to respond to CMS with a Plan of Correction (PoC) for each cited deficiency. Once the PoC is accepted by CMS, it is ultimately made available publicly through the Freedom of Information Act. Even though an organization may fail to comply with one or more of the subsidiary standards during any given survey, it cannot participate in Medicare unless it meets every condition. If the healthcare organization does not come into compliance with all conditions within the period accepted as reasonable by CMS, it is certified as "noncompliant" and a termination process begins for the Medicare and Medicaid programs. Termination means the healthcare entity cannot receive federal reimbursement for services, which typically represents a financial loss for organizations.

Healthcare quality professionals are familiar with the National Practitioner Data Bank (NPDB),[109] which is a federal data bank created because of the Medicare and Medicaid Patient and Program Protection Act of 1987 to serve as a repository of information about healthcare providers in the United States. The NPDB was designed to protect program beneficiaries from unfit healthcare practitioners and required reporting of adverse licensure, hospital privilege, and professional society actions against physicians and dentists related to quality of care. In addition, the NPDB tracks malpractice payments made for all healthcare practitioners.

The HIPAA of 1996 led to the creation of the Healthcare Integrity and Protection Data Bank (HIPDB). HIPDB served as a tracking system to alert users that a comprehensive review of the practitioner, provider, or supplier's past actions may be prudent. It was suggested that HIPDB's information be used in combination with information from other sources in making determinations on employment, affiliation, certification, or licensure decisions. Section 6403 of the ACA authorized the Secretary of HHS to cease the operation of the HIPDB and to consolidate the operation of the HIPDB with the NPDB. The goal was to eliminate duplication between the NPDB and HIPDB. In May 2013, the NPDB and HIPDB merged into one database—NPDB.[110] This databank was established with strict confidentiality protections; the HHS Office of Inspector General has the authority to impose civil money penalties on those who violate the confidentiality provisions.[110]

The NPDB authorizes the government to collect information concerning sanctions taken by state licensing authorities and entities against healthcare practitioners. In 1990, Congress amended the law by broadening the language to include any negative action or finding by these authorities, not just sanctions. Intended to improve the quality of healthcare, this law encourages state licensing boards, hospitals, professional societies, and healthcare organizations to identify and discipline those who engage in unprofessional behavior, to report medical malpractice payments, and to restrict the ability of incompetent physicians, dentists, and other healthcare practitioners to move between states without disclosure or discovery of their previous history. Examples of adverse actions include revocation or alteration to licensure, clinical privileges, and professional society membership, and exclusions from Medicare and Medicaid. Government peer-review organizations and private accreditation organizations are required to report negative actions taken against healthcare practitioners or organizations.

Federal Resources

Finding information about federal regulations is becoming progressively easier because the government invested in publicly available electronic databases accessed through the Internet. Healthcare quality professionals are encouraged to take advantage of the Internet in seeking the most up-to-date federal regulations through the review of information posted on official governmental sites. The *Federal Register* is the official daily publication for rules, proposed rules, and notices of federal agencies and organizations, as well as presidential executive orders. The *Code of Federal Regulations* (*CFR*) is the codification of these rules published in the *Federal Register*, which is divided into 50 titles that represent broad areas subject to federal regulation. It is updated by amendments that appear daily in the *Federal Register*. Each volume of the *CFR* is updated once each calendar year.

Twice a year, federal agencies publish a Regulatory Agenda.[111] This agenda can be very helpful for healthcare quality professionals to understand the direction for selected federal agencies in the coming year. As an example, the HHS plan provides not only the annual priorities for the fiscal year as an overview but also the detailed information about each of the priorities (if the priority is an unfunded mandate, legal authority, statement of need, legal basis, alternative, cost and benefit, risk, timetable, and contact information). These documents are useful communication tools for healthcare quality professionals to understand future directions for regulations.

The process to change regulations can be slow and frustrating, resulting in outdated regulations. There are many challenges to keeping evidence-based regulatory standards current.[112] Federal, state, and local government regulators must provide due process to those affected by their actions—this provides the healthcare industry the opportunity to review proposed changes with any known supporting evidence and to provide written feedback or testimony prior to changes in the regulation. Individuals as well as members of professional associations, like the NAHQ, have the opportunity to comment on proposed regulations.

State Regulations

State governments maintain state health departments that operate licensing programs for healthcare providers and organizations. Licensing requires organizations, providers, and practitioners to meet legal requirements to practice or provide services. In addition to providing licensing services, these departments usually operate enforcement programs for both state licensing requirements and federal certification requirements. In some states, local governments, such as counties and municipalities, can also have their own health departments (which may be branches of the state health department). Licensure for practitioners may be the responsibility of state health departments or separate entities accountable for disciplinary investigations and actions.

State regulations vary greatly in content, detail, and organization of regulations. This requires regulatory professionals to possess state-specific knowledge to guide organizations within the given state. Corporate healthcare entities that operate in multiple states depend on regulatory and quality professionals who play a critical role to navigate requirements within each state.

State healthcare surveys appear much like federal surveys and likely have the same personnel performing the survey. State regulators survey healthcare organizations for licensure, for enforcement of regulations, and in response to complaints made to the agency by consumers of the healthcare service, their family members, or concerned staff. Licensure visits may be routine inspections within defined time periods or may be random unannounced visits conducted based on the resources available to the state agency. State laws may dictate reporting requirements of licensed organizations for unusual occurrences or adverse events, and the law may require the state agency to investigate certain self-reports within a given time frame. Discretion may be allowed on how the agencies respond to and investigate complaints, based on the nature of the complaint and the severity of the allegation.

As with federal surveys, state agencies provide organizations with deficiency reports and require written responses (corrective actions) within a defined period. If organizations are not able to become compliant with state regulations, they risk loss of both licensure within the state and the ability to provide healthcare services. In addition, states report their actions to CMS and accrediting bodies that may initiate their own investigations. Reports of investigations and the organization's response to citations may also become public information or released upon request. Healthcare quality professionals are encouraged to become familiar with relevant state healthcare regulations impacting their practice setting. Most state regulatory agencies post an abundance of relevant information on the Internet.

Regulations and Managed Care

Managed care is "a health care delivery system organized to manage cost, utilization, and quality."[113] Health plans pay the cost of medical care. Healthcare quality professionals working with health plans will want to understand the regulations specific to their situation in the state where business is conducted and healthcare delivery occurs. The federal government regulates managed care and other health plans sponsored by the private sector. However, the states regulate the business of insurance, which includes managed care organizations (MCOs) such as health maintenance organizations (HMOs) that offer managed care policies to individuals, employers, or other purchasers. To add to the complexity, if a private sector employer sponsors a plan that is not purchased from an MCO (i.e., the plan is self-insured), then the plan is regulated solely by the federal government. If that employer contracts with an MCO to provide managed care services to employees, then the regulation depends on who bears the risk: if it is the MCO, the plan is regulated by the state; if the risk is borne

to any degree by the employer, then the plan is subject to federal law only.

This complex division of regulatory responsibilities between the federal and state governments resulted from provisions of several federal laws and subsequent decisions of federal courts. The Employee Retirement Income Security Act of 1974 (ERISA) preempted the states from regulating health plans of private sector employers but left to the states the regulation of the business of insurance. Although the HMO Act of 1973 established certain federal standards for HMOs that elected to operate under federal law, almost all other regulatory authority over the business of health insurance remained with the states. This deferral to state regulation of insurers was altered with the HIPAA of 1996 (P.L. 104-191), which applied federal minimum requirements to state-regulated insurers as well as to employer-sponsored plans, including managed care plans.

Managed care regulations vary state by state, although there are many state laws and regulations based on the National Association of Insurance Commissioners' (NAIC) HMO Model Act. NAIC published model laws on quality assessment and improvement, provider credentialing, network adequacy, grievance procedures, and standards for utilization review.

Private Quasi-Regulators

Although regulation is primarily a government role, there are also private organizations that serve as quasi-regulators in healthcare. Field[114] provides a rich historical perspective on regulation in healthcare, as well as an introduction to private regulators. The American Medical Association (AMA) may be the most well-known organization. The AMA sponsored creation of organizations with oversight roles for the medical profession to supplement government regulators, such as organizations that accredit medical schools, administer licensure examinations, and certify specialists. State medical boards, for example, use privately administered examinations in granting medical licenses, and the Medicare program relies on specialty certification as an indicator of physician quality.

Accreditation and Certification

Accreditation and *certification* are terms used in many organized industries in the United States, including healthcare. The terms are often used incorrectly or interchangeably, which creates confusion, plus they can be used differently in various segments of the industry. *Accreditation* within the context of *accredit* is defined as "official authorization or approval, or recognition for conforming to standards, or to recognize as outstanding,"[115] whereas *certification* is defined within the context of certify as "recognition for meeting special qualifications within a field."[116] In healthcare, accreditation commonly refers to a process reviewing an entire organization's operations, whereas certification commonly refers to a review of part of the organization's operations or care for a specific population. But certification may also be a reference to an individual's competency or the determination of an organization's eligibility to participate in a government program. Accreditation is voluntary and granted by private sector organizations (trade associations, professional societies, or independent businesses). Certification can be provided by either private sector organizations or government agencies.

Federal certification requirements are found across the healthcare continuum. For example, a federal certification requirement is the CMS regulation for all laboratory testing performed on humans through CLIA.[117] All clinical laboratories must be certified to receive Medicare or Medicaid payments. The CLIA maintains a list of CMS-approved accrediting organizations that may perform laboratory inspections, whose requirements are deemed as being equivalent to or more stringent than CMS's regulatory requirements (CMS accepts the accrediting organization's inspection in lieu of its own inspection). Another federal certification requirement is found in the Mammography Quality Standards Act, which requires that all facilities providing mammography must be certified by the FDA.[118] To become certified, a facility must be accredited; the FDA designates the acceptable accrediting bodies. As of January 1, 2017, there are over 8,700 mammography facilities certified.

Accreditation Terms and Concepts

These terms and concepts of accreditation, certification, and the accreditation process are explained to serve as context for understanding the overall accreditation and certification processes.

Standards. Like regulatory requirements, accreditation and certification standards are published and available to organizations that are applying for review or considering pursuit of accreditation or certification. These standards are developed based on evidence for practice, expert opinion and consensus, or research. Accrediting agencies wishing to provide CMS deemed status are preapproved by CMS to assure their minimum standards meet or exceed the CoP or CfC. The requirements or standards that are not tied to the CMS requirements evolve over time with industry knowledge and technology and are more responsive with changes than government regulations. Standards may focus on the infrastructure of the organization, the processes of care delivery, or the outcomes of the care delivery system.

Compliance. Organizations must be able to demonstrate that they are following or adhering to all the elements outlined in the standard. Some accrediting agencies will include elements

of performance as part of their standards to provide further guidance to the organization to ensure that the organization is meeting the expectation. Compliance may be demonstrated in a variety of ways and is not limited to survey processes through regulatory or accrediting agency visits or surveys. However, on-site surveys conducted by accrediting agency surveyors are the most visible mechanisms for demonstrating compliance as part of the accreditation process. Some healthcare organizations consult with experts in the field to conduct mock surveys to identify gaps in compliance to ensure readiness for the official survey.

Application. Accreditation cycles begin with an application requesting an initial or follow-up review or reaccreditation. The accrediting agency reviews the application to determine the scope of the review by evaluating the size and scope of the organization and services to be reviewed. In accordance with the requirements of HIPAA Privacy and Security Rules, and modified by the Health Information Technology for Economic and Clinical Health (HITECH) provisions of the American Recovery and Reinvestment Act of 2009, a healthcare organization and the accrediting agency sign a Business Associate Agreement (BAA) before the organization's survey can begin. A BAA outlines the access, use, and disclosure of any patient-protected health information between the accrediting agency and the healthcare organization.

Costs. Accreditation comes at significant cost to an organization. Not only are staff resources required to maintain compliance and continuous readiness, but fees are also associated with the accreditation process. Fees often are on a sliding scale, reflecting the size and complexity of the organization. For on-site surveys, the number of surveyor hours or days required for the review affects pricing. There are often annual participation fees as well. Costs for survey preparation, hosting the survey team for the on-site survey process, intracycle monitoring, and fees assessed for the regular survey cycle are also factors considered as organizations choose an accreditation agency. Because these fees can be substantial, they must also be included in operating budgets.

Review Cycle. The review cycle varies with each accreditation agency and type of accreditation or certification. However, many are 2- or 3-year cycles.

Survey Duration. The length of the survey is dependent on the type of survey, the size of the organization, the number of surveyors, and the complexity of services offered. Certification surveys for small programs can be as few as one surveyor for 1 day; accreditation surveys for large organizations can be as large as five surveyors or more for 5 days or more. CMS validation surveys at large organizations can involve as many as

20 or more surveyors for up to 2 weeks or longer, depending on findings.

Performance Measures. Performance measures are often a required element of accreditation and certification, and are frequently publicly reported. Measures may be developed by the review organization, by professional organizations through consensus, or through national organizations such as the National Quality Forum (NQF). NQF was created in 1999 by a coalition of public- and private sector leaders after the President's Advisory Commission on Consumer Protection and Quality in the Healthcare Industry identified the need for an organization to promote and ensure patient protections and healthcare quality through measurement and public reporting. As of 2017, about 300 NQF-endorsed measures are used in more than 20 federal public reporting and pay-for-performance programs as well as in private sector and state programs and are often used by accreditation agencies to judge quality.[119]

Performance measurement may be an ongoing review for accreditation, with quarterly or annual performance ratings sometimes included on public websites. For example, in the hospital industry, TJC was one of the first accreditation agencies to include on its public website not only the organization's accreditation status, but also comparative performance with respect to "National Patient Safety Goals" and "National Quality Improvement Goals" (e.g., emergency department throughput measures, venous thromboembolism, immunization). In the health plan industry, National Committee for Quality Assurance (NCQA) reports its accreditation decisions on its public website. It includes plan-specific information about performance on the Healthcare Effectiveness and Data Information Set (HEDIS®) grouped into five consumer-friendly categories (Access and Service, Qualified Providers, Staying Healthy, Getting Better, and Living with Illness). HEDIS is designed to provide purchasers and consumers with the information they need to reliably compare the performance of health plans. HEDIS results are included in Quality Compass, an interactive, web-based comparison tool that allows users to view plan results and benchmark information.

Serious Reportable Events. Some state agencies and accrediting organizations require or strongly encourage healthcare organizations to report SREs. For example, through Massachusetts law (Chapter 305 of the Acts of 2008), hospitals and ASCs are required to report SREs to the Massachusetts Department of Public Health (DPH). In Massachusetts, the list includes 28 of NQF SREs, which are adverse events that are of concern to both the public and healthcare professionals and providers; clearly identifiable and measurable, and thus feasible to include in a reporting system; and of a nature such that the risk of occurrence is significantly influenced by the policies and procedures of the healthcare facility. Reported events are posted on the DPH website for public review. The law also prohibits hospitals from charging for these events or seeking reimbursement for SRE-related services.[120] TJC adopted a formal Sentinel Event Policy in 1996 to help hospitals that experience serious adverse events improve safety and learn from those sentinel events. *Sentinel events* include any patient safety event that reaches the patient and causes death, permanent harm, or severe temporary harm and intervention required to sustain life. Each accredited organization is strongly encouraged, but not required, to self-report sentinel events to TJC.[121] Healthcare quality professionals work with organizational leaders to develop policies and procedures for the reporting of SREs. More on this topic can be found in *Patient Safety*.

Surveyors. On-site accreditation surveys are completed by professionals from within the field of review. In addition to document review (reports, management plans, risk assessments, evaluations, etc.), which may take place in advance of the on-site review, interviews with staff, patients, and providers are a normal part of a survey.

Observations and Summation. Depending on the healthcare services under review, on-site surveys will also encompass observations of routine care delivery and the associated medical record documentation (hard copy and electronic), staff performing procedures, and visits to home care patients. Most reviews conclude with a summation conference by the review team to inform leadership of compliance findings.

Accreditation Decision. Following review of all the data and evidence sources, an accreditation decision is determined for the organization. The decision usually includes an overall assessment of the organization or service that reflects a full accreditation decision, or a decision with limitations or restrictions that the organization must resolve within a designated time frame.

Deficiencies and Findings. Depending on the number and scope of deficiencies cited, follow-up surveys may be part of the accreditation decision. Cited deficiencies or requirements for improvement must be corrected and documentation submitted to the reviewing organization within predetermined time frames. The organization's leaders often receive in-depth information that can be used internally to prioritize performance improvement activities to enhance care quality and patient safety, with the implicit expectation that the organization will use this feedback in its continuous quality, safety, and performance improvement programs. The accreditation decision is also shared with interested parties such as consumers, patients, purchasers, and government agencies that require accreditation or certification for participation. The level of detail shared outside the organization ranges from a simple list of organizations that were successful (with no indication of organizations that failed) to detailed information on performance.

Intracycle Requirements. In an effort for the accreditation review to be an ongoing process and for organizations to be continuously ready, accreditation agencies may require intracycle activities to confirm sustained compliance. Requirements for a periodic self-assessment or performance review between surveys may require submission of data to the agency or for public reporting or attestations of process completion.

Voluntary or Required. In the healthcare industry, the act of accreditation involves an objective or impartial review of an organization by an external agency against recognized and published standards or requirements. (*Agency* is used as a generic term to represent accreditation organizations or bodies, or certification organizations or bodies.) This impartial accreditation review is conducted by industry professionals (e.g., physicians, nurses, pharmacists, dieticians,

administrators, life safety code specialists) who, through direct observation summarized in reports, publicly attest to the resulting accreditation status. The review is "voluntary," as compared to "required" like licensure; however, the review may be required for participation in reimbursement programs such as Medicare or for participation in contracts to provide care and receive reimbursement through insurance programs. In competitive markets, accreditation or certification may be viewed by the public as an endorsement for providing a minimum level of quality or standard of care, and therefore as a business "requirement" even if it is "voluntary."

Deeming. Accreditation may also be accepted as evidence of meeting state and federal regulatory requirements. During the CMS deeming process, discussed earlier, accredited organizations would be deemed to meet CMS CoP requirements when accredited through CMS-approved agencies (see **TABLE 1-9**). Per CMS,[101] the total number of Medicare-participating certified healthcare facilities across all program types increased 40% from 24,752 in FY 2008 to 34,583 in FY 2014. Deemed status is attractive to many organizations because it may negate the

Table 1-9 CMS-Approved Accreditation Organizations

Organization	Program Type	Website
Accreditation Association for Ambulatory Health Care (AAAHC)	ASC	www.aaahc.org
Accreditation Commission for Health Care, Inc. (ACHC)	HHA Hospice	www.achc.org
American Association for Accreditation of Ambulatory Surgery Facilities (AAAASF)	ASC Outpatient physical therapists (OPT) RHC	www.aaaasf.org
American Osteopathic Association/Healthcare Facilities Accreditation Program (AOA/HFAP)	ASC CAH Hospital	www.hfap.org
Center for Improvement in Healthcare Quality (CIHQ)	Hospital	www.cihq.org
Community Health Accreditation Program (CHAP)	HHA Hospice	www.chapinc.org
DNV GL Healthcare	Hospital CAH	www.dnvglhealthcare.com
The Compliance Team (TCT)	RHC	www.thecomplianceteam.org
The Joint Commission	ASC CAH HHA Hospice Hospital Psychiatric hospital	www.jointcommission.org

ASC, ambulatory surgery center; CAH, critical access hospital; CMS, Centers for Medicare & Medicaid Services; HHA, home health agency; RHC, Rural Health Clinics.
Note: For the most current contact information for these organizations, visit https://www.cms.gov/Medicare/Provider-Enrollment-and-Certification/SurveyCertificationGenInfo/Downloads/Accrediting-Organization-Contacts-for-Prospective-Clients-.pdf.
Adapted from Centers for Medicare & Medicaid Services. CMS-approved accrediting organization contacts for prospective clients. 2015.

need for an additional survey by state personnel on behalf of federal CMS regional offices. However, CMS randomly selects deemed status accredited facilities for 60-day validation surveys as part of its oversight of accrediting organizations with approved Medicare accreditation programs. In addition, some states accept accreditation to meet regulatory requirements for state licensure.

Value of Accreditation

Although many hospitals and many health plans are accredited, accreditation is not uniformly adopted across all segments of the healthcare industry. Home care and hospice agencies, one of the fastest growing segments of the continuum, may also be accredited. Nursing home accreditation is limited. There are not the same financial incentives to seek accreditation since legislation does not authorize deemed status in Medicare or Medicaid for private accrediting bodies to substitute for government oversight. CMS (Medicare and Medicaid) and the states (Medicaid) developed regulatory standards and government survey and certification programs to enforce nursing home regulations. In the primary care setting, an increased focus is placed on attainment of patient-centered medical home (PCMH) recognition or certification. This signifies that patient treatment is coordinated through a primary care physician who ensures the patient receives the necessary care when and where needed and in a manner that the patient can understand.[122]

As the healthcare industry faces ongoing pressure for cost containment, questions surface as to the "value" of accreditation in relation to the cost. Literature continues to grow about the benefits of accreditation. One of the most extensive reviews of accreditation value is a literature review published by Accreditation Canada,[123] which summarizes literature findings on the value and impact of healthcare accreditation. This information may be helpful to articulating the value proposition for quality and safety. The review includes results and conclusions from research, gray literature, and experience-based articles. Accreditation is an integral part of healthcare services in more than 70 countries, as either a voluntary or government-mandated requirement. See **TABLE 1-10** for a summary of cited benefits of accreditation with expanded discussion of several below.

External Credibility. Consistent with the historical view in the United States, accreditation is cited as improving an organization's reputation among end-users and enhancing awareness and perception of quality care. It is also cited as improving communication and collaboration internally and with external stakeholders. All of this is thought to demonstrate credibility and a commitment to quality and accountability, which are hallmarks of healthcare reform.

Improved Quality. Accreditation is cited as leading to improved patient outcomes. The improved outcomes may result from

accreditation, which provides a framework to create and implement systems and processes to improve operational effectiveness. Accreditation is also cited as providing healthcare organizations with a well-defined vision for sustainable quality improvement initiatives. This vision and framework enable organizations to sustain improvements in quality and organizational performance, enabled ongoing self-analysis of performance in relation to standards, and ensured an acceptable level of quality among healthcare providers. These quality improvements are realized as the accreditation process achieves the following:

- increases healthcare organization's compliance with quality and safety standards;
- decreases variance in practice among healthcare providers and decision makers by standardizing core processes;
- codifies organizational policies and procedures; and
- continuously raises the bar regarding quality improvement initiatives, policies, and processes.

Organizational Learning. Accreditation is cited as promoting capacity building, professional development, and organizational learning. The accreditation process itself could highlight practices that were working well and may have a spillover effect, whereby the accreditation of one service helps to improve the performance of others. Accreditation is also cited as enhancing an organization's understanding of the continuum of care. Healthcare industry benefits are also realized through sharing policies, procedures, and best practices among accredited healthcare organizations.

Staff Effectiveness. Accreditation is cited as contributing to the effectiveness of organizations' staff in the following ways: strengthening interdisciplinary team effectiveness; promoting an understanding of how each person's job contributes to the healthcare organization's mission and services; providing a team-building opportunity for staff and improving their understanding of their coworkers' functions; and contributing to increased job satisfaction among physicians, nurses, and other providers.

Reduced Costs. Accreditation is cited as decreasing liability costs and mitigating the risk of adverse events, which would ultimately reduce costs as well. Accreditation could also impact costs by helping to identify an organization's areas that need additional funding and then providing a platform for negotiating this funding.

Accreditation, Certification, and Recognition Agencies

Accreditation agencies continue to evolve and grow, and now represent a significant segment of the healthcare industry. Not only has the number of organizations that

Table 1-10 Benefits of Accreditation

Better Care

Improves patient's health

Improves the organization's reputation among end-users and enhances their awareness and perception of quality care as well as their overall satisfaction level

Provides a framework to help create and implement systems and processes that improve operational effectiveness and advance positive health outcomes

Organizational Effectiveness

Promotes a quality and safety culture

Increases healthcare organization's compliance with quality and safety

Demonstrates credibility and a commitment to quality and accountability

Supports the efficient and effective use of resources in healthcare services

Sustains improvements in quality and organizational performance

Promotes the sharing of policies, procedures, and best practices among healthcare organizations

Provides healthcare organizations with a well-defined vision for sustainable quality improvement

Enhances the organization's understanding of the continuum of care

Stimulates sustainable quality improvement efforts and continuously raises the bar regarding quality improvement initiatives, policies, and processes

Leads to the improvement of internal practices

Enhances the reliability of laboratory testing

Workforce

Ensures an acceptable level of quality among healthcare providers

Promotes capacity building, professional development, and organizational learning

Decreases variances in practice among healthcare providers and decision makers

Improves communication and collaboration internally and with external stakeholders

Enables ongoing self-analysis of performance in relation to standards

Strengthens interdisciplinary team effectiveness

Provides opportunity for team building with staff and improves their understanding of coworkers' job and responsibilities

Promotes an understanding of how each person's job contributes to the healthcare organization's mission and services

Contributes to increased job satisfaction among physicians, nurses, and other providers

Risk Management

Decreases liability costs; identifies areas for additional funding for healthcare organizations; and provides a platform for negotiating this funding

Mitigates the risk of adverse events

Source: Table constructed using information from Accreditation Canada. The value and impact of health care accreditation: a literature review. https://accreditation.ca/sites/default/files/value-and-impact-en.pdf. Accessed May 5, 2017:1–3.

offer services increased, but the services provided have also expanded. Agencies no longer offer one program as their single service line but offer diversified products across the healthcare continuum with both accreditation and certification programs. Most offer associated education or consultation programs to assist organizations with survey readiness activities.

Several accrediting bodies are summarized below with an overview of the services they offer. Healthcare quality professionals are encouraged to explore agency websites to learn specific information about agencies that accredit or certify their own organizations. Survey cycles vary by accrediting agency. Many of the organizations provide tools or resources on their websites to help consumers understand or evaluate compliance or quality of care when considering the services of an organization. Healthcare providers or other industry organizations may also find assessment or evaluation tools made available by these agencies in their effort to improve the quality and safety of care across the industry.

AABB. Formerly the American Association of Blood Banks, AABB accreditation is granted for collection, processing, testing, distribution, and administration of blood and blood components; hematopoietic progenitor cell activities; cord blood activities; perioperative activities; relationship testing activities; and immunohematology reference laboratories.

Accreditation Association for Ambulatory Health Care. Accreditation Association for Ambulatory Health Care (AAAHC) is a private, not-for-profit organization formed in 1979. Its standards advance and promote patient safety, quality care, and value for ambulatory healthcare through peer-based accreditation processes, education, and research. AAAHC accredits ambulatory healthcare settings including ambulatory healthcare clinics, ASCs, birthing centers, office-based surgery centers, community health centers, medical home practices, MCOs, as well as Indian health centers and military healthcare facilities, among others.

Accreditation Commission for Health Care. In existence since 1985, Accreditation Commission for Health Care (ACHC) began offering accreditation services nationally in 1996. ACHC offers seven different accreditation programs. Accreditation and deeming authority are offered for Home Health; Hospice; and Durable Medical Equipment, Prosthetics, Orthotics, and Supplies (DMEPOS). Accreditation programs are offered for Private Duty, Pharmacy, Sleep, Behavioral Health, and Hospital Accreditation. ACHC and DNV GL Healthcare partnered together to provide a single-source accreditation solution for hospitals and health systems with ancillary services.

American College of Radiology. Since 1987, the American College of Radiology (ACR) has accredited more than 38,000 facilities in 10 different imaging modalities. The ACR offers accreditation programs in computed tomography, magnetic resonance imaging (MRI), breast MRI, ultrasound, breast ultrasound, mammography, stereotactic breast biopsy, and radiation oncology practice, as well as nuclear medicine and positron emission tomography.

American College of Surgeons. American College of Surgeons (ACS) is a scientific and educational association of surgeons that was founded in 1913 to improve the quality of care for the surgical patient by setting high standards for surgical education and practice. ACS offers surgical accreditation and verification programs, such as the Commission on Cancer, and the Committee on Trauma, which verifies the presence of resources consistent with varying trauma level designation, as well as bariatric and breast center accreditation programs.

American Nurses Credentialing Center. The American Nurses Credentialing Center (ANCC), a subsidiary of the American Nurses Association, aims to promote excellence in nursing and healthcare globally through credentialing programs. ANCC's credentialing programs certify and recognize individual nurses in specialty practice areas; recognize healthcare organizations for promoting safe, positive work environments; and accredit continuing nursing education organizations. ANCC developed and leads the Magnet Recognition Program,[124] which recognizes healthcare organizations for quality patient care, nursing excellence, and innovations in professional nursing practice.

College of American Pathologists (CAP). CAP Laboratory Accreditation Program accredits a variety of laboratory settings from complex university medical centers to physician office laboratories. It covers a complete array of disciplines and testing procedures. CMS granted the CAP Laboratory Accreditation Program deeming authority. It is also recognized by TJC and can be used to meet many state certification requirements. CAP also provides laboratory accreditation to forensic drug testing facilities, biorepository facilities, and reproductive laboratories, in collaboration with the American Society for Reproductive Medicine.

Commission of Office Laboratory Accreditation. Completing the Commission of Office Laboratory Accreditation (COLA) program demonstrates that a clinical laboratory is following CLIA; COLA is recognized by TJC. It accredits different types of laboratories, such as physicians' offices, community hospitals, mobile clinics, Veterans Administration, and the

Department of Defense. In addition, COLA is approved by CMS to accredit laboratories for certain specialties such as chemistry, hematology, microbiology, immunology, and immunohematology/transfusion services.

CARF International. CARF International surveyed hundreds of thousands of programs throughout North and South America, Europe, Africa, and Asia since it was founded as an independent, nonprofit accreditor in 1966. Accreditation programs are offered in the following areas across the healthcare continuum: Aging Services, Behavioral Health, Continuing Care Retirement Communities, Child and Youth Services, DMEPOS, Employment and Community Services, Medical Rehabilitation, Opioid Treatment Programs, and Vision Rehabilitation Services.

Community Health Accreditation Partner. Community Health Accreditation Partner (CHAP) is an independent, not-for-profit, accrediting body for community-based healthcare organizations. Created in 1965 as a joint venture between the American Public Health Association and the National League for Nursing, CHAP was the first accrediting body for home and community-based healthcare organizations in the United States. Through deeming authority granted by the CMS, CHAP has the regulatory authority to survey agencies providing home health, hospice, and home medical equipment services to determine if they meet the Medicare CoP and CMS Quality Standards.

DNV GL Healthcare. The National Integrated Accreditation for Healthcare Organizations (NIAHO) requirements combines hospital accreditation with ISO 9001. The core of DNV GL hospital accreditation in the United States and internationally is the NIAHO standards platform, created by DNV GL in 2008 for U.S. hospitals. DNV's platform is that accreditation is not an inspection but rather a catalyst for quality and patient safety. The organization follows a collaborative approach to help healthcare providers identify, assess, and manage risk while ensuring sustainable business practices. DNV GL's NIAHO assesses both Medicare CoP and ISO 9001 Standards for the formation and implementation of quality and performance improvement systems. DNV GL formed an alliance with the ACHC to meet an organization's ancillary accreditation needs. ACHC has Medicare Deeming Authority for Home Health, Hospice, and DMEPOS, and additional services include Pharmacy, Private Duty, Behavioral Health, Convenient Care Clinics, and Sleep. DNV GL also provides Managing Infection Risk, Primary Stroke Center, Comprehensive Stroke Center, Acute Stroke Ready, and Hip & Knee Replacement Program Certifications.

Healthcare Facilities Accreditation Program. Originally created in 1945 to conduct an objective review of services

provided by osteopathic hospitals, Healthcare Facilities Accreditation Program (HFAP) received its deeming authority from CMS in 1965. It meets or exceeds the standards required by CMS/Medicare to provide accreditation to all hospitals, ambulatory care/surgical facilities, mental health facilities, physical rehabilitation facilities, clinical laboratories, and CAHs. HFAP also provides certification reviews for primary stroke centers.

The Joint Commission. Founded in 1951, TJC is an independent, not-for-profit organization that accredits and certifies nearly 21,000 healthcare organizations and programs in the United States. TJC accreditation and certification is recognized nationwide as a symbol of quality that reflects an organization's commitment to meeting certain performance standards. TJC accredits different types of healthcare organizations including but not limited to Ambulatory Care, Behavioral Health Care, CAH, Home Care, Hospital, Office-Based Surgery, and Opioid Treatment Program. Certification is offered for such programs as Palliative Care, Health Care Staffing Services, Patient Blood Management, Perinatal Care, and Primary Care Medical Home.[125]

National Committee for Quality Assurance. Founded in 1990, National Committee for Quality Assurance (NCQA) is a private, not-for-profit organization which accredits and/or certifies healthcare organizations. NCQA offers different accreditation programs such as Health Plans, Disease Management, Case Management, and Managed Behavioral Healthcare Organizations. Certifications are available for Credentials Verification Organizations, Disease Management, Multicultural Health Care, and Wellness & Health Promotion, to name a few.

URAC. Formerly known as the Utilization Review Accreditation Commission, URAC accredits many types of healthcare organizations depending on the specific functions they carry out with a portfolio of programs that spans the healthcare industry. URAC accreditations, certifications, and designations address healthcare management, healthcare operations, health plans, pharmacy quality management, and providers. The following are examples of accreditation and certification programs offered: Accountable Care; Clinical Integration; Community Pharmacy; Dental Network; Drug Therapy Management; Health Plan with Health Insurance Marketplace; PCMH Certification; Telehealth Accreditation; and Workers Compensation and Property, and Casualty Pharmacy Benefit Management Accreditation.

Accreditation or Recognition Program Selection

There are usually several choices in how an organization fulfills mandatory external validation requirements and the quality professional needs to understand the various options available for meeting these requirements. In addition, there might be several options for attaining optional disease-specific and specialty certifications from one or more different accrediting or certifying bodies. The healthcare quality professional is typically responsible for ensuring that the organization meets expectations for all mandatory external regulatory and accreditation programs.

Depending on the size, scope, and complexity of the organization, the responsibility of meeting these expectations may belong solely to the healthcare quality professional or may be shared with other department or service leaders (Chief Nursing Officer, etc.). The nature and scope of external requirements typically depend upon the type of organization, the specific services provided, and the state-specific regulatory requirements that are usually tied to licensure. Healthcare quality professionals may be asked to take the lead in quantifying the specific accreditation-related costs, both external directly related to the accreditation agency and internal related to the staff, time, and resources required to meet accreditation standards and achieve compliance.

Organizational Approaches to Continuous Survey Readiness

Organizational leaders and healthcare quality professionals set the approach to ensuring that an organization is compliant with external standards and regulations. Full compliance involves ensuring that leaders, staff, and physicians across the organization are meeting all elements of the standards and regulations on a consistent basis, not only at the time of survey.

Just-in-Time Readiness

Organizations that are not far along in the journey to high reliability may employ just-in-time regulatory or accreditation readiness models, which come with great financial and personnel costs. When organizations use just-in-time programs with ramp-up activities in the months prior to anticipated surveys, tremendous additional resources are required to demonstrate regulation or standard compliance. Extra staff or extra time is required for self-assessments or gap analyses; corrective actions to assure compliance; meetings for policy revision approvals; and frontline staff education on policy revisions, operational process improvements, and expected survey procedures.

These organizations experience tremendous relief when surveys are completed and may commit to a vision that the next 2- to 3-year cycle will be different. However, organizational memory can be short, and competing priorities may replace the vision of continuous readiness. Organizations that experience unplanned surveys with numerous citations may also experience a crisis-management cycle, which requires tremendous unplanned additional resources. Compliance issues can be costly to organizations in terms of financial outlays for corrections, public reputation damage that leads to further financial losses in competitive markets, and staff turnover, as the work environment is no longer healthy. Many organizations started to embrace a continuous readiness approach when on-site surveys became unannounced. Some work to embed continuous readiness into the structure and culture of the organization.

Continuous Readiness

The goal of continuous readiness programs is to break crisis-management cycles and just-in-time cultures to provide continuous safe, high-quality patient care and sustained compliance with regulations, standards, evidence-based practices, and professional standards. Benefits to continuous readiness include increased likelihood that the organization is meeting expectations for high-quality and safe care as well as a safe environment on a consistent basis. Key components of successful continuous readiness programs include leadership commitment, manager accountability, survey readiness oversight, requirement oversight, organizational assessment, staff education, survey procedure planning, presurvey activities, on-site survey activities, postsurvey activities, and staff recognition (FIG. 1-21).

Leadership Commitment

The expectation and support for continuous readiness must come from the highest levels of leadership. It is then up to the healthcare quality professional to translate the expectation into action. To understand the role of leadership in creating a culture of continuous readiness, it is useful to first examine the words of the concept individually. *Culture* is defined as "the set of shared attitudes, values, goals, and practices that characterizes an institution or corporation."[31] *Continuous* is defined as "marked by uninterrupted extension in space, time, or sequence"[126]; *readiness* is defined as the state of being prepared mentally or physically for some experience or action, immediately available, or prepared for immediate use.[127] The outcome of these activities is the demonstration of *compliance*, which is defined as "conformity in fulfilling official requirements."[128]

Drawing on these definitions, one sees that a culture of continuous readiness is an attitude and value demonstrated throughout the organization in goals and practices that yield an uninterrupted state of mental preparedness by demonstrating that staff throughout the organization are immediately

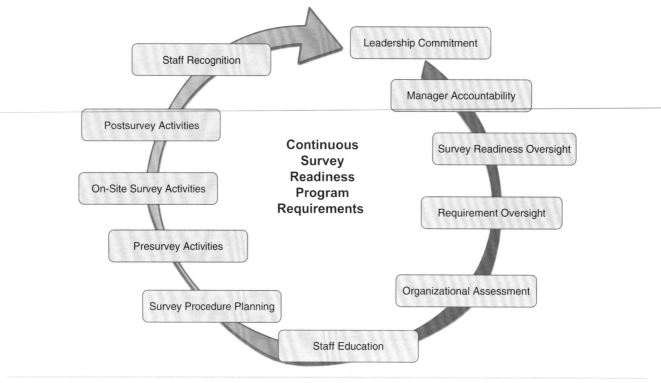

Figure 1-21 **Continuous survey readiness program requirements.**

physically ready or available to demonstrate compliance. Given the current healthcare environment and public expectations for safe patient care, discrete "survey readiness" is not a central focus in this definition. This is because each patient, rather than each survey, deserves continuous care and service that meets regulatory and accreditation requirements—every day.

Leadership commitment to continuous readiness must be in place for programs to be successful and sustained. Leaders must be willing to change their organization's culture to one of readiness, which requires the leaders to commit to personal change and create an environment where the values, ways of thinking, managerial styles, paradigms, and approaches to problem solving support a culture of readiness. Leaders must be patient and persistent to see this transformation through by defining what readiness looks like within their organization, aligning staff with that vision, and inspiring staff despite obstacles that will surface.

To commit, leaders must understand the business case for compliance and the costs of noncompliance. Costs may be known from previous ramp-up activities or noncompliance situations, or there may be potential costs from adverse media attention and loss of business. With the expanding culture of transparency and public reporting of performance measures, organizations are subject to scrutiny from a variety of perspectives once media attention is drawn to them. The business case for continuous readiness also includes the impact of ramp-up activities and crisis compliance management.

Staff and managers can experience frustration and burnout with crisis compliance management and seek employment elsewhere, thus depleting organizations of experienced employees and those who possess crucial institutional memory.

Leaders must include continuous readiness within organizational strategic priorities to change the culture. It must be part of the operational budgeting process and key leadership activities, as well as a foremost topic that leaders inquire about in routine discussions (briefings and huddles) with staff and managers during rounding. Leaders also must be willing to hold managers accountable for readiness responsibilities.

Management Accountability

Managers play a key role in continuous readiness activities. Compliance is evaluated by what happens at the point of care delivery, for which managers are accountable. Policies and procedures need to be aligned with the most current standards and regulations to provide the guidance and structure for those providing or supporting care delivery. However, actual practice and policies must be aligned to achieve compliance. It is the manager's role to determine when practice and policies are inconsistent, understand root causes of variance, and take corrective action required for either policy adjustments or staff behavior adjustments. Managers are also responsible for ensuring that individuals within their span of control are held accountable to regulatory and accreditation expectations.

Managers evaluate individuals while they are doing their work to ensure that key process and policy expectations are always met. Individuals need to be held answerable for their performance, and the manager's role is to provide coaching and feedback, positive reinforcement for behavior that meets policy expectations, and escalating to progressive discipline as appropriate.

Healthcare quality professionals in leadership roles cannot be the lone voices requiring compliance in complex organizations. The management team provides operational oversight within an organization and is the key to ensuring continuous compliance within its areas of accountability. Healthcare quality professionals must provide the program structure and education to help managers understand the requirements. New managers have steep learning curves to understand not only their departmental operations but also functional interrelations associated with regulatory and accreditation requirements. As managers learn to juggle operations, fiscal accountabilities, staffing, and the patient experience (satisfaction and engagement), they must also incorporate sustained compliance into their busy days. Unfortunately, it may be easier to allocate time to the faces and duties of the given day rather than to proactive readiness responsibilities. Thus, the culture of the organization and the leaders' strategic priorities will be determining factors in the success of readiness programs.

Survey Readiness Oversight

Continuous survey readiness (CSR) is the goal rather than ramp-up process. Since most surveys are unannounced, the CSR model is ideal. Healthcare quality professionals may hold a role with primary responsibility for survey readiness oversight. One effective way of providing survey readiness oversight is through the formation of interdepartmental and multidisciplinary workgroups or ongoing committees representing the full scope of services included in the anticipated survey(s) whose composition will vary depending on the type of organization and services provided (e.g., hospital, MCO, long-term care facility, HHA, ambulatory care center). Some organizations create workgroups for related clusters of accreditation standards and others have a single multidisciplinary group to evaluate readiness on the standards across the entire organization. At a minimum, each workgroup consists of the healthcare quality professional and appropriate departmental representatives with sufficient knowledge to identify gaps in compliance and the authority to modify organizational practices and processes to become compliant with expectations.

Departments consistently requiring representation include nursing, medical staff, pharmacy, facilities, and infection control. Membership on these workgroups will further depend on the size and scope of the organization as well as the scope of the individual workgroup (when more than one workgroup

is formed). In a hospital setting, other members might include the safety officer, risk manager, and director of health information management. In an MCO, additional members might include a customer relations representative, physician relations or medical staff coordinator, network coordinator, information systems or data processing representative, and benefits administrator. Medical staff play a significant role and bear the responsibility of accountability for compliance and performance improvement; however, it may be challenging to schedule time for their participation in planning activities and to clear their schedules when the actual survey process commences. Medical staff participation requires constant communication as information becomes available.

The frequency with which survey readiness groups meet will vary depending on the outcome of ongoing self-assessments and available resources to complete identified tasks. If the oversight and planning groups perform this work in a continuous fashion and the organization created an adaptable CSR culture, the last-minute rush and accompanying stress will be lessened as the survey window approaches. Publications and commercial education programs are available with suggested checklists to assist with survey preparation. The most important element, however, is a coordinated, ongoing effort to meet the intent of the regulations or standards.

Requirements Oversight

A critical component of a CSR program is a defined process to ensure the organization is aware of changes and emphasis in standards or regulations. Changes may be in the form of additions, deletions, or clarifications. Most regulatory or accreditation agencies define processes for changes in requirements and standards. This usually involves notification to the affected organizations; there is a period during which comments or feedback on proposed changes is accepted prior to their publication. Comment periods allow healthcare organizations the opportunity to provide feedback on proposed changes in regulations. Comments can be submitted individually or as an organization. Once official changes are released, clarifications may be found in FAQ documents as well. Healthcare quality professionals check with the agencies and organizations that survey their facilities to understand the relative frequency with which changes are made; the process for assimilating public feedback and comments from affected organizations; and the notification process to the affected organizations, including the medium (e.g., e-mail, paper letter, website announcements) and to whom in the affected organization communications are directed (e.g., the chief executive officer versus the regulatory professional).

Once changes are identified, gap analyses must be completed to understand implications to the organization. Operational leaders and oversight committees will need guidance as to the scope and urgency of required changes. It is helpful to create a notification list of individuals within the organization who receive communications related to standards. These communications are most effective when they are put into context for the recipient. For example, the communication can include a description of the change, the agency making the change, actions required on the part of the various stakeholders within the organization (leadership, managers, employees), risk assessment of the change, identification of resources required (if any) to implement the change, and deadlines associated with required actions.

Evaluating Organizational Compliance

Periodic and ongoing self-assessment is a cornerstone of CSR programs. The ability to evaluate the state of compliance with key regulatory and accreditation requirements is a critical step in this process. Accreditation and regulatory requirements cover a broad scope, including clinical practice, service quality, documentation, patient experience, quality assessment, performance improvement, patient safety, and management of adverse events. In the just-in-time preparation model, compliance is not sustained but fluctuates in response to known survey cycles—compliance improves immediately before a survey and gradually declines after each survey. The goal of CSR programs is the opposite—sustained compliance. To do this, an organization must evaluate its compliance state on a regular basis and maintain an infrastructure that sustains the effort.

With an annual self-assessment, organizations plan for a thorough assessment once a year, often at the beginning of the budget planning cycle for the new fiscal year, with the results used to drive a compliance work plan with adequate resources for the upcoming fiscal year. Resources are dedicated for the review, whether conducted internally or by an external consultant, because time is required for content experts to conduct actual reviews and document their findings. In this model, an assessment is completed and presented to leadership and quality, safety, and performance improvement oversight committees, and often to the governing body as part of the annual quality plan or annual budget presentation. Ideally, the outcome of the assessment is formatted in a report that includes a gap analysis related to specific standards, with findings and recommendations written in a manner that facilitates corrective action planning with key department leaders identified as responsible for each action with specific timelines for milestone actions leading to full compliance.

With an ongoing assessment, organizations plan for a thorough assessment during the year, often dividing the workload into smaller monthly activities. Although some organizations may dedicate individuals or departments to CSR through the designation of specific roles for annual and ongoing self-assessment, action planning, and overall accreditation activity management, not all organizations are able to do this. The advantage of an ongoing assessment is that the assessment can be resourced and integrated into operational activities and reported over an ongoing (but defined) period, allowing for action plan development, implementation, and monitoring throughout the year. A disadvantage of this model is that it requires focused project management with sufficient coordination to ensure completion of the entire assessment and to ensure monitoring and oversight of required corrective actions. There is a risk of not completing the entire assessment; it may be difficult for the organization to have a "snapshot" of compliance to understand performance.

Regardless of how the organization is staffed or structured to support ongoing self-assessment, as the assessment components are completed, findings are presented to leadership and oversight committees. Presentation to the organization's governing body, as appropriate, can be periodically delivered as a summary of the assessment components, rather than a single completed report. This type of report is also most useful when in the format of a gap analysis related to specific standards, with findings and recommendations written in a manner that facilitates rapid corrective action planning. Once the findings are presented, corrective action plans must be developed and monitored on an ongoing basis. Monitoring schedules, however, are more complex because they must incorporate scheduled assessments to be completed as well as follow-up activities on those already completed. Assigning accountability is critical in any action planning activity.

Many organizations find that a minimum of monthly status reports is required on assessment components and the corrective actions to provide the oversight necessary to achieve compliance. Quarterly status reports are not recommended because there is a high risk that the organization will not be aware of slippage soon enough to take appropriate action.

Tools and Strategies for Assessment

Regulatory or accrediting agencies offer tools to help organizations manage self-assessment activities. Access to information such as easy-to-use checklists may be readily available on websites. Additional paper-based or computer-based project management programs designed specifically for the identified regulations, accreditation, or certification programs also may be purchased directly from the agencies or from third-party entrepreneurs. External consulting organizations will also provide educational programs or tools for evaluation or preparation activities on a fee-for-service basis.

Checklists. Organizations develop checklists to help monitor ongoing compliance as well as day of survey activity. As an example, a survey readiness tool for department managers serves as standard work for managers to use when rounding in their departments. The content is developed to meet accreditation expectations and organizational circumstances. A hospital survey readiness document may include clinical rounding, infection control, patient safety, and environmental rounding elements. Clinical rounding elements may include a review of restraint records, high-risk fall patients, care plan review, code blue cart checklists, and pain assessment/reassessment documentation. Infection control elements may include items such as direct observation of hand hygiene, linen cart coverings, dirty and clean utility room observations, and cleaning procedures. And, environmental elements for review may include fire procedures, door wedges, medical gas storage, and staff identification badges.

Work Plans. Organizations are encouraged to develop specific work plans to outline key activities that need to take place to support the survey process. For example, a work plan for an unannounced survey would include key activities that need to occur when a survey team shows up at the organization. In addition to each action, key responsible individuals including alternates are identified.

Tracers. A key part of many on-site surveys and survey self-assessment processes is the tracer methodology. The tracer methodology follows the experience of care, treatment, or services for several patients through the organization's entire healthcare delivery process. Tracers allow surveyors during survey and staff or consultants during self-assessment processes to identify performance issues in one or more steps of the process, or interfaces between processes. The types of tracers used by various accrediting and regulatory agencies during the on-site survey are as follows:

- Individual tracer activity: These tracers are designed to "trace" the care experiences that a patient had while at an organization. It is a way to analyze the organization's system of providing care, treatment or services using actual patients as the framework for assessing standards compliance. Patients selected for these tracers will likely be those in high-risk areas or whose diagnosis, age, or type of services received may enable the best in-depth evaluation of the organization's processes and practices.
- System tracer activity: Includes an interactive session with relevant staff members in tracing one specific "system" or process within the organization, based on information from individual tracers. Although individual tracers follow a patient through his or her course of care, the system tracer evaluates the system or process, including the integration of related processes, and the coordination and communication among disciplines and departments in those processes. Examples of topics evaluated by system tracers during accreditation surveys

include data management, infection control, and medication management.
- Focused tracers: The goal of these tracers is to identify risk points and safety concerns within different levels and types of care, treatment, or services. Program-specific tracers focus on important issues relevant to the organization, such as clinical services offered and high-risk, high-volume patient populations.

Leading the Survey Process

Survey procedures are planned based on what is expected with anticipated surveys. Healthcare quality professionals may have the responsibility to develop and manage survey procedures for the organization because they serve as internal experts and consultants. An accreditation or regulatory site visit requires organization and preparation and is the culmination of CSR activities. **TABLE 1-11** lists the components of a visit for presurvey activities, on-site survey activities, and postsurvey activities.

The coordination required to achieve favorable accreditation or certification status or successful regulatory licensing or certifications must be delegated to those individuals with the most knowledge about healthcare quality, regulations, and standards interpretation and implementation. This coordination role can be delegated to a leader or manager within the quality area or to a designated role in larger organizations or health systems, such as a director of accreditation and regulatory readiness. Important preparation tasks for organizations to complete are generally outlined in survey manuals and can be planned for each anticipated survey.

Formal plans are recommended, with multiple staff and leaders familiar with the process. The organization's general survey procedure planning will likely include the components described in the following section. **TABLE 1-12** provides additional examples of survey readiness activities to prepare for anticipated surveys.

Survey Outcomes

Most accreditation organizations improved the timeliness of processes that result in an accreditation or certification decision. Some organizations use proprietary software that captures surveyor observations and translates observations into an overall survey decision outcome, whereas others provide written reports back to the accrediting organization where further internal review occurs before a final survey outcome decision is made. Individual accreditation agencies have procedures for disputing survey outcome decisions and healthcare quality professionals are familiar with processes available to challenge or dispute findings both during and after the on-site survey.

Table 1-11 Accreditation or Regulatory Survey Visit Activities

Space Planning and Hosting Considerations

- Surveyors' workroom
- Command center
- Other conference rooms for surveyor meetings with staff
- Hosting considerations
- Documentation preparation

Presurvey Activities (12 Months After Last On-Site)

- Opportunities from last survey addressed and hardwired
- Maintaining improvements of corrective action plans
- Keeping staff apprised of key standards and regulations and changes
- Self-assessment compliance gap analyses
- Educational programs re: building skills related to regulatory, accreditation, or performance and quality improvement
- Activities to prepare staff and leadership for anticipated survey activities
- Survey planning documents current and relevant

On-Site Survey Activities

- Surveyor Arrival
  - Welcome surveyor(s)
  - Obtain photo identification
  - Assemble individuals and teams (use phone tree)
  - Assign escorts and scribes
  - Assign central point of contact
- Organizational Notification
  - "XYZ organization would like to welcome XXX organization to our facility today."
- Survey Command Centers
  - Survey coordinator is in charge
  - Defined staff roles and key information tracked
- Other considerations
  - Office supplies: chart pads, easels, grease boards, clipboards, projectors, etc.
  - Communications equipment: phones and facsimile lines
  - Computers
  - Tracking system for surveyor requests
  - Key documents of folders for easy access
    - current organizational charts,
    - program descriptions,
    - plans for the provision of care,
    - governing body structures,
    - professional staff bylaws,
    - copies of licenses,
    - governing body minutes, and
    - key quality and administrative reports.
- Identification of Deficiencies using Survey Analysis for Evaluating Risk (SAFER)
  - areas of noncompliance at an aggregate level compared to Evidence of Standard Compliance (ESC)
  - require organizational follow-up activity and corrective action within 60 days
  - Immediate Threats to Life (ITLs)
  - *Immediate jeopardy (IJ)* is a mechanism to escalate crisis survey issues immediately
    - Such a deficiency will automatically result in a condition-level deficiency under the applicable Medicare Condition(s) of Participation

(continued)

Table 1-11 Accreditation or Regulatory Survey Visit Activities (*continued*)

• Survey Exit Conferences: Surveyors summarize the findings and deficiencies that will be cited and disclose anticipated next steps in the survey process
  ○ Organization conducts its own debriefing as soon as possible to evaluate the survey process.
    ▪ Evaluate how the organization managed the survey process
    ▪ Decide whether to accept or dispute outcome
    ▪ Senior leaders (CEO, CNO, CMO) consider a special communication to the organization's staff to share survey outcome appreciation

Postsurvey Activities
• Sustain compliance, especially opportunities for improvement identified in survey
• Develop corrective action plans
  ○ the topic or standard cited,
  ○ compliance issues for correction,
  ○ planned actions,
  ○ the target deadline for completion, and
  ○ the name of the person accountable for the action.
• Staff recognition
  ○ personal words of thanks,
  ○ notes of appreciation, or
  ○ public acknowledgment in committees or meetings are all effective means of recognition.

Sources: Table developed by Luc R. Pelletier, MSN, APRN, PMHCNS-BC, FAAN, CPHQ, FNAHQ, using the following sources: Brown DS. Regulation, accreditation, and continuous readiness. In: Pelletier LR, Beaudin CL, eds. *Q Solutions: Essential Resources for the Healthcare Quality Professional*. 3rd ed. Chicago, IL: National Association for Healthcare Quality; 2012; Center for Improvement in Healthcare Quality. Accreditation policies for acute care hospitals, Effective January 2016. 2015. http://www.cihq.org/home.asp. Accessed January 13, 2017; Centers for Medicare & Medicaid Services. State operations manual: Appendix Q: Guidelines for determining immediate jeopardy. 2004. cms.hhs.gov/Regulations-and-guidance/Guidance/Manuals/downloads//som107ap_q_immedjeopardy.pdf. Accessed January 14, 2017; The Joint Commission (2016). The SAFER™ Matrix and changes to the post-survey process. https://www.jointcommission.org/assets/1/18/The_Safer_Matirx_and_Changes_to_Post_Survey_Process.pdf. Accessed January 13, 2017.

Postsurvey Activities

The focus of this period is achieving and sustaining compliance, especially in areas where the survey identified opportunities for improvement. The facility's self-assessment gap analysis and follow-up on corrective action plans drive the educational program, as well as awareness of changing regulations and standards. When deficiencies are cited or even suspected from a survey, the organization designs and implements corrective actions immediately in anticipation of the final report. Final reports can be delayed when they require a state agency to submit a report to a federal agency for final approval of the survey decisions, or if accreditation agencies wish a review of challenging findings by their central office. When the report is delayed, it may be difficult to remember the details of the survey citation or leadership attention may be on new matters, making corrective action planning more difficult. Even with delayed reports, a short deadline may be mandated (e.g., 10 days) to submit corrective actions. Survey findings form the basis for future leadership oversight on appropriate committee and leadership meeting agendas.

Education and Training in a Learning Organization

Senge's concept of the learning organization can be applied to healthcare. His definition of a *learning organization* is one "where people continually expand their capacity to create the results they truly desire, where new and expansive patterns of thinking are nurtured, where collective aspiration is set free, and where people are continually learning to see the whole together."[6(p3)] A *learning healthcare system* "is designed to generate and apply the best evidence for the collaborative healthcare choices of each patient and provider; to drive the process of discovery as a natural outgrowth of patient care; and to ensure innovation, quality, safety, and value in health care."[129(pix)] The most pressing needs for change identified by the IOM roundtable are those related to adaptation to the pace of change; the stronger synchrony of efforts; a culture of shared responsibility; a new clinical research paradigm; clinical decision support systems; universal electronic health records; and tools for database linkage, mining, and use, among others.[129(p5)]

Table 1-12 Examples of Survey Readiness Activities

- Clarify vacation expectations of key staff and leaders based on known survey windows.

- Assign survey roles for key staff duties such as command center operations, space planning, surveyor escorts, runners, or scribes. Determine both a primary and a back-up person for each role and provide an overview of expectations for the role in advance.
  - The *Escort's* primary function is to remain with the surveyor always so the surveyor is not unattended. Escorts develop a relationship with an individual surveyor and should be consistent throughout the survey, unless there is not a good match with the surveyor's personality. Escorts should be matched to surveyors with similar skill sets, for example, a physician with a physician or a nurse with a nurse. In some organizations, executives such as the CNO and CMO will serve as escorts to demonstrate the organization's commitment to the accreditation process.
  - *Runners* are responsible for contacting the command center to provide a brief report of activity, surveyor location, and specific surveyor requests.
  - *Scribes* are responsible for documenting the activities of the surveyor, taking notes, and keeping information organized.
  - *Sweep teams* are groups of individuals who round in advance of the surveyors to answer questions that staff may have and ensure compliance with standards.

- Determine if confidentiality releases, security codes, access cards, or additional name badges will be needed and be sure both scribes and escorts have access to all required clinical areas.

- Update organizational charts that can be attached to the phone lists to facilitate location of key staff during a survey.

- Update lists of phone numbers and create distribution lists for survey communications that include the organization's most common communication methods (e-mail, telephone, or pagers) to facilitate rapid communication during the survey. Set up a digital messaging structure when text pager or phone systems are available.

- Review previous regulatory or accreditation survey reports and the respective corrective action plans to evaluate sustained compliance.

- Ensure that the most current licenses, certificates, patient rights posters, and required signage are posted.

- Assemble required documents to ensure easy access to the most current documents.

- Review policies and procedures to ensure all are current.

- Test systems to quickly produce required lists of patients, residents, or clients including scheduled procedures or visits.

- Sweep care areas and departments for outdated policies, procedures, guidelines, order sets, forms, and privilege binders.

- Prepare surveyor orientation materials to prepare for documentation reviews for medical records that introduce electronic records or components of hybrid electronic and paper systems.

- Conduct medical record reviews of open records to ensure compliant records for vulnerable topics. If paper records are in use and a record has been thinned, ensure the appropriate information is included in the new volume and that the previous volumes are available if requested.

- Audit the human resources (HR) file system to ensure access to the complete HR file is readily available on site and that required documentation for education and training is available.

- Check education materials and brochures to ensure availability in the common languages for the populations served by the organization.

- Monitor the environment to ensure that it is clean and compliant with applicable fire and life safety codes.

- If the organization is spread out over a large geographic area, determine whether drivers or shuttles are needed to take surveyors to distant clinical areas. If employees are using their own vehicles, be sure vehicles are clean inside and out.

- Determine surveyor parking plans. Designated spaces close to the main entrance can be identified once a survey has begun. Parking vouchers may be provided. There may also need to be reserved parking spaces for employees driving surveyors or those coming in during the day for key interviews.

- Prepare packets to be given to surveyors upon arrival that include a map of the facility, facility contact list with phone numbers and pagers, organizational chart for the senior leadership team, parking information, and guest ID badges, if required. Information or brochures on local area restaurants and attractions also may be appreciated after the survey if the team has traveled to the survey location.

In a learning organization, learning needs to be embedded in the way the organization operates. When learning is embedded, it means that learning is a regular part of work and results in solving problems at their source (root cause). Building and sharing knowledge is deployed throughout the organization; and is driven by opportunities to effect significant, meaningful change and to innovate. Sources for learning include staff and physicians' ideas; research findings; patient and other customer input; best-practice sharing; and benchmarking.

Organizational learning has multiple benefits. It can result in increased value to patients through new and improved healthcare services as well as the development of new healthcare business opportunities. Organizational learning can lead to the development of evidence-based approaches and new healthcare delivery models. Patient safety can be enhanced through reduced errors, defects, waste, and related costs. Finally, organizational learning can lead to greater agility in managing change and disruption in the current healthcare environment.[11]

Staff Knowledge and Competency

To evaluate needs and ensure general staff knowledge and competency, the healthcare quality professional needs first to evaluate his or her own knowledge and competency for the area of education and training being offered. NAHQ offers *HQ Essentials* as a framework to support healthcare quality professionals in assessing and expanding their professional knowledge and abilities across six essential healthcare quality professional competency areas:

- Health Data Analytics
- Population Health and Care Transitions
- Performance and Process Improvement
- Regulatory and Accreditation
- Quality Review and Accountability
- Patient Safety.

For the topics covered in this section, healthcare quality professionals are encouraged to review the *HQ Essentials: Essential Competencies: Regulatory & Accreditation*[130] to gain a better understanding of the key competency descriptors to identify the extent to which current skill sets and professional experience align with the competency elements as well as the level of proficiency in each topical area.

Quality, Safety, and Performance Improvement Education and Training

Providing training on quality, safety, and performance improvement is often a collaborative effort between healthcare quality professionals as the subject matter experts and educators as the experts on teaching and learning modalities. Education to achieve varying levels of understanding of principles related to quality, safety, and performance improvement has been incorporated into the basic training programs for many different health professions. Healthcare quality professionals should work with organizational leaders to gain an understanding of which health professions have students in their organizations, and work with key leaders to align, to the extent possible, quality training projects with organizational quality priorities. Many health professions have professional associations or societies that offer education and training in healthcare quality and safety. The healthcare quality professional may be called upon to assist leaders and clinicians in assessing the value of available offerings.

There are multiple approaches to education using adult learning principles and accelerated learning methods, including the following:

- Engage multiple senses to enhance learning (auditory, visual, kinesthetic).
- Use concepts and principles, then add application into practice.
- Allow "toys" to activate the brain to facilitate learning.
- Allow students to teach each other key concepts; acting as a teacher promotes a stronger focus on learning.
- Cluster learning material into key categories and teach in segments, building on easier concepts and then adding more difficult ones.

The use of simulation and case studies to apply concepts or tools is another effective way to enhance training. Most types of hands-on experience and practice will make the learning fun and more relevant and increase muscle memory for the task.

Training on quality, safety, and performance improvement must address the current employee base, physicians, new employees, and students/trainees. Although core concepts and tools can be taught and reemphasized to embed the improvement philosophy into the culture, there will be degradation in memory unless the information is clearly integrated into daily work and used often. For this reason, just-in-time training is often used for teams or projects.

By building a learning organization, leaders foster an environment conducive to learning about quality, safety, and performance improvement. This opens boundaries across departments, disciplines, and professions and stimulates the exchange of ideas. The way to foster this development is to create learning forums, which may take many forms to achieve innovation and learning. The learning organization will excel in a culture of performance excellence and improvement because the cultural foundation will support ongoing learning, change, and improvement. AHRQ[35] provides free continuing education events in the areas of comparative effectiveness, quality and patient safety, and prevention/care management. These continuing education opportunities are described in detail in their website.

Staff Education for Continuous Survey Readiness

One strategy as part of the ongoing organizational assessment process is just-in-time staff education. As areas of opportunity are identified and addressed, staff are reminded of regulatory and accreditation expectations in an educational and coaching manner. Wherever possible, the healthcare quality professional relates the specific desired behavior as expected in the regulation or standard back to the impact on high-quality and safe patient care. CSR programs require solid organization-wide education programs with staff participation from all levels within an organization. Healthcare quality professionals must develop an effective and efficient education and training that targets defined levels within the organization:

- Leadership must receive information to prioritize resources for readiness, to model required changes in behavior, and to speak to key leadership and other relevant standards when surveyors visit their facilities.
- Managers must have information related to care delivery requirements and structure or process requirements, as well as required documentation that must be immediately available to surveyors. Managers need to participate in staff education programs, often becoming the staff educator after train-the-trainer programs.
- Frontline staff must receive information to comply with standards and regulations related to direct care delivery, which will be found in policies and procedures related to their work. There will also be documentation requirements they must understand and comply with, such as specific care documentation, equipment checks for maintenance or performance within defined parameters (i.e., test results or temperature ranges), communication documentation with transitions in care, or required education and training that must be documented.

Effective education plans must target defined departments within an organization, but must also acknowledge interprofessional interdependencies. For example, key messages for large care delivery departments such as nursing may be different from key messages for smaller ancillary departments or specialty departments. If programs are not designed specifically for an intended audience, participants may believe most of the material applies to another department or may be unable to apply the message to its own department.

Education departments can help organizations design targeted programs and provide the structure for delivery. Because CSR is ongoing, a variety of approaches and learning methods are used, including the following:

- face-to-face education,
- rounds of work areas with environment assessment and staff knowledge assessment (briefings, huddles),
- questions and answer tools (daily, weekly, and monthly),
- resource books of common standards updated at least annually,
- self-assessment tools to identify gaps in comparison to standards and education and other action plans to address the gaps,
- visual tools or cognitive aids such as posters on safety goals or performance improvement model,
- content experts to respond one-on-one to questions or interpretation of standards,
- mock surveys to assess compliance with standards in an ongoing manner,
- tools for tracer activities, and
- just-in-time training.

Successful CSR education programs are the outcome of creative education modalities that reach staff and leaders alike and effectively impart key messages and reinforce them across the organization. Healthcare quality professionals must be creative in developing effective ongoing programs, because the workforce is constantly changing as healthcare staff change roles or organizations. Although healthcare quality professionals work to maintain a continuous state of readiness for survey activity, education calendars are planned as part of a cohesive program. Creating an ongoing series will be more effective than a sporadic offering of seemingly unrelated topics. Educational programs may best be long-range programs designed around multiyear survey cycles.

Training Effectiveness

Kirkpatrick's foundational principles for evaluating effectiveness of training were first published in 1959, but continue to be relevant and used by healthcare quality professionals today. The focus was a return on expectations as the ultimate indicator of value, and value must be created before it can be measured. The framework for evaluation can be envisioned as a compelling chain of evidence that demonstrates the bottom-line value to the organization.

Framework for Evaluating the Results of Training. As an expert in the field of training, Kirkpatrick[131] perceived three reasons for evaluating training programs, namely,

1. to determine how to improve future training,
2. to determine whether the current training continues, and
3. to justify the existence of the training department.

To the extent trainers can demonstrate important outcomes from training, they will be important to the quality and safety movement and the organization itself. Kirkpatrick[131] suggests there are four important levels of training evaluation: reaction, learning, behavior, and results. This model is often used to describe various levels of measuring training effectiveness.

Reaction. This is the extent to which the participants are satisfied with training. Because negative attitudes toward the program can interfere with learning, this is an important measurement. Reactions are often measured at the end of the training program or soon after the program ends through use of a questionnaire about what participants thought and felt about the training. For example, here are two ways of measuring reactions:

1. Customer (trainee) satisfaction, or their opinion (What did they like? What did they learn? Was anything missing?), using a Likert rating scale for feedback.
2. Good facilitator, interesting or useful subject, adequate facilities, opinion of atmosphere, scheduling, additional comments.

Learning. When participants change attitudes, improve knowledge, or increase skill because of the program, learning occurred. Unless one of these parameters changes, it is unlikely that behavior will change. Learning is best measured both before and after training and, where possible, includes some type of control group as a basis of comparison. The type of measure used will depend on what is being evaluated. For example, increased skill may need to be evaluated by a specialist in that area, whereas a change in attitude can be measured using a before-and-after questionnaire. For example, learning can be measured by a change in attitude, skills, or knowledge and using pre- and posttests, test performance, demonstrations/simulation, or role play.

Behavior. This level refers to behavioral change because of training. It focuses on the transfer of knowledge, skills, or attitudes from the classroom to the job. Although positive reactions may produce a desire to change behavior, and learning may give participants the skills to know how and what to change, it does not necessarily follow that behavior will change. In addition to positive reactions and learning, employees must work in a climate supportive of change, and they must see some reward associated with changing their behaviors. These do not have to be tangible rewards; intangible rewards such as a feeling of achievement are important motivators for change. The climate depends heavily on the support of the supervisor, further supporting the importance of all levels of management being involved in quality, safety, and performance improvement education and training.

Ideally, behaviors are measured both before and after training, allowing ample time for behavioral change to occur. Pretraining and posttraining information can be collected by questionnaires, interviews, and from those who can observe participants' behaviors (e.g., immediate supervisor, customers, peers). Some relevant examples of behavioral changes relating to quality and safety may include the extent to which

- department heads deploy quality, safety, and performance improvement concepts, methods, and tools;
- staff report variances in processes and near misses;
- senior leaders communicate the organization's values (measured by employee questionnaires and focus groups); and
- leadership practices reflect employee involvement, engagement, and participation.

Results. This is the last—and probably the most important—level of program evaluation described by Kirkpatrick. Indicators used to measure results are tied to the driving force behind conducting training in the first place. For example, did quality of care improve, and was this a function of quality, safety, and performance improvement training? Were overall errors reduced through organization-wide quality and safety training? As with evaluation of behavioral changes, result evaluation is conducted before and after training, uses a control group, allows ample time for results to be achieved, monitors results over time, and compares the cost of the training program with the benefit. In some cases, a direct link between training and results will be difficult to prove because many other factors might influence an outcome. However, evidence that supports the link should be gathered. Examples of results may include

- final overall change for the business because of the training program;
- improved quality, improved production, or decreased costs; and
- increased job satisfaction, reduced problems or accidents, or increased sales.

Return on Investment. Phillips suggested a fifth level of evaluation: ROI evaluation, in which the fourth level of the standard model is compared with the overall costs of training.[132,133] The ROI evaluation addresses how the bottom line changed because of training. The ROI asks the question "Were the benefits greater than the cost?"[132] Phillips describes methods for isolating the effects of the program or process, methods of converting data to monetary values, cost categories, intangible benefits, and communication targets. For quality, safety, and performance improvement, are staff using the tools and methods (e.g., more improvement projects being initiated) and are outcomes improving and if so is value being demonstrated beyond the cost of the training?

Section Summary

Organizational leadership and management of quality and safety are the linchpin to effective continuous quality, safety, and performance improvement programs. This section discussed healthcare organizations as CASs, leadership fundamentals, organizational infrastructure required to support quality and safety, strategic planning, leadership and organizational culture, and key concepts of regulatory, accreditation, and external recognition programs that impact healthcare quality and safety. Change management, innovation and creativity, a business case for quality and continuous readiness are reviewed. The healthcare quality professional's role is defined and described as essential to an organization's success in maintaining a quality and safe environment for patients and families. The healthcare quality professional's role in making operational the principles of leadership and management can be found in other sections of *HQ Solutions* and NAHQ products.

Recent changes in the healthcare reimbursement landscape make the role of the healthcare quality professional even more critical as value, translated in part through high-quality, reliable care and service delivery, becomes the focus for healthcare transformation. Armed with principles, tools, and techniques, the healthcare quality professional is an invaluable resource to the healthcare enterprise as it strives, through leadership and management, and education, training and communication to provide essential, safe, and effective healthcare services.

References

1. Institute of Medicine. *Medicare: A Strategy for Quality Assurance* (Vol. 2). Washington, DC: National Academy Press; 2000.
2. Institute of Medicine, Committee on Quality of Health Care in America. *Crossing the Quality Chasm: A New Health System for the 21st Century*. Washington, DC: National Academies Press; 2001.
3. Stamatis DH. *Total Quality Management in Healthcare: Implementation Strategies for Optimum Results*. Chicago, IL: Irwin; 1996.
4. Dentzer S. Still crossing the quality chasm—or suspended over it? *Health Aff.* 2011;30(4):554–555.
5. Merriam-Webster. System. https://www.merriam-webster.com/dictionary/system. Accessed January 15, 2017
6. Senge PM. *Fifth Discipline: The Art and Practice of the Learning Organization*. New York, NY: Doubleday; 1990.
7. Ginter PM, Swayne LE, Duncan WJ. *Strategic Management of Health Care Organizations*. 4th ed. Oxford, England: Blackwell.
8. Wiltz C. 5 principles of systems thinking for a changing healthcare ecosystem. In: *Medical Device and Diagnostic Industry*. 2013. http://www.mddionline.com/article/5-principles-systems-thinking-changing-healthcare-ecosystem.
9. Begun J, Zimmerman B, Dooley K. Health care organizations as complex adaptive systems. In: Mick S, Wyttenbach M, eds. *Advances in Health Care Organization Theory*. San Francisco, CA: Jossey-Bass; 2003:253–258.
10. Zimmerman B, Lindberg C, Plsek P. *Edgeware: Insights From Complexity Science for Health Care Leaders*. Irving, TX: VHA; 2001.
11. Deming WE. *Out of the Crisis*. Cambridge, MA: MIT Press; 2000.
12. Juran JM. *The Juran on Leadership for Quality: An Executive Handbook*. New York, NY: Free Press; 1989.
13. Plsek PE. Redesigning healthcare with insights from the science of complex adaptive systems. In: *Crossing the Quality Chasm: A New Health System for the 21st Century* (Appendix B). Washington DC: National Academies Press, Institute of Medicine, Committee on Quality of Healthcare in America; 2001.
14. Plsek PE. *Harnessing Disruptive Innovation in Health Care*. Rockville, MD: Agency for Healthcare Research and Quality. https://innovations.ahrq.gov/perspectives/harnessing-disruptive-innovation-health-care. Accessed May 6, 2017.
15. Plsek PE, Kilo CM. From resistance to attraction: a different approach to change. *Physician Exec.* 1999;25(6):40–46.
16. Inozu B, Chauncey D, Kamataris V, Mount C. *Performance Improvement for Healthcare: Leading Change With Lean, Six Sigma, and Constraints Management*. New York, NY: McGraw-Hill; 2012.
17. Kotter JP. What leaders really do. *Harv Bus Rev.* 1990;68:103–111.
18. Robbins S, Judge TA. *Organizational Behavior*. 16th ed. Upper Saddle River, NJ: Prentice Hall; 2015.
19. Kelly D. *Applying Quality Management in Healthcare: A Process for Improvement*. Chicago, IL: Health Administration Press; 2003.
20. Donabedian A. *The Definition of Quality and Approaches to its Assessment*. Ann Arbor, MI: Health Administration Press; 1980.
21. Ayanian JZ, Markel H. Donabedian's lasting framework for health care quality. *N Engl J Med.* 2016;375(3):205–207. doi:10.1056/NEJMp1605101
22. Mullan F. A founder of quality assessment encounters a troubled system firsthand. *Health Aff (Millwood)*. 2001;20(1):137–141.
23. Baldrige Performance Excellence Program. *2017–2018 Baldrige Excellence Framework: A Systems Approach to Improving Your Organization's Performance*. Gaithersburg, MD: U.S. Department of Commerce, National Institute of Standards and Technology; 2017. https://www.nist.gov/baldrige. Accessed June 27, 2017.
24. Institute for Healthcare Improvement. A framework for leadership of improvement. www.ihi.org/knowledge/Pages/Tools/IHIFrameworkforLeadershipforImprovement.aspx. Accessed January 20, 2017.
25. Swensen S, Pugh M, McMullan C, Kabcenell A. High-impact Leadership: Improve Care, Improve the Health of Populations, and Reduce Costs. IHI White Paper. Cambridge, MA: Institute for Healthcare Improvement. Also available at ihi.org.
26. Institute for Healthcare Improvement. IHI Triple aim initiative. http://www.ihi.org/engage/initiatives/tripleaim/pages/default.aspx Accessed January 20, 2017.
27. Swensen SJ, Dilling JA, McCarty PM, Bolton JW, Harper CM. The business case for health-care quality improvement. *J Patient Saf.* 2013;9(1):44–52. doi:10.1097/PTS.0b013e3182753e33
28. Burns JM. *Leadership*. New York, NY: Harper and Row; 1978.
29. Goleman D. Leadership that gets results. *Har Bus Rev.* 2000:78–90.
30. Kouzes JM, Posner BZ. *Leadership: The challenge*. San Francisco: Jossey-Bass; 2002.
31. Merriam-Webster. Culture. https://www.merriam-webster.com/dictionary/culture. Accessed January 15, 2017.
32. Siehl L, Martin J. *Learning Organizational Culture*. Palo Alto, CA: Stanford University, Graduate School of Business; 1982.
33. Rokeach M. *The Nature of Human Values*. New York, NY: Free Press; 1973.
34. Watkins MD. What is organizational culture? And why should we care? *Harv Bus Rev.* 2013. https://hbr.org/2013/05/what-is-organizational-culture.

35. Agency for Healthcare Research and Quality. Patient safety primer: Safety culture. www.psnet.ahrq.gov/primer.aspx?primerID=5. Accessed January 20, 2017.

36. Schein EH. *Organizational Culture and Leadership: A Dynamic View.* 2nd ed. San Francisco, CA: Jossey-Bass; 1992

37. Schneider B, ed. *Organizational Culture and Climate.* San Francisco, CA: Jossey-Bass; 1990.

38. Agency for Healthcare Research and Quality. Surveys on patient safety culture. Rockville, MD: Agency for Healthcare Research and Quality. http://www.ahrq.gov/professionals/quality-patient-safety/patientsafetyculture/index.html. Accessed January 15, 2017. Published July 2012. Updated October 2016.

39. Sexton JG, Helmreich RL, Neilands TB, et al. The Safety Attitudes Questionnaire: psychometric properties, benchmarking data, and emerging research. *BMC Health Serv Res.* 2006. http://bmchealthservres.biomedcentral.com/articles/10.1186/1472-6963-6-44. Accessed April 24, 2017.

40. Shortell SM, Morrison E, Robbins S. Strategy-making in health care organizations: a framework and agenda for research. *Medical Care Rev.* 1985;2:219–266. doi:10.1177/107755878504200203

41. Luthans F, Hodgetts R, Thompson K. *Social Issues in Business: Strategic and Public Policy Perspectives.* 6th ed. Upper Saddle River, NJ: Prentice Hall.

42. Baldrige Performance Excellence Program. *2011-2012 Baldrige Excellence Framework: A Systems Approach to Improving Your Organization's Performance.* Gaithersburg, MD: U.S. Department of Commerce, National Institute of Standards and Technology; 2011.

43. SSM Health Care. Our mission: SSM Health Care home page. http://www.ssmhealth.com/sluhospital/our-mission/. Accessed May 8, 2017.

44. Charleston Area Medical Center. About us. www.camc.org. Accessed May 8, 2017.

45. Minnesota Department of Health. SMART objectives. http://www.health.state.mn.us/divs/opi/qi/toolbox/print/objectives.pdf. Accessed January 14, 2017.

46. Business Dictionary. Goal congruence. http://www.businessdictionary.com/definition/goal-congruence.html. Accessed January 14, 2017.

47. Campanella P, Vukovic V, Parente P, et al. The impact of public reporting on clinical outcomes: a systematic review and meta-analysis. *BMC Health Serv Res.* 2016;16:296. doi:10.1186/s12913-016-1543-y

48. Leapfrog Group. About us and our mission. http://www.leapfroggroup.org/about. Accessed January 19, 2017.

49. Healthgrades. About us. https://www.healthgrades.com/about/. Accessed January 19, 2017.

50. Fung CH, Lim YW, Mattke S, Damberg C, Shekelle PG. Systematic review: the evidence that publishing patient care performance data improves quality of care. *Ann Intern Med.* 2008;148(2):111–123.

51. Silow-Carroll S, Alteras T, Meyer JA. Hospital quality improvement: strategies and lessons learned from U.S. hospitals. http://www.commonwealthfund.org/publications/fund-reports/2007/apr/hospital-quality-improvement--strategies-and-lessons-from-u-s--hospitals. Accessed January 15, 2017.

52. Gaucher EJ, Coffey RJ. *Total Quality in Healthcare: From Theory to Practice.* San Francisco, CA: Jossey-Bass; 1993.

53. Hutchins D. *Hoshin Kanri: The Strategic Approach to Continuous Improvement.* Surrey, United Kingdom: Gower; 2016.

54. Garman A, Scribner L. Leading for quality in healthcare: development and validation of a competency model. *J Healthc Manag.* 2011;56(6):373–382.

55. Botwinick L, Bisognano M, Haraden C. *Leadership Guide to Patient Safety.* IHI Innovation Series White Paper. Cambridge, MA: Institute for Healthcare Improvement. http://www.ihi.org/resources/Pages/IHIWhitePapers/LeadershipGuidetoPatientSafetyWhitePaper.aspx. Accessed January 14, 2017.

56. Taitz JM, Lee TH, Sequist TD. A framework for engaging physicians in quality and safety. *BMJ Qual Saf.* 2012;21:722–728. doi:10.1136/bmjqs-2011-000167

57. Pelletier LR, Stichler JE. Patient-centered care and engagement: nurse leaders' imperative for health reform. *J Nurs Adm.* 2014;44(9):473–480. doi:10.1097/NNA.0000000000000102

58. Conway J. Getting boards on board: engaging governing boards in quality and safety. *Jt Comm J Qual Patient Saf.* 2008;34(4):214–220. doi:10.1016/S1553-7250(08)34028-8

59. The Governance Institute. *Maximizing the Effectiveness of the Board's Quality Committee: Leading Practices and Lessons Learned.* San Diego, CA: The Governance Institute; 2015.

60. Institute for Healthcare Improvement. High impact leadership: improve care, improve the health of populations, and reduce costs. http://www.ihi.org/resources/pages/ihiwhitepapers/highimpactleadership.aspx. Accessed May 8, 2017.

61. National Association for Healthcare Quality and Institute for Healthcare Improvement. Quality structure and functions at half the expense. http://www.nahq.org/uploads/IHI_RD_Report_W26_NAHQ_Quality_Department_Final_Feb_27_2013.pdf. Accessed January 22, 2017.

62. Evans JR, Dean JW. *Total Quality: Management, Organization and Strategy.* 3rd ed. Mason, OH: Thomson South-Western; 2003.

63. Mosby's Medical Dictionary. Change agent. http://medical-dictionary.thefreedictionary.com/change+agent. Accessed January 23, 2017.

64. Schein EH. Kurt Lewin's change theory in the field and in the classroom: notes toward a model of managed learning. *Syst Pract.* 1996;9:27. doi:10.1007/BF02173417

65. Smith MK. *Kurt Lewin: groups, experiential learning and action research.* www.infed.org/thinkers/et-lewin.htm. Accessed May 8, 2017.

66. Palmer B. *Making Change Work: Practical Tools for Overcoming Human Resistance to Change.* Milwaukee, WI: ASQ Quality Press; 2004.

67. Palmer B. Overcoming resistance to change. *Quality Progress.* 2004;37(4):35–39.

68. DeWeaver M, Gillespie L. *Real World Project Management.* New York, NY: Quality Resources; 1997.

69. Galpin TJ. Connecting culture to organizational change. *HR Magazine.* 1996;41(30):84–89.

70. Galpin TJ. *The Human Side of Change.* San Francisco, CA: Jossey-Bass; 1996.

71. Kotter JP, Cohen DS. *The Heart of Change.* Boston, MA: Harvard Business Publishing; 2002.

72. Kotter JP. *Leading Change.* Boston, MA: Harvard Business Publishing; 1996.

73. Cancer Prevention Research Center. Transtheoretical model. http://web.uri.edu/cprc/detailed-overview/. Accessed January 20, 2017.

74. De Zuelta PC. Developing compassionate leadership in healthcare: an integrative review. *J Healthcare Leadership.* 2015;8:1–10. doi:10.2147/JHL.S93724

75. Institute for Healthcare Improvement. Changes for improvement. www.ihi.org/knowledge/Pages/Changes/default.aspx. Accessed January 20, 2017.

76. Pew Research Center. *Women and Leadership: Public Says Women are Equally Qualified, But Barriers Persist.* Washington, DC: Pew Research Center; 2015. www.pewresearch.org. Accessed May 8, 2017.

77. Olivo T. The profile of an effective healthcare leader. *Becker's Hospital Review.* http://www.beckershospitalreview.com/hospital-management-administration/the-profile-of-an-effective-healthcare-leader.html. Accessed May 8, 2017.

78. American Psychological Association. The road to resilience: what is resilience? www.apa.org/helpcenter/road-resilience.aspx. Accessed January 14, 2017.

79. Institute for Healthcare Improvement. How to improve. www.ihi.org/knowledge/Pages/HowtoImprove/default.aspx. Accessed January 20, 2017.

80. Institute for Healthcare Improvement. How to improve. www.ihi.org/knowledge/Pages/HowtoImprove/default.aspx. Accessed 2008.

81. Langley GL, Nolan KM, Nolan TW, Norman CL, Provost LP. *The Improvement Guide: A Practical Approach to Enhancing Organizational Performance.* 2nd ed. San Francisco, CA: Jossey-Bass; 2009.

82. NEJM Catalyst Insights Council. Disconnects in transforming health care delivery: how executives, clinical leaders, and clinicians must bridge their divide and move forward together. http://catalyst.nejm.org/insights/. Accessed February 24, 2017.

83. Merriam-Webster. Best practice. https://www.merriam-webster.com/dictionary/best practice. Accessed January 22, 2017.

84. Maher L, Plsek P, Bevan H. *Creating the culture for innovation: guide for executives.* Coventry, UK: NHS Institute for Innovation and Improvement. http://www.nhsiq.nhs.uk/media/2760655/creating_the_culture_for_innovation_-_guide_for_executives.pdf. Accessed May 8, 2017.

85. Plsek PE. *Working Paper: Models for the Creative Process.* www.directedcreativity.com/pages/WPModels.html. Accessed January 20, 2017.

86. Horth DM, Vhear J. *Becoming a Leader Who Foster Innovation* (White Paper). Greensboro, NC: Center for Creative Leadership; 2014.

87. Christensen CM, Bohmer RMJ, Kenagy J. Will disruptive innovations cure health care? *Harv Bus Rev.* 2000;78(5):102–112, 199.

88. Plsek P. AHRQ innovations exchange: creating a culture of innovation. https://innovations.ahrq.gov/article/creating-culture-innovation. Accessed May 8, 2017.

89. Pradhan P, Pradhan K. Emerging health-care innovations. In: Singh VK, Lillrank P, eds. *Innovations in Healthcare Management: Cost-Effective and Sustainable Solutions.* Boca Raton, FL: CRC Press.

90. Singh VK, Lillrank P. *Innovations in Healthcare Management: Cost-Effective and Sustainable Solutions.* Boca Raton, FL: CRC Press; 2015.

91. Plsek PE. Complexity and the adoption of innovation in health care. http://nihcm.org/pdf/Plsek.pdf. Accessed January 14, 2017.

92. Rogers E. *The Diffusion of Innovations.* 5th ed. New York, NY: Free Press; 1995.

93. Institute for Healthcare Improvement. Linking tests of change. www.ihi.org/IHI/Topics/Improvement/ImprovementMethods/HowToImprove/rampsofchange.html. Accessed January 20, 2017.

94. Institute for Healthcare Improvement. Spreading changes. www.ihi.org/knowledge/Pages/HowtoImprove/ScienceofImprovementSpreadingChanges.aspx. Accessed January 20, 2017.

95. Berwick DM. Disseminating innovations in health care. *JAMA.* 2003;289(15):1969–1975. doi:10.1001/jama.289.15.1969

96. Institute for Healthcare Improvement. Tips for testing changes. www.ihi.org/knowledge/Pages/HowtoImprove/ScienceofImprovementTipsforTestingChanges.aspx. Accessed January 20, 2017.

97. Leatherman S, Berwick D, Illes D, et al. The business case for quality: case studies and an analysis. *Health Aff.* 2003;22(2):17–30. doi:10.1377/hlthaff.22.2.17

98. Bailit M, Dyer M. *Beyond Bankable Dollars: Establishing A Business Case for Improving Healthcare.* New York, NY: Commonwealth Fund; 2004.

99. Centers for Medicare & Medicaid Services. Emergency Medical Treatment & Labor Act (EMTALA). www.cms.gov/Regulations-and-Guidance/Legislation/EMTALA/index.html?redirect=/EMTALA. Accessed January 20, 2017.

100. Centers for Medicare & Medicaid Services, Office of Civil Rights. Health information privacy. www.hhs.gov/ocr/privacy. Accessed January 20, 2017.

101. Centers for Medicare & Medicaid Services. Clinical Laboratory Improvement Amendments (CLIA). www.cms.hhs.gov/clia. Accessed January 20, 2017.

102. Centers for Medicare & Medicaid Services. About us. https://www.cms.gov/About-CMS/About-CMS.html. Accessed January 20, 2017.

103. U.S. Department of Health & Human Services. Regional offices. https://www.hhs.gov/about/agencies/iea/regional-offices/. Accessed May 8, 2017.

104. Centers for Medicare & Medicaid Services. Regulations & guidance. www.cms.hhs.gov/Regulations-and-Guidance/Regulations-and-Guidance.html. Accessed January 20, 2017.

105. U.S. Government Publishing Office. Code of Federal Regulations Title 42: Public health: Part 482—Conditions of Participation for hospitals. https://www.gpo.gov/fdsys/pkg/CFR-2015-title42-vol5/xml/CFR-2015-title42-vol5-part482.xml. Accessed January 13, 2017.

106. National Archives and Records Administration. *Code of Federal Regulations,* Title 42, Volume 3, Part 482. http://www.ecfr.gov/cgi-bin/text-idx?tpl=/ecfrbrowse/Title42/42tab_02.tpl. Accessed February 8, 2017.

107. Centers for Medicare & Medicaid Services. State operations manual: appendix A—survey protocol, regulations and interpretive guidelines for hospitals. https://www.cms.gov/Regulations-and-Guidance/Guidance/Manuals/downloads/som107ap_a_hospitals.pdf. Accessed January 20, 2017.

108. Customs Mobile. All Titles. Title 42. Chapter IV. Part 488. Subpart A—General Provisions. https://www.customsmobile.com/regulations/expand/title42_chapterIV_part488_subpartA_section488.7#title42_chapterIV_part488_subpartA_section488.10. Updated November 23, 2016. Accessed January 27, 2017.

109. U.S. Department of Health & Human Services, Office of the Inspector General. National Practitioner Data Bank: malpractice reporting requirements (OIE-01-90-00521). Accessed December 10, 2016. https://oig.hhs.gov/oei/reports/oei-01-90-00521.pdf

110. U.S. Department of Health & Human Services, Health Resources and Services Administration. *NPDB Guidebook.* Rockville, MD: U.S. Department of Health & Human Services; 2015. https://www.npdb.hrsa.gov/resources/aboutGuidebooks.jsp. Accessed January 13, 2017.

111. Regulations.gov. Regulatory agenda. https://resources.regulations.gov/public/component/main?__dmfClientId=1484422488197&__dmfTzoff=300. Accessed January 14, 2017.

112. Conway P, Berwick D. Improving the rules for hospital participation in Medicare and Medicaid. *JAMA.* 2011;306(20):2256–2257. doi:10.1001/jama.2011.1611

113. Medicaid.gov. Managed care. https://www.medicaid.gov/medicaid/managed-care/index.html. Accessed May 8, 2017.

114. Field RI. *Healthcare Regulation in America: Complexity, Confrontation and Compromise.* New York, NY: Oxford University Press; 2007.

115. Merriam-Webster. Accredit. https://www.merriamwebster.com/thesaurus/accreditation. Accessed January 15, 2017.

116. Merriam-Webster. Certify. https://www.merriam-webster.com/dictionary/certify. Accessed January 15, 2017.

117. Centers for Medicare & Medicaid Services. FY 2015 Report to Congress (RTC): Review of Medicare's Program Oversight of Accrediting Organizations (AOs) and the Clinical Laboratory Improvement Amendments of 1988 (CLIA) Validation Program. https://www.cms.gov/Medicare/Provider-Enrollment-and-Certification/SurveyCertificationGenInfo/Downloads/Survey-and-Cert-Letter-16-07.pdf. Dated January 29, 2016. Accessed January 23, 2017.

118. Food & Drug Administration. Radiation-emitting products: Mammography Quality Standards Act regulations. www.gov/Radiation-EmittingProducts/MammographyQualityStandardsActandProgram/Regulations/ucm110906.htm. Accessed January 14, 2017.

119. National Quality Forum. NQF's history. http://www.qualityforum.org/about_nqf/history/. Accessed December 20, 2016.

120. Massachusetts Department of Health and Human Services. Serious reportable events. http://www.mass.gov/eohhs/gov/departments/dph/programs/hcq/serious-reportable-event-sres.html. Accessed January 27, 2017.

121. The Joint Commission. Sentinel event policy and procedure. https://www.jointcommission.org/sentinel_event_policy_and_procedures/. Accessed January 27, 2017.

122. American College of Physicians. What is patient centered medical home? https://www.acponline.org/practice-resources/business/payment/models/pcmh/understanding/what-pcmh. Accessed May 6, 2017.

123. Accreditation Canada. The value and impact of health care accreditation: a literature review. https://accreditation.ca/sites/default/files/value-and-impact-en.pdf. Accessed May 5, 2015.

124. American Nurses Credentialing Center. Magnet Recognition Program Overview. http://www.nursecredentialing.org/Magnet/ProgramOverview. Accessed January 23, 2017.

125. The Joint Commission. Facts about the Joint Commission. www.jointcommission.org/facts_about_the_joint_commission. Accessed 2016.

126. Merriam-Webster. Continuous. https://www.merriam-webster.com/dictionary/continuous. Accessed January 15, 2017.

127. Merriam-Webster. Ready. https://www.merriam-webster.com/dictionary/ready. Accessed January 15, 2017.

128. Merriam-Webster. Compliance. https://www.merriam-webster.com/dictionary/compliance. Accessed January 15, 2017.

129. Institute of Medicine, Roundtable on Evidence-Based Medicine. *The Learning Healthcare System: Workshop Summary*. Washington, DC: National Academies Press; 2007.

130. National Association for Healthcare Quality. *HQ essentials: essential competencies: regulatory & accreditation*, 2017.

131. Kirkpatrick DL. *Another Look at Evaluating Training Programs*. Alexandria, VA: American Society for Training & Development; 1998.

132. Phillips JJ. ROI. *Training Dev.* 1996;50:42–47.

133. Phillips JJ, Phillips PP. *ROI at Work: Best-Practice Case Studies From the Real World*. Alexandria, VA: American Society for Training and Development (now the Association for Talent Development); 2005.

Suggested Readings

Brown SL, Eisenhardt KM. *Competing on the Edge: Strategy as Structured Chaos*. Boston, MA: Harvard Business School Publishing; 1998.

Centers for Medicare & Medicaid Services. CMS Quality Strategy 2016. https://www.cms.gov/Medicare/Quality-Initiatives-Patient-Assessment-Instruments/QualityInitiativesGenInfo/Downloads/CMS-Quality-Strategy.pdf. Accessed January 14, 2017.

Centers for Medicare & Medicaid Services. Key milestones in Medicare and Medicaid history, selected years: 1965–2003. *Health Care Financ Rev.* 2005;27(2):1–3. www.cms.gov/Research-Statistics-Data-and-Systems/Research/HealthCareFinancingReview/downloads//05-06Winpg1.pdf

Gaucher EJ, Coffey RJ. *Breakthrough Performance: Accelerating the Transformation of Health Care Organizations*. San Francisco, CA: Jossey-Bass; 2000.

Greenhalgh T, Plsek PE. Four-part special series on complex science. *BMJ.* 2001;323:625–628.

Hadelman J. *The Impact of Strategic Healthcare Leadership: Top Ten Leadership Trends in Health Care in the 21st Century*. Oak Brook, IL: Witt/Kieffer; 2000.

Henry J. Kaiser Family Foundation. The states. www.statehealthfacts.org. Accessed 2017.

Horak BJ. *Strategic Planning in Healthcare: Building a Quality-Based Plan Step-by-Step*. Portland, OR: Book News; 1999.

The Joint Commission. Accreditation Survey Activity Guide for Health Care Organizations. https://www.jointcommission.org/assets/1/18/2016_Organization_SAG_August_Release_Corrected.pdf. Published August 2016. Corrected November 2016. Accessed January 20, 2017.

Katzenbach JR. *Teams at the Top*. Cambridge, MA: Harvard Business Publishing; 1998.

Kotter JP. Why transformation efforts fail. *Har Bus Rev.* 1995 (March–April):59–67.

Kouzes JM, Posner BZ. *Leadership Challenge: How to Get Extraordinary Things Done in Organizations*. San Francisco, CA: Jossey-Bass; 2012.

Mackenzie SJ, Goldmann DA, Perla RJ, Parry GJ. Measuring hospital-wide mortality—pitfalls and potential. *J Healthc Qual.* 2016;38(3):187–194.

Marx D. *Whack-a-Mole: The Price We Pay for Expecting Perfection*. Plano, TX: By Your Side Studios; 2009.

Mignano JL, Miner L, Cafeo C, et al. Routinization of HIV testing in an inpatient setting: a systematic process for organizational change. *J Healthc Qual.* 2016;38(3):e10–e18.

Mitchell SE, Martin J, Holmes S, et al. How hospitals reengineer their discharge processes to reduce readmissions. *J Healthc Qual.* 2016;38(2):116–126.

Nash DB. Improving health outcomes through population health practice. *J Healthc Qual.* 2016;38(2):64–65.

Palleschi MT, Sirianni S, O'Connor N, Dunn D, Hasenau SM. An interprofessional process to improve early identification and treatment for sepsis. *J Healthc Qual.* 2014;36(4):23–31.

Perla RJ, Bradbury E, Gunther-Murphy C. Large-scale improvement initiatives in healthcare: a scan of the literature. *J Healthc Qual.* 2013;35(1):30–40.

Perlin JB, Horner SJ, Englebright JD, Bracken RM. Rapid core measure improvement through a "Business Case for Quality." *J Healthc Qual.* 2014;36(2):50–61.

Plsek PE, Greenhalgh T. The challenge of complexity in healthcare. *BMJ.* 2001;323:625–628. doi:10.1136/bmj.323.7313.625

Ridling DA, Magyary D. Implementation science: describing implementation methods used by pediatric intensive care units in a national collaborative. *J Healthc Qual.* 2015;37(2):102–116.

Schein EH. *Organization Culture and Leadership*. San Francisco, CA: Jossey-Bass; 2004.

Shields JA, Jennings JL. Using the Malcolm Baldrige "Are We Making Progress" survey for organizational self-assessment and performance improvement. *J Healthc Qual.* 2013;35(4):5–15.

Social Security Administration. Use of state agencies to determine compliance by providers of services with Conditions of Participation. www.ssa.gov/OP_Home/ssact/title18/1864.htm. Accessed January 15, 2017.

Stacey RD. *Complexity and Creativity in Organizations*. San Francisco, CA: Berrett-Koehler; 1996.

Waldrop MM. *Complexity: The Emerging Science at the Edge of Order and Chaos*. New York, NY: Simon and Schuster; 1992.

Online Resources

AABB
www.aabb.org

Accreditation Association for Ambulatory Health Care (AAAHC)
www.aaahc.org

Accreditation Commission for Health Care (ACHC)
www.achc.org

Agency for Healthcare Research and Quality (AHRQ)
- **Quality & Patient Safety Resources**
www.ahrq.gov/qual/patientsafetyculture
- **Education & Training for Health Professionals**
https://www.ahrq.gov/professionals/education/index.html
- **AHRQ-Sponsored Continuing Education Activities**
https://www.ahrq.gov/professionals/education/continuing-ed/index.html

American College of Radiology (ACR)
www.ACRAccreditation.org

American College of Surgeons (ACS)
www.facs.org

American Nurses Credentialing Center (ANCC)
www.nursecredentialing.org

CARF International
www.carf.org

Centers for Disease Control and Prevention
www.cdc.gov

Centers for Medicare & Medicaid Services
www.cms.hhs.gov

Clinical Laboratory Improvement Amendments
www.cms.hhs.gov/clia

Code of Federal Regulations
https://www.gpo.gov/

College of American Pathologists (CAP)
www.cap.org

Commission of Office Laboratory Accreditation (COLA)
www.cola.org

Community Health Accreditation Partner (CHAP)
www.chapinc.org

DNV GL Healthcare
www.dnvglhealthcare.com

Emergency Medical Treatment and Active Labor Act
www.cms.gov/EMTALA

Federal Register
www.federalregister.gov

Health Insurance Portability and Accountability Act
www.hhs.gov/ocr/privacy

Healthcare Facilities Accreditation Program (HFAP)
www.hfap.org

Institute for Healthcare Improvement
- **Education Resources**
http://www.ihi.org/education/Pages/default.aspx
- **General Resources**
http://www.ihi.org/resources/Pages/default.aspx

The Joint Commission (TJC)
www.jointcommission.org

National Association for Healthcare Quality (NAHQ) HQ Essentials Competencies
http://www.nahq.org/education/Q-Essentials/q-essentials.html

National Committee for Quality Assurance (NCQA)
www.ncqa.org

National Quality Forum: Field Guide to NQF Resources
http://www.qualityforum.org/Field_Guide/

National Practitioner Data Bank
www.npdb.hrsa.gov

Occupational Safety and Health Administration
www.osha.gov

The Henry J. Kaiser Family Foundation
www.kff.org

U.S. Department of Health & Human Services
www.hhs.gov

U.S. Food & Drug Administration
www.fda.gov

URAC
www.urac.org

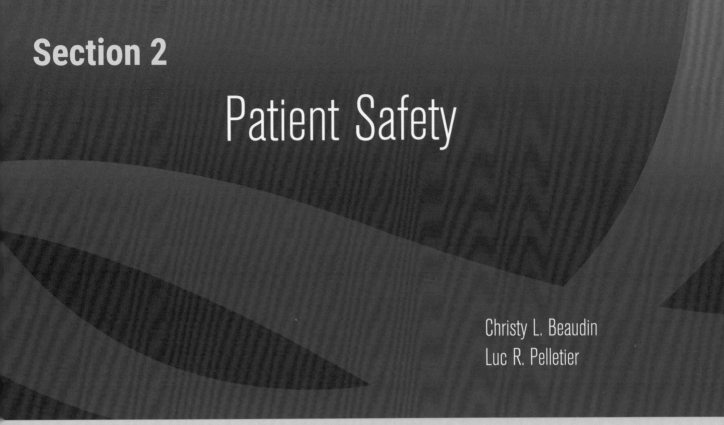

Section 2

Patient Safety

Christy L. Beaudin
Luc R. Pelletier

SECTION CONTENTS

Abstract

Ensuring patient safety is imperative for the healthcare quality professional. The duty of any healthcare professional is to work with others to provide safe care, treatment, and services using current evidence-based principles, practices, and tools. This section offers a comprehensive overview of safety principles and practices relevant to healthcare delivery across the continuum of care. The safety imperative is discussed and various patient safety programs are described. Patient safety culture approaches and systems thinking principles are examined. Practical tools for assessment, planning, implementation, and evaluation that healthcare quality professionals can use in daily practice are reviewed. The successful integration of safety concepts and practices results from leadership commitment and the healthcare workforce understanding about what works (and what does not) in healthcare structure and processes. A culture of safety thrives in a learning organization with effective leadership, an engaged and intentional healthcare workforce, and activated patients.

Learning Objectives

1. Provide leadership in the creation and maintenance of a safety culture throughout the organization by assessing needs, developing and deploying the organizational safety plan, and spreading safety concepts using principles such as human factors engineering, high reliability, just culture and systems thinking.

2. Understand how systems of safety, safety culture, reliability, and continuous learning put the patient at the center of safe healthcare delivery.

3. Promote effective risk management strategies through use of safety practices, tools and technology such as incident reporting, sentinel/adverse event review, root cause analysis, failure mode and effects analysis, and checklists.

4. Facilitate the ongoing evaluation and improvement of patient safety using tools and health information technology for identifying risks and harm reduction.

The Patient Safety Imperative

Eliminating errors and reducing harm are imperative to deliver on the promise of the delivery of care, treatment, and services in a safe environment free of errors and harm. The provision of care, treatment, or services across the continuum is composed of various elements including assessing, planning, providing, and coordinating care to address patient needs. This section synthesizes current knowledge related to patient safety, preventing errors, and reducing harm across the continuum of care. Strategic and operational components of developing a patient safety program are presented.

To build an organization's safety culture means tackling the most important patient safety issues facing healthcare organizations today, which include the following:

- Adopting and sustaining a culture of safety
- Identifying organizational champions
- Deploying and sustaining patient safety strategies
- Determining key drivers for patient safety programs
- Sustaining the gains of implementing safety innovations
- Ensuring the adoption of current and evolving safety-related technologies.

There are many aspects of patient safety that are important such as leadership and the mindful integration of safety concepts into an organization's vision, mission, strategic plan, goals, and objectives. These aspects are discussed in this section. Patient safety practices and approaches to reduce harm and preventable errors are presented. Guidance is offered for using tools and integrating safety into the healthcare organization's operations and processes. Comprehensive references, resources, and suggested readings are also provided. Note that the term "patient safety" is used throughout but "patient" represents any label for the user of healthcare services across the continuum such as patient, client, resident, consumer, customer, stakeholder, recipient, or partner.

Transforming Patient Safety in the 21st Century

Medical errors have economic and emotional consequences that are recognized by regulatory requirements for patient safety and error reduction identified in federal, state, and local mandates, standards for practice in accreditation standards (e.g., The Joint Commission [TJC], National Committee for Quality Assurance, and CARF International), and guidance for safe practices using evidence-based guidelines (e.g., the

National Quality Forum [NQF] and AHRQ Patient Safety Network).

The national imperative and patient safety call for action emerged in the first decade of the 21st century. In 1999, the Healthcare Research and Quality Act of 1999 was enacted and the call to action released in the Institute of Medicine's (IOM) *To Err Is Human: Building a Safer Health System*. In 2000, there was the first National Summit on Medical Errors. Federal actions to reduce medical errors began to appear (e.g., patient safety grants and a national agenda). In 2001, evidence was published about what providers could do to make healthcare safer.

By 2007, Patient Safety Indicators were developed, the National Resource Center formed, and the Agency for Healthcare Research and Quality (AHRQ) Patient Safety Network launched.[1]

In 2008, the Centers for Medicare & Medicaid Services (CMS) announced a proposed rule to update payment policies and rates for hospitals under the inpatient prospective payment system (PPS). The rule included new additions of hospital-acquired infections for fiscal year 2009, including several conditions identified by the NQF as "serious reportable adverse events" (also called "never events"). The complete list of 29 serious reportable events was updated in 2011 is shown in **TABLE 2-1**.[2(pp iii–iv)] CMS

Table 2-1 Serious Reportable Events in Healthcare—2011 Update

1. Surgical or Invasive Procedure Events

   a. Surgery or other invasive procedure performed on the wrong site

   b. Surgery or other invasive procedure performed on the wrong patient

   c. Wrong surgical or other invasive procedure performed on a patient

   d. Unintended retention of a foreign object in a patient after surgery or other invasive procedure

   e. Intraoperative or immediately postoperative/postprocedure death in an American Society of Anesthesiologists Physical Status Classification System Class 1 patient

2. Product or Device Events

   a. Patient death or serious injury associated with the use of contaminated drugs, devices, or biologics provided by the healthcare setting

   b. Patient death or serious injury associated with the use or function of a device in patient care, in which the device is used or functions other than as intended

   c. Patient death or serious injury associated with intravascular air embolism that occurs while being cared for in a healthcare setting

3. Patient Protection Events

   a. Discharge or release of a patient/resident of any age who is unable to make decisions to anyone other than an authorized person

   b. Patient death or serious injury associated with patient elopement (disappearance)

   c. Patient suicide, attempted suicide, or self-harm that results in serious injury while being cared for in a healthcare setting

4. Care Management Events

   a. Patient death or serious injury associated with a medication error (e.g., errors involving the wrong drug, wrong dose, wrong patient, wrong time, wrong rate, wrong preparation, or wrong route of administration)

   b. Patient death or serious injury associated with unsafe administration of blood products

   c. Maternal death or serious injury associated with labor or delivery in a low-risk pregnancy while being cared for in a healthcare setting

   d. Death or serious injury of a neonate associated with labor or delivery in a low-risk pregnancy

   e. Patient death or serious injury associated with a fall while being cared for in a healthcare setting

   f. Any Stage III, Stage IV, and unstageable pressure ulcers acquired after admission/presentation to a healthcare setting

   g. Artificial insemination with the wrong donor sperm or wrong egg

   h. Patient death or serious injury resulting from the irretrievable loss of an irreplaceable biological specimen

   i. Patient death or serious injury resulting from failure to follow up or communicate laboratory, pathology, or radiology test results

5. Environmental Events

   a. Patient or staff death or serious injury associated with an electric shock in the course of a patient care process in a healthcare setting

   b. Any incident in which systems designated for oxygen or another gas to be delivered to the patient contain no gas, the wrong gas, or are contaminated by toxic substances

   c. Patient or staff death or serious injury associated with a burn incurred from any source in the course of a patient-care process in a healthcare setting

   d. Patient death or serious injury associated with the use of physical restraints or bedrails while being cared for in a healthcare setting

(continued)

Table 2-1 Serious Reportable Events in Healthcare—2011 Update (*continued*)
6. Radiologic Events
a. Death or serious injury of a patient or staff associated with the introduction of a metallic object in the MRI area
7. Potential Criminal Events
a. Any instance of care ordered or provided by someone impersonating a physician, nurse, pharmacist, or other licensed healthcare provider
b. Abduction of a patient/resident of any age
c. Sexual abuse/assault on a patient or staff member within or on the grounds of a healthcare setting
d. Death or serious injury of a patient or staff member resulting from a physical assault (i.e., battery) that occurs within or on the grounds of a healthcare setting

Reprinted from National Quality Forum. Serious Reportable Events in Healthcare—2011 Update: A Consensus Report; 2011. Copyright 2011 by National Quality Forum, with permission.

withholds payment to hospitals if any of these events occurs in an acute-care facility.

In 2010, the Affordable Care Act (ACA) legislation directed the U.S. Department of Health & Human Services (HHS) National Quality Strategy (NQS) "to better meet the promise of providing all Americans with access to healthcare that is safe, effective, and affordable."[3(p2)] The development of the NQS would occur with input from various stakeholders to influence a realistic, achievable strategy. Thus, the NQF convened the multi-stakeholder National Priorities Partnership comprising 48 public and private sector partners to provide input as HHS developed the NQF goals, measures, and strategic opportunities.[3(p2)]

In 2016, the *CMS Quality Strategy* pursued the NQS aims (Six Aims and The Triple Aim). The HHS NQS's aims and priorities outlined in the strategy are displayed as FIGURE 2-1.[3(p11)] The CMS Quality Strategy Goal 1 is to "make care safer by reducing harm caused in the delivery of care."[4(p5)] For this goal, different foundational principles are used to support change and improvement including eliminating disparities, strengthening data structures and systems, enabling local innovations, and fostering learning organizations.[4(pp10–11)] Alternative payment structures in 2016 to 2018 promote quality goal attainment as Medicare will increasingly be making payments to providers that are tied to quality or value.

In September 2016, CMS furthered its commitment to patient safety when it awarded $347 million to continue progress toward a safer healthcare system. Awards were made to 16 national, regional, or state hospital associations, quality improvement organizations (QIOs), and health system organizations for efforts in reducing hospital-acquired conditions (HACs) and readmissions in the Medicare program. This is only part of broader efforts to transform the healthcare system into one that works better for the American people

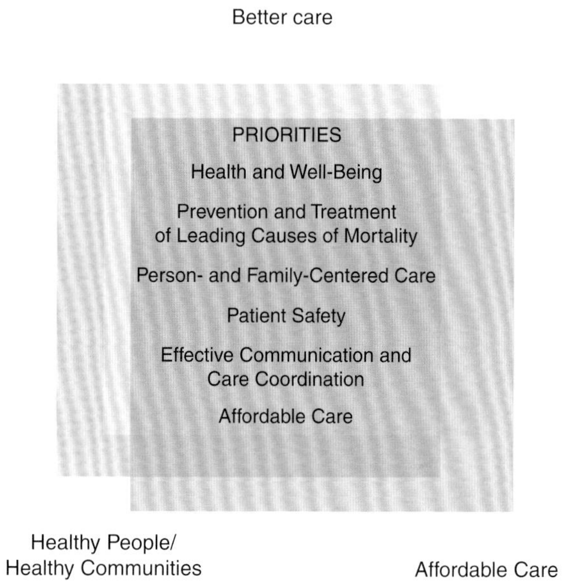

Figure 2-1 **National quality strategy aims and priority areas.** (Reprinted from National Priorities Partnership. *Input to the Secretary of Health and Human Services on priorities for the National Quality Strategy.* Washington, DC: National Quality Forum; Copyright 2011, with permission.)

by delivering better care, spending smartly, and focusing on improved health status.

National Strategy for Quality Improvement

The *National Strategy for Quality Improvement in Health Care*[5] describes three broad aims of an NQF: better care, healthier people/healthy communities, and affordable care (i.e., The Triple Aim). The NQF also considers six priority areas for an NQF, one of which is to make care safer. The goals include the following:

- Improve patient, family, and caregiver experience of care related to quality, safety, and access across settings.

- In partnership with patients, families, and caregivers—using a shared decision-making process—develop culturally sensitive and understandable care plans.
- Enable patients and their families and caregivers to navigate, coordinate, and manage their care appropriately and effectively.[3]

The NPP envisions "healthcare that honors each individual patient and family, offering voice, control, choice, skills in self-care, and total transparency, and that can and does adapt to individual and family circumstances, and to differing cultures, languages, and social backgrounds."[6(p17)] The NPP partners vowed to ensure all patients

- provide feedback on the experience of care that healthcare organizations will use to improve care;
- access tools and support systems to the effective navigation and management of care; and
- access information and assistance that enables informed decisions about treatment options.[6(p8)]

Addressing the need to improve the safe delivery of healthcare, Congress passed public and private sector efforts and generated landmark regulations and reports such as the Patient Safety and Quality Improvement Act of 2005, in response to the IOM's groundbreaking report, *To Err Is Human*. The IOM was renamed in 2016. It is now the Health and Medicine Division, which is a division of the National Academies of Sciences, Engineering, and Medicine (The National Academies).

Patient Safety Organizations

At the turn of the century, the IOM sparked national attention to avoidable medical errors. Patient Safety Organizations (PSOs) evolved from public and private sector concerns. The Patient Safety and Quality Improvement Act of 2005[7] conferred privilege and confidentiality protections for providers who choose to work with PSOs. This promotes shared learning from medical errors and improves patient safety across the nation.

To implement the Patient Safety Act, HHS issued the Patient Safety and Quality Improvement final rule.[8] The Patient Safety Act and the Patient Safety Rule authorized the creation of PSOs to improve quality and safety through the collection and analysis of data on patient events.[9] Now many organizations such as the NQF, AHRQ, and CMS are working together to ensure the success of the work accomplished by PSOs. As of December 2016, there are 86 active PSOs in 29 states and the District of Columbia currently listed by AHRQ.[10]

PSOs are organizations with the shared goal of improving the quality and safety of healthcare delivery. Eight patient safety activities are carried out by, or on behalf of PSOs or healthcare providers, namely,

1. efforts to improve patient safety and the quality of healthcare delivery;
2. collection and analysis of patient safety work product (PSWP);
3. development and dissemination of information regarding patient safety, such as recommendations, protocols, or information regarding best practices;
4. use of PSWP to encourage a culture of safety and provide feedback and assistance to effectively minimize patient risk;
5. maintenance of procedures to preserve confidentiality with respect to PSWP;
6. provision of appropriate security measures with respect to PSWP;
7. use of qualified staff; and
8. activities related to the operation of a patient safety evaluation system and the provision of feedback to participants in a patient safety evaluation system.[10]

Organizations eligible to become PSOs include public or private entities, profit or not-for-profit entities, provider entities such as hospital chains, and other entities that establish special components to serve as PSOs. By providing privilege and confidentiality, PSOs create a secure environment in which clinicians and healthcare organizations can collect, aggregate, and analyze data. Privileged information is not subject to disclosure or discovery and cannot be asked about in testimony thereby permitting more candid discussions about quality of care that may reduce the risks and hazards associated with patient care.

Public Reporting

Public reporting in healthcare moved from its starting point with voluntary and/or regulatory agency-driven reporting to mandatory and improvement-focused. Beginning with the reporting of mortality rates by CMS in the 1980s, over the decades more public and private sector reporting development has occurred producing comparable data and science-based methodology. These developments were also framed by stakeholder expectations for accountability, transparency, and improvement. Stakeholders include a host of healthcare providers and payers—government at all levels, health plans, hospitals, ambulatory care, long-term care, physicians and group practices to name a few. Accreditation agencies and private interest groups are stakeholders. And most important, the public and consumer interests and involvement has grown.

As the stakeholder base for public reporting expands and diversifies, Halpern et al. suggest that "public reporting should be used to hold systems accountable to their own goals."[11(p32)] In linking quality and patient safety efforts, information should be published on what was learned, recommendations and changes made, and the responsiveness of the institution to patient safety issues. There is no doubt that public reporting offers value related to the allocation of the healthcare dollars but work is still needed to better understand what value is brought to the consumer in choosing a healthcare provider or health plan.[12]

Twenty-seven states plus the District of Columbia had passed legislation or regulation supporting adverse event reporting to a state agency. The laws and regulations were intended to raise accountability in healthcare organizations. Public reporting has the potential to improve patient safety through event analysis and by disseminating lessons learned.[13] Eight states use the NQF reportable adverse incident list in their reporting systems; seven states use a modified or partial NQF list, and twelve states use their own non-NQF list.[13(p8)] The effectiveness of reporting systems is not yet fully understood. However, many reporting system administrators experienced an "impact on communication among facilities, provider education, internal agency tracking or trending, and/or implementation of facility processes to address quality of care. Nine states report increased levels of provider and facility transparency and awareness of patient safety because of their reporting systems."[13(p3)]

Examples of current public and private sector reporting efforts are described below.

Reporting and Tracking. An array of reporting and tracking programs related to patient safety have been deployed by the federal government. The Center for Food Safety and Applied Nutrition (CFSAN) Adverse Event Reporting System is a database that contains information on adverse event and product complaint reports. These are submitted to the Food & Drug Administration (FDA) for foods, dietary supplements, and cosmetics. It is designed to support the safety surveillance program. The Vaccine Adverse Event Reporting System (VAERS) is a national safety surveillance program co-sponsored by the Centers for Disease Control and Prevention (CDC) and the FDA. VAERS collects information about adverse events that occur after the administration of vaccines licensed for use in the United States.

The National Healthcare Safety Network (NHSN) is far reaching in its tracking and reporting for patient safety. Attention to infection prevention and control began to grow as part of the national effort to achieve "zero" in HAIs. Public reporting of infection rates became the "new clinical mandate."[14(p3)] The NHSN also plays a leadership role in promoting patient safety by providing a secure, Internet-based

safety surveillance system. Through its efforts, it applies quality and safety improvement methods by

- collecting and reporting on national and state-specific standardized infection ratios;
- providing facilities, states, regions, and the nation with data needed to identify problem areas, measure progress of prevention efforts, and ultimately eliminate healthcare-associated infections (HAIs); and
- allowing healthcare facilities to track blood safety errors and important healthcare process measures (e.g., healthcare personnel influenza vaccine status and infection-control adherence rates).[15]

In October 2014, CMS began reducing Medicare payments for certain hospitals that ranked in the worst performing quartile with respect to HACs. The measures reflect a composite of NHSN data and AHRQ Patient Safety Indicators.

Expectations about voluntary and mandatory incident reporting systems (IRS) at organizational and system levels are still evolving. In 1999, the IOM advocated the use of IRS. The IOM recommended that "a nationwide mandatory reporting system should be established that provides for the collection of standardized information by governments about adverse events that result in death or serious harm. Reporting should initially be required of hospitals and eventually be required of other institutional and ambulatory care delivery settings."[16] According to a 2014 study by the National Academy for State Health Policy, state-level event reporting systems were launched but have not changed since 2007. As of January 2015, there were 28 states with mandates (see **TABLE 2-2**). Accreditation organizations, like TJC, have voluntary and mandatory event reporting.

Hospital and Outpatient Ratings. CMS began its hospital and outpatient rating and reporting systems with Hospital Compare in 2002. This was a joint effort between Medicare and the Hospital Quality Alliance (HQA). Over 10 years, CMS and the Alliance worked together to grow public reporting efforts in a meaningful way and beyond structural measures of quality including the Hospital Consumer Assessment of Healthcare Providers and Systems (HCAHPS). The HQA ceased in 2012 after accomplishing its goals.

With Hospital Compare and HCAHPS serving as both foundation and experience, CMS continued its development efforts launching other "Compare" programs for healthcare providers across the continuum of care—Physician Compare, Nursing Home Compare, Home Health Compare, Dialysis Facility Compare, and Long-Term Care Hospital Compare. In addition, there are Quality Reporting Systems and Programs for End-Stage Renal Disease,

Table 2-2 Authorized Event Reporting Systems (2000, 2007, and 2015)

	2000	2007	2015
Number of states with authorized event/event reporting systems	15	27	28
Areas of focus	• Adverse events/patient safety • Several focused solely on abuse, neglect or clinical outcomes	• Focus on adverse events with intent to improve patient safety	• Focus on adverse events with intent to improve patient safety
States with systems	• Colorado • Florida • Kansas • Massachusetts • Nebraska • New Jersey • New York • Ohio • Pennsylvania • Rhode Island • South Carolina • South Dakota • Tennessee • Texas • Washington	• California • Colorado • Connecticut • District of Columbia • Florida • Georgia • Illinois • Indiana • Kansas • Maine • Maryland • Massachusetts • Minnesota • Nevada • New Jersey • New York • Ohio • Oregon • Pennsylvania • Rhode Island • South Carolina • South Dakota • Tennessee • Utah • Vermont • Washington • Wyoming	• California • Colorado • Connecticut • District of Columbia • Florida • Georgia • Illinois • Indiana • Kansas • Maine • Maryland • Massachusetts • Minnesota • Nevada • New Hampshire • New Jersey • New York • Ohio • Oregon • Pennsylvania • Rhode Island • South Carolina • South Dakota • Tennessee • Texas • Utah • Vermont • Washington

Table adapted and modified from Hanlon C, Sheedy K, Kniffin T, Rosenthal J. *2014 Guide to State Adverse Event Reporting Systems*. Washington, DC: National Academy for State Health Policy; 2015. http://www.nashp.org/2014-guide-state-adverse-event-reporting-systems/. Accessed April 17, 2017.

ambulatory surgical centers, PPS-exempt cancer hospitals, inpatient hospitals, inpatient psychiatric facilities, inpatient rehabilitation facilities, outpatient hospitals, physicians, and QIOs. These programs offer payers and consumers valuable tools for value-based purchasing and selecting providers for personal healthcare services and treatment. Performance on safety measures such as readmissions and HAIs are available.

Heath Plan Performance. The National Committee for Quality Assurance (NCQA) develops standards and measures that hold health plans accountable for the care provided to their constituents. Their performance measurement system, Healthcare Effectiveness Data and Information Set (HEDIS), is one of the most widely used performance measure data sets that is targeted toward health plans, wellness and health promotion, and disease management programs. This tool is used by more than 90% of America's health plans to measure performance on important dimensions of care and service. Because so many plans collect HEDIS data, there is comparability and acceptability by third-party payers. Some patient safety areas addressed by HEDIS include the following:

- Safe and judicious antipsychotic use in children and adolescents
- HAIs
- Follow up after an emergency visit for mental illness, alcohol, and other drug dependence
- Falls risk management (RM).

HEDIS data are publicly reporting with available benchmarks. The results are used by consumers to select the best health plan for their needs by looking at the plan performance and comparing plan performance with other plans.[17] HEDIS reporting is third-party payer requirement for health plans.

Safety Grades. The Leapfrog Group is a voluntary initiative that serves to mobilize employer purchasing power to guide America's health industry in adopting "giant leaps" in patient safety. The group's mission is "to trigger giant leaps forward in the safety, quality and affordability of U.S. healthcare by using transparency to support informed healthcare decisions and promote high-value care."[18(¶6)] In 2001, Leapfrog launched a hospital survey to collect data on three "leaps" (computerized physician order entry, Intensive Care Units [ICUs] appropriately staffed with intensivists, and ensuring enough surgical volume to safely perform certain high-risk procedures). Initially participating hospitals were ranked, but in 2012 Leapfrog began assigning A, B, C, D, and F letter grades. By 2016, the Leapfrog Hospital Survey represented 1,859 hospitals in the United States (60% of hospital beds). Employers and other purchasers as well as health plans and community leaders are using Leapfrog Hospital Survey results and Leapfrog Hospital Safety Grades for payment reform and public reporting.

Partnership for Patients

Partnership for Patients: Better Care, Lower Costs is a public–private partnership to help improve the quality, safety, and affordability of healthcare for all Americans. Using as much as $1 billion in new funding provided by the ACA and leveraging several ongoing programs, the DHHS works with a wide variety of public and private partners to achieve the two core goals of this partnership: keep patients from getting injured or sicker in the healthcare system, and help patients heal without complication by improving transitions from acute-care hospitals to other care settings, such as home or a skilled nursing facility. Its mission is to help patients take care into their own hands. The partnership uses Hospital

Improvement Innovation Networks that work at the regional, State, national, or hospital system level to sustain and accelerate national progress and momentum toward continued harm reduction in the Medicare program.

Beyond reducing harm caused in hospitals, the Partnership for Patients is an important test of what can occur when the nation acts as one to address a major national health problem. The CMS Innovation Center dedicated more than $500 million to test models of safer care delivery and promote implementation of best practices in patient safety. The Innovation Center "allows the Medicare and Medicaid programs to test models that improve care, lower costs, and better align payment systems to support patient-centered practice."[19(¶1)] In addition, CMS provided $500 million for a community-based care transition program created by the ACA to support hospitals and community-based organizations in helping Medicare beneficiaries at high risk for readmission to the hospital safely transition from the hospital to other care settings. More than 7,300 partners, including more than 3,200 hospitals, physicians, nursing groups, consumer groups, and employers have pledged their commitment to the Partnership for Patients.[5,20]

The Six Aims

The IOM highlighted problems in healthcare delivery. In the seminal IOM report, the Committee on Quality of Health Care in America stated healthcare frequently harms and routinely fails to deliver its potential benefits. It was noted that the American healthcare delivery system needed fundamental change.[21(p1)] In addition, it concluded healthcare was not being provided with the best scientific knowledge. The IOM report suggested an agenda for "crossing the chasm" by changing the healthcare delivery system. Its agenda includes the following components:

- All healthcare constituencies (e.g., purchasers, healthcare professionals, regulators, consumers) can commit to a national statement of purpose for the healthcare system, setting six aims for improvement to raise the quality of care to unprecedented levels.
- Clinicians, patients, and healthcare organizations need to adopt a new set of principles to guide the redesign of care processes.
- Through the DHHS, a set of priorities must be identified to focus initial efforts, provide resources to stimulate innovation, and initiate the change process.
- Healthcare organizations need to design and implement more effective support processes to make change in the delivery of care possible.

An environment needs to be created to foster and reward improvement in the context of ever-expanding knowledge and rapid change. This is accomplished by creating an infrastructure that supports evidence-based practice, uses information technology (IT), aligns incentives with outcomes, and prepares the workforce to better provide care, treatment, and services.

As part of the agenda for change, the IOM outlined six improvement aims to address key dimensions of healthcare quality. At a minimum, healthcare should remain as follows:

1. *Safe*: Avoid injuries to patients from care that is intended to help them.
2. *Effective*: Provide care based on scientific knowledge regarding who will likely benefit, and restrain from providing care when it is not likely to benefit a patient.
3. *Patient-Centered*: Care is respectful and responsive to patient preferences, needs, and values. Furthermore, patient values and preferences guide clinical decisions.
4. *Timely*: Wait times and harmful delays for those who receive and provide care are eliminated.
5. *Efficient*: Care is provided in ways that avoid waste, including waste of equipment, supplies, ideas, and energy.
6. *Equitable*: Care does not vary in quality because of the patient's personal characteristics such as gender, ethnicity, geographic location, and socioeconomic status.[21]

Since the IOM started delivering reports on patient safety in 2000, various national organizations, state and federal agencies, accreditation organizations, and professional associations have focused on the identification of safe practices and strategies for organizational or system-wide implementation. In addition, many states have established coalitions to promote patient safety. For example, the Connecticut Center for Patient Safety promotes "high quality, safe healthcare and the rights of patients by promoting person-centered care, best practices and transparency in healthcare."[22(¶2)] Originally organized by residents who had been harmed by the healthcare system, it provides useful tools and resources for consumers. The Oregon Patient Safety Commission (OPSC) was one of the first legislatively mandated organizations to reduce the risk of serious adverse events occurring in Oregon's healthcare system and encourages a culture of patient safety through patient safety reporting, early discussion and resolution, and quality improvement initiatives.[23]

The Triple Aim

The Triple Aim was introduced by Berwick et al.[24]—improving the experience of care, improving the health of populations, and reducing per capita costs of healthcare. Since it was introduced, thinking about the Triple Aim continues to evolve. A fourth aim or quadruple aim was proposed by Sikka et al.[25] who suggest adding improving the experience of providing care, including workforce engagement and workforce safety. Bodenheimer and Sinsky[26] suggest that the goal be added of improving the worklife of healthcare providers, including clinicians and staff.

Organizations such as the American Hospital Association (AHA) continue advancing work in patient safety using the Triple Aim to frame principles for practice. In 2016, the AHA reaffirmed its commitment to creating safe and highly reliable healthcare organizations through a culture of high reliability whereby hospitals improve quality and patient safety.[27] CMS reframed the aims simply as *Better Care, Smarter Spending, Healthier People* as the federal government extends financial support for innovation and efforts continue to improve the healthcare delivery system in the United States. In fact, health outcomes are improving and adverse events are decreasing as patient safety improved dramatically, thanks in part to the Partnership for Patients. Patient harm fell by 17%, saving 50,000 lives and billions of dollars.[28]

Patient-Centered Outcomes

Established in 2012, the Patient-Centered Outcomes Research Institute (PCORI) has "a sizeable and growing portfolio of projects designed to improve patient care and outcomes through patient-centered comparative clinical effectiveness research (CER). The research fund is guided by the PCORI five National Priorities for Research and Research Agenda. The work under these priorities is managed by our scientific programs, which track it and evaluate its effectiveness."[29,30(¶1)] PCORI established national priorities for patient-centered comparative clinical effectiveness that include the following:

- Assessment of Prevention, Diagnosis, and Treatment Options: Comparing the effectiveness and safety of alternative prevention, diagnosis, and treatment options to see which one works best for different people with a health problem.
- Improving Healthcare Systems: Comparing health system–level approaches to improving access, supporting patient self-care, innovative use of health IT, coordinating care for complex conditions, and deploying workforce effectively.
- Communication and Dissemination Research: Comparing approaches to providing comparative effectiveness research information, empowering people to ask for and use the information, and supporting shared decision-making between patients and their providers.
- Addressing Disparities: Identifying potential differences in prevention, diagnosis, or treatment effectiveness, or preferred clinical outcomes across patient populations and the healthcare required to achieve best outcomes in each population.
- Accelerating Patient-Centered Outcomes Research and Methodological Research: Improving the nation's capacity to conduct patient-centered outcomes research, by building data infrastructure, improving analytic methods, and training researchers, patients, and other stakeholders to participate in this research.[30(¶2)]

Contextualizing Patient Safety

Patient safety reflects science, encompasses practices and interventions, and aims to reduce the occurrence of preventable events. It requires intention, vigilance, and trust to build a culture of safety. These are important as one considers the person and the healthcare delivery system. Patient safety and quality improvement are intertwined. Different techniques can be used to assess performance with the findings used to inform change. "It is important to adopt various process-improvement techniques to identify inefficiencies, ineffective care, and preventable errors, and influence changes associated with systems."[31(p3-1)] Through the work of various government, quasi-government, and voluntary groups, different definitions emerged that address the prevention of errors and the reduction of harm, such as the following:

- *Patient safety* is the "freedom from accidental injury due to medical care or medical errors."[16(p4)]
- *Patient safety* is "indistinguishable from the delivery of quality health care,"[32(p5)] in a culture of safety where ". . . caregivers are encouraged to report medical errors, 'near misses,' or adverse events, where they can be discussed in an atmosphere of trust and mutual respect without fear of blame or retribution."[33(p195)]
- *Patient safety* refers to the "freedom from accidental or preventable injuries produced by medical care. Thus, practices or interventions that improve patient safety are those that reduce the occurrence of preventable adverse events."[34(¶1)]
- *Patient safety* is "a discipline in the health care sector that applies safety science methods toward the goal of achieving a trustworthy system of health care delivery.

Patient safety is also an attribute of health care systems; it minimizes the incidence and impact of, and maximizes recovery from, adverse events."[35(p6)]
- *Patient safety* is "the prevention and mitigation of harm caused by errors of omission or commission that are associated with healthcare, and involving the establishment of operational systems and processes that minimize the likelihood of errors and maximize the likelihood of intercepting them when they occur."[36]
- *Patient safety* is a public health issue. It is "the absence of preventable harm to a patient during the process of health care. The discipline of patient safety is the coordinated efforts to prevent harm, caused by the process of health care itself, from occurring to patients."[37(¶3)]

Considering any one of these definitions, one can quickly recognize that there are myriad of patient safety issues across the continuum of care that demand consideration (e.g., hazards and patient complexities in behavioral health environments or the outpatient settings). Some issues may be less obvious but just as serious. Some issues are experienced by most types of healthcare organizations. However, there are issues unique to the setting where care, treatment, and services are provided. The healthcare quality professional will want to be familiar with these to direct patient safety activities in their setting and help define what patient safety means in the organization. **TABLE 2-3** offers examples of the kinds of safety concerns that the healthcare quality professional might encounter in different healthcare settings.

See *Performance and Process Improvement* and *Organizational Leadership* sections for more information about frameworks and tools used in quality and performance improvement.

Table 2-3 Examples of Patient Safety Concerns Across the Continuum of Care

Organization Type	Safety Concerns	
Any Healthcare Organization	*Safety Culture* • Just culture (fair and blame-free) • Failure to embrace a culture of safety *Care and Treatment* • Patient identification errors • Care coordination and transitions (within facility, between facilities, to community) • Delay in treatment • Falls • Inadequate management of behavioral health issues • Leaving /terminating treatment against medical advice • Inadequate test result reporting and follow-up • Unsafe injection practices	*Medication-Related* • Medication errors related to pounds and kilograms • Medication errors • Adverse drug events *Infection Prevention & Control* • Inadequate antimicrobial stewardship • Superbugs *Environmental Safety* • Facility safety *Health Information* • Patient safety event/data transparency • Disclosure of private or confidential health information • Data integrity

(continued)

Table 2-3 Examples of Patient Safety Concerns Across the Continuum of Care (*continued*)

Organization Type	Safety Concerns	
	Care and Treatment (cont'd)	*Health Information (cont'd)*
	• Inadequate monitoring for respiratory depression in patients on opioids • Readmissions	• Unrecognized patient deterioration • Health IT configurations and organizational workflow that do not support each other • Misuse of USB ports causing devices to malfunction • Cybersecurity
Acute Care—General Medical	• Diagnostic errors • Healthcare-acquired infections • Medication errors • Handoffs • Inadequate cleaning of flexible endoscopes • Missed alarms	• Drug shortages • Inadequate surveillance of monitored patients • Inappropriate patient ventilation • Test results reporting errors
Acute Care—General Surgical	• Wrong patient, wrong site, wrong procedure • Reprocessing issues • Operative/postoperative complication • Unintended retention of a foreign body • Failure to effectively monitor postoperative patients for opioid-induced respiratory depression	• Insufficient training of clinicians in OR technology • Gamma camera mechanical failures • Healthcare-acquired infections • Sepsis • Test results reporting errors • Unintentional retained objects during surgery even with correct count
Acute Care—Pediatric	• Perinatal death/injury • Falls • Inadequate management of behavioral health issues • Medication errors • Readmissions • Test results reporting errors	• Catheter-Associated Urinary Tract Infections (CAUTI) • Central line-associated blood stream infection (CLABSI) • Pressure Injuries • Surgical site infections • Ventilator-associated pneumonia • Venous thromboembolism
Acute Care—Psychiatric	• Suicide attempt/successful suicide	• Test results reporting errors • Elopement
Nursing Home/Long-Term Care	• Missed alarms; alarm hazards • Patient/resident violence	• Handoffs • Communication • Staffing
Primary Care	• Diagnostic errors and test results (missed or delayed) • Delay in proper treatment or preventive services	• Communication and information flow processes • Inadequate management of behavioral health issues
Home Health	• Needlestick and sharps injuries • Violence • Mismatch of physical space, equipment and supplies • Home oxygen fires	• Falls in home • Lack of preparation, training, and support of caregivers • Caregiver's health and wellbeing neglected by self and others

Table constructed from the following references: Agency for Healthcare Research and Quality. Improving patient safety in nursing homes: a resource list for users of the AHRQ Nursing Home Survey on Patient Safety Culture; 2016. http://www.ahrq.gov/sites/default/files/wysiwyg/professionals/quality-patient-safety/patientsafetyculture/nursing-home/resources/nhimpptsaf.pdf. Accessed April 17, 2017; Barnet S, Green M, Punke H. 10 top patient safety issues for 2016. Becker's Infection Control & Clinical Quality; 2016. http://www.beckershospitalreview.com/quality/10-top-patient-safety-issues-for-2016.html. Accessed April 17, 2017; Children's Hospital Association Solutions for Patient Safety. SPS prevention bundles; 2016. http://www.solutionsforpatientsafety.org/for-hospitals/hospital-resources/. Accessed April 17, 2017; Cocchi R. Top 5 patient safety concerns all hospitals should review. Healthcare Bus Technol. 2014. http://www.healthcarebusinesstech.com/patient-safety-hospitals/. Accessed April 17, 2017; ECRI Institute. Executive brief: top 10 patient safety concerns for healthcare organizations 2016; 2016. https://www.ecri.org/EmailResources/PSRQ/Top10/2016_Top10_ExecutiveBrief_final.pdf. Accessed April 17, 2017; ECRI Institute. Executive brief: top 10 health technology hazards for 2015; 2015. https://www.ecri.org/Resources/Whitepapers_and_reports/2016_Top_10_Hazards_Executive_Brief.pdf. Accessed April 17, 2017; Hoban S. 3 safety concerns to consider in long-term care. Long-term Living; 2015. http://www.ltlmagazine.com/news-item/3-safety-concerns-consider-long-term-care. Accessed April 17, 2017; The Joint Commission. Summary data of sentinel events reviewed by The Joint Commission; 2016. https://www.jointcommission.org/assets/1/18/Summary_2Q_2016.pdf; Lang A, Toon L, Cohen SR, et al. Client, caregiver, and provider perspectives of safety in palliative home care: a mixed method design. Saf Health. 2015;1:1–14. https://safetyinhealth.biomedcentral.com/articles/10.1186/2056-5917-1-3. Accessed April 17, 2017; National Academies of Science, Engineering, and Medicine. Improving diagnosis in health care; 2015. http://www.nationalacademies.org/hmd/reports/2015/improving-diagnosis-in-healthcare. Accessed April 17, 2017; National Patient Safety Foundation. Important patient safety issues: What you can do; 2016. http://www.npsf.org/?page=safetyissuespatfam. Accessed April 17, 2017; The National Institute for Occupational Safety and Health (NIOSH). NIOSH fast facts: home healthcare workers: how to prevent needlestick and sharps injuries; 2012. http://www.cdc.gov/niosh/docs/2012-123/pdfs/2012-123.pdf. Accessed April 17, 2017; The National Institute for Occupational Safety and Health (NIOSH). NIOSH fast facts: home healthcare workers: how to prevent violence on the job; 2012. http://www.cdc.gov/niosh/docs/2012-118/pdfs/2012-118.pdf. Accessed April 17, 2017; Webster JS, King HB, Toomey LM, et al. Understanding quality and safety problems in the ambulatory environment: seeking improvement with promising teamwork tools and strategies; 2008. http://www.ahrq.gov/downloads/pub/advances2/vol3/advances-webster_76.pdf; WHO Collaborating Centre for Patient Safety Solutions. Patient Identification, Patient Safety Solutions, Volume 1, Solution 2; 2007. http://www.who.int/patientsafety/solutions/patientsafety/PS-Solution2.pdf. Accessed May 17, 2017.

Systems Thinking and Patient Safety

Whereas "do no harm" was previously an individual responsibility, a paradigm shift makes "safety a system priority."[21(p67)] When patient harm occurs, the cause is frequently traced to flaws in the system of care. Adopting "systems" thinking requires a healthcare organization to think beyond the person and beyond blame. Whereas individual behavior can result in an error, looking at health delivery from a systems perspective enables the organization to identify and manage errors differently. Using a systems approach, the conditions under which an individual works and the complexity of the process are the foci. By recognizing human and process variability in a systemic way, leadership and healthcare personnel can work together to avert errors or mitigate their effects. This is foundational to high-reliability organizations (HROs), which will be discussed later in this section.

Patient Safety Culture

The current era of patient safety ushered in thinking such as achieving zero defects, pursuing perfection, and transforming healthcare.[38–40] This thinking influences how organizations create the strategy for culture of safety goals and objectives. Although everyone in the healthcare enterprise is responsible for quality and safety, an organization's leadership must emphasize safety as a core component of culture, ongoing strategy planning, and of their quality and performance improvement program. Designing an organizational structure for patient safety is like designing a house:

> Like the physical structure of a house, organizational structure identifies and distinguishes the individual parts of an organization and ties these pieces together to define an integrated whole. Organizational structure differs from the physical structure of a house, however, in that it encompasses more than inanimate characteristics of walls, doors, and windows. Organizational structure includes the interaction patterns that link people to people and people to work, and unlike a house, structural dimensions of organizations frequently change and evolve.[41(p399)]

In creating the organizational structure, leadership should not be preoccupied with failure but recognize that their "leadership is the critical element in a successful patient safety program and is non-delegable."[42(p1)] Leadership works to ensure that patient safety is supported by a strong but flexible foundation with straight walls, working doors, and opaque windows. In 2017, TJC explained that the role of leadership is essential in developing the safety culture and described 11 tenets that help an organization achieve and sustain a safety culture.[43] See FIGURE 2-2 for a description of these tenets.

The readiness of an organization needs to be assessed for the implementation of patient safety practices. This may typically start at the strategic planning stage with the mission and vision statements, core values, and strategic goals. Reason[44,45] suggested that different safety culture elements can be considered:

- Informed culture: Culture in which everyone is clear about acceptable and unacceptable actions. Being informed is supported by the availability of safety data that is actively disseminated.
- Reporting culture: Errant behaviors can be reported without fear of punishment or blame.
- Learning culture: An organization can learn from its mistakes and make changes.
- Flexible culture: The organization and the people in it can adapt effectively to changing demands.
- Just culture: Errors and unsafe acts are not punished if the error was unintentional. Those who act recklessly or take deliberate and unjustifiable risks are still be subject to disciplinary action.

Healthcare organizations committed to a just culture identify and correct the systems or processes of care contributing to the medical error, adverse events, near miss, or close call—they do not assign blame. It is important that the organization is clear about terms used for identifying, investigating, reporting, and disclosure of safety events. Errors, adverse events, preventable adverse events, and sentinel events are described as follows:

- Medical error: An error is defined as the failure of a planned action to be completed as intended or the use of a wrong plan to achieve an aim. Errors can include problems in practice, products, procedures, and systems.[46]
- Adverse event: An injury caused by something that happened in the delivery of medical care rather than by the underlying disease or condition of the patient. How adverse events might be categorized could be determined by setting (e.g., hospital, skilled nursing facility). Adverse events are sometimes further categorized as follows:
  ○ Preventable adverse events: Those that occurred due to error or failure to error or system design flaw.
  ○ Ameliorable adverse events: Events that, while not preventable, could have been less harmful if care had been different.
  ○ Adverse events due to negligence: Those that occurred due to care that falls below the standards expected of clinicians in the community.[47]
- Sentinel event: A sentinel event is a patient safety event that reaches a patient and results in death, permanent harm, severe temporary harm, and/or intervention required to sustain life. An event can also be considered

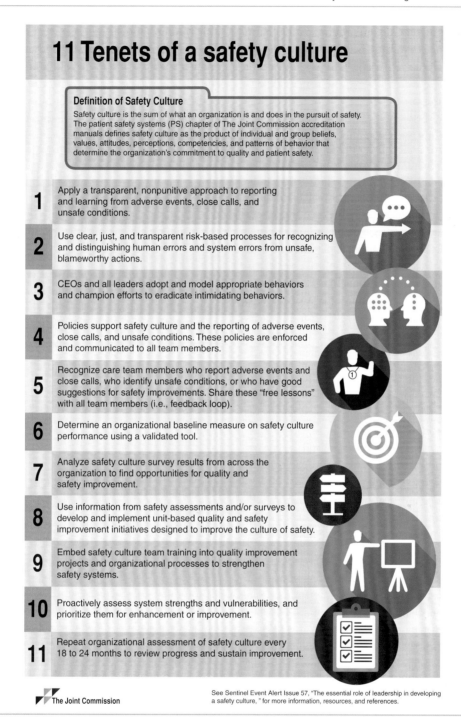

Figure 2-2 **11 tenets of a safety culture.** (Reprinted from The Joint Commission. Addition resources. Sentinel Event Alert 57: the essential role of leadership in developing a safety culture; 2017. https://www.jointcommission.org/sea_issue_57/. Accessed April 27, 2017. ©2017 The Joint Commission, All Rights Reserved, with permission.)

sentinel if the event signaled the need for immediate investigation and response.[48]

Close calls and near misses are those that never reached a patient, may have reached a patient or reached a patient with no serious harm. Near misses and close calls may be recognized and defined as follows:

- An event, situation, or error that took place but was captured before reaching the patient.[49]
- An act of commission or omission that had the potential to harm a patient but did not occur due to a planned/unplanned recovery or corrective action and timely intervention.[50,51]

- An event or situation that did not produce patient harm due to either chance or capture before reaching the patient or if it did reach the patient, a timely and robust intervention occurred with no subsequent patient harm.[52]
- An error of commission or omission that could have harmed the patient but serious harm did not occur due to chance, prevention, or mitigation.[53]

Understanding errors and feeling protected by a nonpunitive culture, more healthcare professionals will report errors, near-misses, and close calls. This in turn will improve patient safety through opportunities for improvement identified and lessons learned.[54,55] In a just culture, there is awareness throughout the organization that medical errors are inevitable—humans make errors, systems can be flawed. Just Culture can make the system safer by recognizing competent professionals make mistakes. It also acknowledges that even competent professionals develop unhealthy norms (shortcuts or routine rule violations); nevertheless, this culture has zero tolerance for reckless behavior. Three principles of a just culture are described here:

1. Just culture is not an effort to reduce personal accountability and discipline. It is a way to emphasize the importance of learning from mistakes, near misses, and close calls to reduce future preventable errors.
2. An individual is accountable to the system and the greatest error is to not report a mistake. Doing so prevents the system and others from learning.
3. Policies discouraging any healthcare provider from self-reporting errors are at odds with the goals of a fair and just culture. Even those errors that do not result in harm or injury are reported and serve as learning opportunities.

Success occurs when everyone in a healthcare organization serves as a safety advocate regardless of their position or role. Providers and consumers will feel safe and supported when they report medical errors or near misses and voice concerns about patient safety. How are the human/emotional aspects associated with patient safety balanced with how the system reflects and responds to those human emotions? In building a safety culture, Botwinick and colleagues[42] noted when leaders begin asking *what happened* instead of *who made the error*, the culture within their healthcare institutions begin to change.

Patient-Centered Care

Consumers are becoming more engaged in healthcare decision-making and more willing to tell their stories to the public when things do not go right. One of the most poignant was the Josie King incident. In 2001, King was 18 months old when she died in a hospital as the result of a cascade of errors including hydration and receiving enough fluids, use of narcotics, and listening to the family when additional assistance was requested for concern about Josie's condition.

Josie's mother, Sorrel King, later went public with the findings about the breakdowns leading to her daughter's death at a premier medical system in Baltimore, MD. The Josie King Foundation was established with the mission to "encourage a culture of safety by providing tools that allow health care organizations the ability to communicate, collaborate, improve and share."[56(¶3)] Together with the hospital and provider groups, King also founded the Patient Safety Group in 2004, which upholds the mission to "encourage a culture of safety by providing tools that allow healthcare organizations the ability to communicate, collaborate, improve, and share."[57(¶1)]

Healthcare professionals respect and include patients and families in decision-making. They keep the patient and the family at the center of all that they do. Research suggests that clinicians working with patients and their families can contribute to a better understanding of their role and responsibilities related to safety. A Cochrane systematic review including 115 controlled studies representing 34,444 research participants reported that providing patients with decision aids

- improves knowledge regarding their options,
- reduces the decisional conflict,
- increases active role in decision-making,
- improves accurate risk perceptions of possible benefits and harms among patients,
- increases the likelihood that choices are more consistent with their informed values, and
- enhances communication between the patient and the clinicians.[58(¶15)]

Activated patients—those who manage their own care by having the knowledge, skills, and confidence—are shown to achieve better clinical outcomes.[59] The healthcare quality professional's role includes support of a person-centered approach in developing safety programs and fostering patient and staff engagement. Safety can be advanced through the consideration of different aspects of clinical excellence such as psychological safety (creating an environment where people are comfortable and have opportunities to raise concerns and questions), leadership (facilitating and monitoring teamwork, improvement, respect, and psychological safety), and transparency (openly sharing data and other information concerning safe, respectful, and reliable care with staff, partners, and families). These and other aspects are shown in the Framework for Clinical Excellence (FIG. 2-3).

As consumers become more empowered through consumer-directed healthcare, they will demand more from healthcare organizations. Examples of initiatives to consider in program development for consumer-directed healthcare include the following:

- SPEAK UP Program. TJC empowers consumers by providing educational materials and tools as navigational aids for complex healthcare systems. In 2002, in response

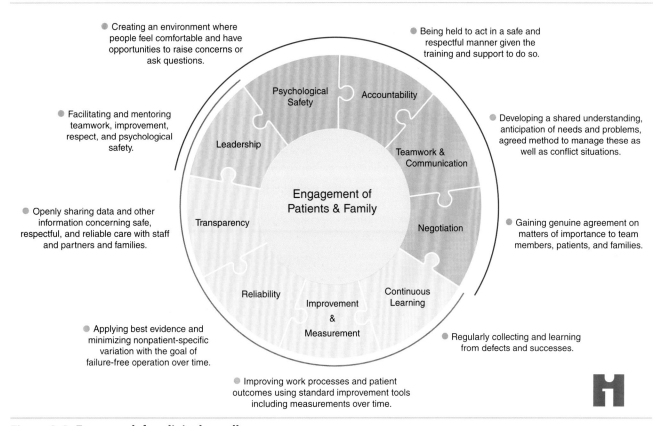

Being held to act in a safe and respectful manner given the training and support to do so.

Creating an environment where people feel comfortable and have opportunities to raise concerns or ask questions.

Facilitating and mentoring teamwork, improvement, respect, and psychological safety.

Developing a shared understanding, anticipation of needs and problems, agreed method to manage these as well as conflict situations.

Openly sharing data and other information concerning safe, respectful, and reliable care with staff and partners and families.

Gaining genuine agreement on matters of importance to team members, patients, and families.

Applying best evidence and minimizing nonpatient-specific variation with the goal of failure-free operation over time.

Regularly collecting and learning from defects and successes.

Improving work processes and patient outcomes using standard improvement tools including measurements over time.

Figure 2-3 **Framework for clinical excellence.** (Reprinted from Frankel A, Haraden C, Federico F, Lenoci-Edwards J. *A Framework for Safe, Reliable, and Effective Care.* White Paper. Cambridge, MA: Institute for Healthcare Improvement; 2017, with permission. www.IHI.org. © Institute for Healthcare Improvement and Safe and Reliable Healthcare.)

to a public outcry regarding unsafe practices, TJC, in collaboration with CMS, launched a national campaign to urge consumers to take an active role in identifying and preventing healthcare errors. The goal of the initiative was to empower consumers to become active, involved, and informed participants on the healthcare team.[60]

• OpenNotes. Since 2010, this national initiative funded by the Robert Wood Johnson Foundation and the Commonwealth Fund, gives patients access to the visit notes written by their doctors, nurses, or other clinicians. Potential positive effects of using an open medical record include catching errors in the notes, preventing diagnostic delay, taking medications as prescribed, encouraging patients to speak up, engaging informal caregivers, and enhancing trust.[61,62] OpenNotes has been adopted by facilities and systems of care such as the Department of Veterans Affairs and Geisinger Health Systems.

What is known is that engagement results in patient safety outcomes.[63] The healthcare quality professional can work with others in the organization to determine how elements of engagement can be incorporated into strategic intent, the safety plan, and other related activities (e.g., structure to support engagement, needed skills, awareness building, and practices).

Health Equity

One of the six aims of a quality healthcare system is equity. In a perfect world, equitable care does not vary based on a patient's individual characteristics such as sex, gender identity, ethnicity, geographic location, or socioeconomic status. However, disparities exist and include (1) the way healthcare systems are organized and operate; (2) patient attitudes and behaviors; and (3) healthcare provider biases, prejudices, and uncertainty when treating minorities.[64(pp2–3)] Medical errors can result from ineffective patient-provider communication and the inability of the treating providers to overcome cultural and linguistic barriers. Effective and safe medical treatment depends on good communication between the healthcare team and patient. Cultural competence is an important component of patient safety. Full buy-in from the organization's senior decision-makers is essential to the success of any cultural competency initiative.

Cross and colleagues defined cultural competence as "a set of congruent behaviors, attitudes and policies that come together in a system, agency, or amongst professionals and enables that system, agency and those professionals to work effectively in cross-cultural situations."[65(p iv)] Lack of cultural competence affects healthcare and patient safety.

Patients with limited English proficiency (LEP) comprise 8.6% of the U.S. population, or 25 million people.[66] Patients with LEP have increased risk for adverse events. Divi et al.[67] found that 49.1% of LEP patients experienced physical harm compared with the 29.5% of non-LEPs. In addition, LEP patients experienced higher levels of physical harm (46.8%) compared with their non-LEP counterparts (24.4%). Communication is the third most common root cause of sentinel events and unexpected events, which cause death or serious physical or psychological injury.[68]

Because of inequities, individuals across the United States are unable to reach their optimal health potential. Inequities in healthcare are influenced by "social determinants of health, or those conditions in which individuals are born, grow, live, work and age."[69(¶1)] One of the most modifiable factors is the lack of CLAS, broadly defined as "care and services that are respectful of and responsive to the cultural and linguistic needs of all individuals."[70(¶1)] Various models are proposed to describe cultural competence as a patient-centered approach. All the models have these dimensions in common: knowledge (e.g., understanding the meaning of culture and its importance to healthcare delivery), attitudes (e.g., having respect for variations in cultural norms), and skills (e.g., eliciting the patient's explanatory models of illness).[71(p2)]

The National Standards for Culturally and Linguistically Appropriate Services in Health and Health Care—the National CLAS Standards—were originally released in 2001 and updated in 2013.[70,72] The 15 National CLAS Standards are intended to advance health equity, improve quality, and help eliminate healthcare disparities by establishing a blueprint for health and healthcare organizations to achieve equity. These standards are increasingly recognized as effective for improving quality of care, patient safety, effectiveness, and patient centeredness.[70(p17)] The Standards and actions that an organization might consider to improve patient safety and cultural competency are shown in **TABLE 2-4**.

Leadership and Patient Safety

National pressures mount and new expectations emerge for healthcare leaders. These come from government agencies (e.g., CMS), public reporting groups (e.g., The Leapfrog Group and *U.S. News & World Report*), accreditation agencies (e.g., TJC and the Accreditation Council for Graduate Medical Education), and third-party payers. Third-party payers are using the practice of nonpayment for certain reasonably preventable conditions (e.g., pressure ulcers) and serious preventable events (e.g., leaving a sponge in a patient during surgery).

Table 2-4 The National CLAS Standards and Patient Safety

CLAS Standard	Actions/Interventions
Principal Standard	
1. Provide effective, equitable, understandable, and respectful quality care and services that are responsive to diverse cultural health beliefs and practices, preferred languages, health literacy, and other communication needs.	• Create a more welcoming, safe and inclusive environment that contributes to improved healthcare quality for lesbian, gay, bisexual, and transgender (LGBT) patients and their families (The Joint Commission, 2011). • Negotiating an understanding within which a safe, effective, and mutually agreeable treatment plan can be implemented.
Governance, Leadership, and Workforce	
2. Advance and sustain organizational governance and leadership that promotes CLAS and health equity through policy, practices, and allocated resources.	• Ensure diversity to reflect shifting demographics and populations served in the composition of the C-Suite executives and Board of Directors to diversity of thought, experience, and background in organization's management and Boardroom. • Create policy whereby interpreters must be provided to patients and/or family members when obtaining informed consent, having discussion about advance healthcare directives, gathering critical clinical information (e.g., patient's medical history), explaining the plan of care (e.g., procedures), and providing updates on the treatment plan (e.g., discharge planning, care transitions).
3. Recruit, promote, and support a culturally and linguistically diverse governance, leadership, and workforce that are responsive to the population in the service area.	• Advertise for vacancies through targeted publications (e.g., the Institute for Diversity in Healthcare). • Develop a board recruitment strategy so the Board is representative of the community.

(continued)

Table 2-4 The National CLAS Standards and Patient Safety (*continued*)

CLAS Standard	Actions/Interventions
Governance, Leadership, and Workforce (cont'd)	

4. Educate and train governance, leadership, and workforce in culturally and linguistically appropriate policies and practices on an ongoing basis.	• Supply clinicians with current information regarding susceptibility of particular racial/ethnic groups to certain diseases and conditions and possible lifestyles and dietary habits that impact health or make it difficult for patients to follow treatment plans.
	• Create core curriculum on cultural competence in healthcare to Improve the safety and quality for onboarding new board members and staff.
	• Improve the ability of clinicians to communicate effectively with their patients directly or via interpreters through training in the following:
	  1. Communication skills (including how to effectively negotiate a treatment plan which the patient will be able and willing to follow)
	  2. Cultural awareness (understanding and acceptance of beliefs and lifestyles different from their own).

Communication and Language Assistance	
5. Offer language assistance to individuals who have LEP and/or other communication needs, at no cost to them, to facilitate timely access to all healthcare and services.	• Readily available interpreters in the Emergency Department for LEP patients to avoid delays in care resulting in adverse consequences in the absence of any language assistance service. • Use Ask Me 3 from NPSF for information and resources to educate patients and providers about health literacy and improving patient-provider communication.
6. Inform all individuals of the availability of language assistance services clearly and in their preferred language, verbally and in writing.	• Signage in public areas describing the organization's language assistance services and how to access interpretation services. • Provide information about language assistance services in admission packets for ambulatory, emergency and acute care.
7. Ensure the competence of individuals providing language assistance, recognizing that the use of untrained individuals and/or minors as interpreters should be avoided.	• Interpreter certification through oral and written proficiency tests of their knowledge of conversational and medical language in both English and the language of interpretation. Untrained interpreters may lack knowledge of medical terminology and confidentiality. Untrained interpreters are more likely to commit errors in interpretation that can lead to adverse clinical consequences. • The presence of interpreters may inhibit discussions of sensitive issues, such as domestic violence, substance use, psychiatric illness, and sexual activity.
8. Provide easy-to-understand print and multimedia materials and signage in the languages commonly used by the populations in the service area.	• Create an indexed resource library of educational materials in threshold and/or preferred languages of patient populations served. Integrate with electronic health record if technology permits. • Use digital health products such as customized medication instruction programs that provide easy-to-understand, ethnically appropriate medical information on prescribed medications and access to videos that demonstrate how to take medications prescribed. • Develop a shared vocabulary.
Engagement, Continuous Improvement, and Accountability	
9. Establish culturally and linguistically appropriate goals, policies, and management accountability, and infuse them throughout the organization's planning and operations.	• Designate a high-ranking administrator with decision-making power as Director of Diversity. • Form a Diversity Council or Committee to oversee the implementation of the cultural competency program. • Include cultural competency as a clearly stated focus in quality plans with measures and goals to evaluate success and progress.

(continued)

Table 2-4 The National CLAS Standards and Patient Safety (*continued*)

CLAS Standard	Actions/Interventions
Engagement, Continuous Improvement, and Accountability (cont'd)	
10. Conduct ongoing assessments of the organization's CLAS-related activities and integrate CLAS-related measures into measurement and continuous quality improvement activities.	• Conduct an annual organizational cultural competency assessment using an established tool. • Self-audit for cultural and linguistic competency prior to embarking upon a cultural competency initiative. Include items related to safety such as incident reporting and use of interpreters. • Develop a Disparities Dashboard.
11. Collect and maintain accurate and reliable demographic data to monitor and evaluate the impact of CLAS on health equity and outcomes and to inform service delivery.	• Create standardized screening, admission and intake forms that reflect CLAS-driven demographic data. • Collect data on race and ethnicity, county of origin, and language. • Stratify data by race/ethnicity, payer proxy, and gender. • Gather and compare outcomes statistics for specific populations served with those of the general or majority population for those who do not complete treatment or greater number of repeat clinical presentations of the same complaints.
12. Conduct regular assessments of community health assets and needs and use the results to plan and implement services that respond to the cultural and linguistic diversity of populations in the service area.	• Use U.S. Census data to create organizational snapshot of communities and populations served. • Equipping the medical center and satellite health centers with interpretation equipment and training for staff. • Creation and distribution of Community Health Indicators highlighting population health and disparities.
13. Partner with the community to design, implement, and evaluate policies, practices, and services to ensure cultural and linguistic appropriateness.	• Develop local partnerships; partnerships with other organizations; developing collaborations. • Having a critical mass of influential investigators interested in disparities. • Focusing on conditions prevalent in the community, such as diabetes and cardiovascular disease. • Developing and implementing community-based programs in an ethnically and culturally diverse community. • Developing partnerships between data analysts and clinical champions to address organizational safety concerns.
14. Create conflict and grievance resolution processes that are culturally and linguistically appropriate to identify, prevent, and resolve conflicts or complaints.	• Embedding disparities issues in the quality and patient safety frameworks for complaints and grievances (e.g., include race/ethnicity and language spoken/preferred language) on the complaint form. This permits analysis of complaints by demographic characteristics. • Creation of Patient and Family Relations Program with representation from patients and family.
15. Communicate the organization's progress in implementing and sustaining CLAS to all stakeholders, constituents, and the general public.	• Develop the business case to address disparities in the healthcare organization or system of care. • Interactive Grand Rounds for clinical staff and faculty to develop skills for culturally competent care delivery. • Reporting equity measures related to relevant safety activities on the organization's website.

CLAS, culturally and linguistically appropriate services; LEP, limited English proficiency; NPSF, National Patient Safety Foundation. Table developed by authors Beaudin and Pelletier from field examples and the following references: Alliance for Board Diversity. Missing pieces report: The 2016 Board Diversity Census of women and minorities on Fortune 500 boards. Deloitte Center for Board Effectiveness; 2017. http://theabd.org/2016%20Board%20Diversity%20Census_Deloitte_ABD_Final.PDF; Betancourt JR, Green AR, King RR, et al. *Improving Quality and Achieving Equity: A Guide for Hospital Leaders.* Boston, MA: The Disparities Solutions Center at Massachusetts; General Hospital; 2008. http://www.rwjf.org/en/library/research/2008/01/improving-quality-and-achieving-equity.html; California Health Care Foundation. Digitizing the Safety Net: High Tech Opportunities for the Underserved; 2016. http://www.chcf.org/publications/2016/02/digitizing-safety-net. Accessed February 23, 2017; The Joint Commission. *Advancing Effective Communication, Cultural Competence, and Patient- and Family-Centered Care for the Lesbian, Gay, Bisexual, and Transgender (LGBT) Community: A Field Guide.* Oak Brook, IL: The Joint Commission; Oct. 2011; National Patient Safety Foundation. Ask Me 3. http://www.npsf.org/?page=askme3. Accessed April 16, 2017; Salimbene S. CLAS A-Z: A practical guide for implementing the national standards for culturally and linguistically appropriate services (CLAS) in health care; 2001. https://minorityhealth.hhs.gov/assets/pdf/checked/CLAS_a2z.pdf. Accessed February 22, 2017; U.S. Department of Health & Human Services, Office of Minority Health. The case of the enhanced national CLAS standards. https://www.thinkculturalhealth.hhs.gov/pdfs/EnhancedNationalCLASStandards.pdf. Accessed April 17, 2017.

Leaders are responsible for driving change and improvement in patient safety practices that address these pressures and expectations. A *patient safety practice* is "a type of process or structure whose application reduces the probability of adverse events resulting from exposure to the healthcare system across a range of diseases and procedures"[73(p13)] Applicability of various safety practices is dependent upon many factors, including the healthcare setting, the populations served, high-risk processes, volume-driven practices, and previous performance data. Organizations can use quality tools such as a prioritization matrix to select safety standards relevant to their populations served.

Leadership works with others in the organization to prioritize needs, select practices for improvement, allocate resources to successfully implement patient safety practices, and ensure commitment to interventions and improvement are sustained over time. The governing board and medical leadership participate in the analysis and prioritization process. Patient safety practices are integrated into the organization's strategic direction. Goals are developed that are both realistic and aspirational. Various national organizations employ consensus-driven processes to identify patient safety practices to be adopted by healthcare organizations. Because there is now an abundance of consensus-driven standards, healthcare quality professionals can look to the tried and true work of others to develop their own safety practices. For example, recommendations can be found in *Safe Practices for Better Healthcare: 2010 Update*.[74] These are summarized in **TABLE 2-5.**

As part of its duties, the governing body or board of directors holds accountability for quality of care and patient safety. The heightened attention to public reporting affects this responsibility. Quality oversight is recognized more clearly as a core fiduciary duty, which is the highest standard of care. This is not just financial health and reputation. Accountability for quality and safety cannot be fully delegated to the medical staff and executive leadership. A purpose- and values-driven board, in partnership with executive leadership and medical staff, set performance expectations to elimination of harm while mitigating risks.

Quality and safety contribute to financial stability and offer capital opportunities for growing healthcare organizations.

Table 2-5 Safe Practices for Better Healthcare—2010 Update

Safe Practice	Practice Statement
Safe Practice 1: Leadership Structures and Systems	Leadership structures and systems must be established to ensure organization-wide awareness of patient safety performance gaps, direct accountability of leaders for those gaps, and adequate investment in performance improvement abilities, and that actions are taken to ensure safe care of every patient served.
Safe Practice 2: Culture Measurement, Feedback, and Intervention	Healthcare organizations must measure their culture, provide feedback to the leadership and staff, and undertake interventions that will reduce patient safety risk.
Safe Practice 3: Teamwork Training and Skill Building	Healthcare organizations must establish a proactive, systematic, organization-wide approach to developing team-based care through teamwork training, skill building, and team-led performance improvement interventions that reduce preventable harm to patients.
Safe Practice 4: Identification and Mitigation of Risks and Hazards	Healthcare organizations must systematically identify and mitigate patient safety risks and hazards with an integrated approach to continuously drive down preventable patient harm.
Safe Practice 5: Informed Consent	Ask each patient or legal surrogate to "teach back," in his or her own words, key information about the proposed treatments or procedures for which he or she is being asked to provide informed consent.
Safe Practice 6: Life-Sustaining Treatment	Ensure that written documentation of the patient's preferences for life-sustaining treatments is prominently displayed in his or her chart.
Safe Practice 7: Disclosure	Following serious unanticipated outcomes, including those that are clearly caused by systems failures, the patient and, as appropriate, the family should receive timely, transparent, and clear communication concerning what is known about the event.
Safe Practice 8: Care of the Caregiver	Following serious unintentional harm resulting from systems failures and/or errors that resulted from human performance failures, the involved caregivers (clinical providers, staff, and administrators) should receive timely and systematic care to include: treatment that is just, respect, compassion, supportive medical care, and the opportunity to fully participate in event investigation and risk identification and mitigation activities that will prevent future events.

(continued)

Table 2-5 Safe Practices for Better Healthcare—2010 Update (*continued*)

Safe Practice	Practice Statement
Safe Practice 9: Nursing Workforce	Implement critical components of a well-designed nursing workforce that mutually reinforce patient safeguards, including the following: • a nurse staffing plan with evidence that it is adequately resourced and actively managed and its effectiveness is regularly evaluated with respect to patient safety; • senior administrative nursing leaders, such as a chief nursing officer, are part of the hospital senior management team; • governance boards and senior administrative leaders that take accountability for reducing patient safety risks related to nurse staffing decisions and the provision of financial resources for nursing services; and • provision of budgetary resources to support nursing staff in the ongoing acquisition and maintenance of professional knowledge and skills.
Safe Practice 10: Direct Caregivers	Ensure that non-nursing direct care staffing levels are adequate, that staff are competent, and that they have had adequate orientation, training, and education to perform their assigned direct care duties.
Safe Practice 11: Intensive Care Unit (ICU) Care	All patients in general ICU (both adult and pediatric) should be managed by physicians who have specific training and certification in critical care medicine ("critical care certified").
Safe Practice 12: Patient Care Information	Ensure that care information is transmitted and appropriately documented in a timely manner and in a clearly understandable form to patients and all of the patient's healthcare providers/professionals within and between care settings who need that information to provide continued care.
Safe Practice 13: Order Read Back and Abbreviations	Incorporate within your organization a safe, effective communication strategy, structures, and systems to include the following: • For verbal or telephone orders or for telephonic reporting of critical test results, verify the complete order or test result by having the person who is receiving the information record and "read back" the complete order or test result. • Standardize a list of "do not use" abbreviations, acronyms, symbols, and dose designations that cannot be used throughout the organization.
Safe Practice 14: Labeling of Diagnostic Studies	Implement standardized policies, processes, and systems to ensure accurate labeling of radiographs, laboratory specimens, or other diagnostic studies so the right study is labeled for the right patient at the right time.
Safe Practice 15: Discharge Systems	A discharge plan must be prepared for each patient at the time of hospital discharge, and a concise discharge summary must be prepared for and relayed to the clinical caregiver accepting responsibility for postdischarge care in a timely manner. Organizations must ensure there is confirmation of receipt of the discharge information by the independent licensed practitioner who will assume responsibility for care after discharge.
Safe Practice 16: Safe Adoption of Computerized Prescriber Order Entry	Implement a computerized prescriber order entry system built upon the requisite foundation of reengineered evidence-based care, an assurance of healthcare organization staff and independent practitioner readiness, and an integrated information technology infrastructure.
Safe Practice 17: Medication Reconciliation	The healthcare organization must develop, reconcile, and communicate an accurate patient medication list throughout the continuum of care.
Safe Practice 18: Pharmacist Leadership Structures and Systems	Pharmacy leaders should have an active role on the administrative leadership team that reflects their authority and accountability for medication management systems performance across the organization.
Safe Practice 19: Hand Hygiene	Comply with current Centers for Disease Control and Prevention (CDC) hand hygiene guidelines.
Safe Practice 20: Influenza Prevention	Comply with current CDC recommendations for influenza vaccinations for healthcare personnel and the annual recommendations of the CDC Advisory Committee on Immunization Practices for individual influenza prevention and control.

(continued)

Table 2-5 Safe Practices for Better Healthcare—2010 Update (*continued*)

Safe Practice	Practice Statement
Safe Practice 21: Central Line–Associated Bloodstream Infection Prevention	Take actions to prevent central line–associated bloodstream infection by implementing evidence-based intervention practices.
Safe Practice 22: Surgical Site Infection Prevention	Take actions to prevent surgical site infections by implementing evidence-based intervention practices.
Safe Practice 23: Care of the Ventilated Patient	Take actions to prevent complications associated with ventilated patients—specifically, ventilator-associated pneumonia, venous thromboembolism, peptic ulcer disease, dental complications, and pressure ulcers.
Safe Practice 24: Multidrug-Resistant Organism (MDRO) Prevention	Implement a systematic MDRO eradication program built on the fundamental elements of infection control, an evidence-based approach, assurance of hospital staff and independent practitioner readiness, and a reengineered identification and care process for patients with or at risk for MDRO infections. *Note*: This practice applies to, but is not limited to, epidemiologically important organisms such as methicillin-resistant *Staphylococcus aureus*, vancomycin-resistant enterococci, and *Clostridium difficile*. Multidrug-resistant gram-negative bacilli—such as *Enterobacter* species, *Klebsiella* species, *Pseudomonas* species, and *Escherichia coli*—and vancomycin-resistant *S. aureus* should be evaluated for inclusion on a local system level based on organizational risk assessments.
Safe Practice 25: Catheter-Associated Urinary Tract Infection Prevention	Take actions to prevent catheter-associated urinary tract infection by implementing evidence-based intervention practices.
Safe Practice 26: Wrong Site, Procedure, and Person Surgery Prevention	Implement the Universal Protocol for Preventing Wrong Site, Wrong Procedure, Wrong Person Surgery™ for all invasive procedures.
Safe Practice 27: Pressure Ulcer Prevention	Take actions to prevent pressure ulcers by implementing evidence-based intervention practices.
Safe Practice 28: Venous Thromboembolism Prevention	Evaluate each patient upon admission, and regularly thereafter, for risk of developing venous thromboembolism. Use clinically appropriate, evidence-based methods of thromboprophylaxis.
Safe Practice 29: Anticoagulation Therapy	Organizations should implement practices to prevent patient harm resulting from anticoagulant therapy.
Safe Practice 30: Contrast Media-Induced Renal Failure Prevention	Use validated protocols to evaluate patients at risk for contrast-media-induced renal failure and gadolinium-associated nephrogenic systemic fibrosis, and use a clinically appropriate method to reduce the risk for adverse events based on the patient's risk evaluations.
Safe Practice 31: Organ Donation	Hospital policies consistent with applicable law and regulations should be in place and address patient and family preferences for organ donation, as well as specify the roles and desired outcomes for every stage of the donation process.
Safe Practice 32: Glycemic Control	Take actions to improve glycemic control by implementing evidence-based intervention practices that prevent hypoglycemia and optimize the care of patients with hyperglycemia and diabetes.
Safe Practice 33: Falls Prevention	Take actions to prevent patient falls and reduce fall-related injuries by implementing evidence-based intervention practices.
Safe Practice 34: Pediatric Imaging	When computed tomography imaging studies are undertaken on children, "child-size" techniques should be used to reduce unnecessary exposure to ionizing radiation.

As decisions are made about bond ratings, agencies such as Standard & Poor's and Moody's Investors Service stress the importance of the healthcare leader's attention to clinical quality outcomes and safety

> From a credit perspective, a not-for-profit hospital's focus on a quality agenda can translate into improved ratings through increased volume and market share, operational efficiencies, better rates from commercial payers, and improved financial performance. Like many strategies, [Moody's] recognize[s] that realizing financial returns from a quality strategy may require large capital costs and incurred operating losses in the short term. However, over the long term, a hospital's focus on quality will be viewed as a credit positive if greater patient demand and financial improvements materialize. Many not-for-profit hospitals are launching strategies to improve evidence-based clinical outcomes and patient safety, which we view as the two key facets of a strategy aimed at improving quality. The effort to improve quality is a major component of most hospitals' mission to provide the best patient care possible.[75(p1)]

These perspectives are critical to the conversations about the business case for quality and safety.

When providing quality care and reducing harm as part of an organization's strategy, the board, executives, and medical staff have the opportunity for continual, transparent, and data-informed deliberations about capital and human resource investments. And in doing so, consider harm and its impact on the bottom-line. This criticality was underscored by a recent Moody's report on for-profit and not-for-profit hospital performance whereby

> technological innovation in healthcare will likely lead to lower patient volumes at both for-profit and not-for-profit hospitals. However, for hospitals at the forefront of healthcare technology, the benefits of innovation will outweigh the reduction in volumes. Telemedicine and remote monitoring, particularly for high-risk populations, will reduce emergency room visits and inpatient admissions because they will improve preventative care. These technologies will also reduce hospital visits by making it more clear when a patient can be effectively managed at home (e.g., heart-burn vs heart attack). Further, advances in medical technologies and minimally invasive surgeries will also lead to more procedures being done in lower-cost settings, such as physician offices or ambulatory service centers, rather than in hospitals. . . . Technological improvements in medical equipment, handheld devices, and electronic health records will also reduce medical errors, which are costly in many ways (including payment penalties, higher insurance and litigation costs).[76(p4)]

Investments in technology that reduce medical errors or more effective care management, also contribute to the hospital or healthcare system's financial stability and growth. Better care, smarter spending, healthier people.

Patient safety must be integrated by leadership into strategic planning. Institute for Healthcare Improvement (IHI)[77] outlines six things all boards can consider in their effort to improve quality and reduce harm:

1. Learning, starting with the board: Develop capability as a board. Learn how the best boards work with executives and physician leaders to reduce harm. Set an expectation for similar levels of education and training for all staff.
2. Establishing executive accountability: Oversee the effective execution of a plan to achieve aims to reduce harm, including executive team accountability for clear performance improvement targets.
3. Setting aims: Set a specific aim to reduce harm this year. Make an explicit public commitment to measurable quality improvement (e.g., a reduction in unnecessary mortality and harm), establishing a clear aim for the facility or system.
4. Establishing and monitoring system-level measures: Identify a small group of organization-wide measures of patient safety (e.g., facility-wide harm, risk-adjusted mortality), update the measures continually, and make them transparent to the entire organization and customers.
5. Gathering data and hearing stories: Select and review progress toward safer care as the first agenda item at every board meeting; progress is grounded in transparency and a desire to put a human face on harm data.
6. Changing the environment, policies, and culture: Commit to establishing and maintaining an environment that is respectful, fair, and just for all who experience pain and loss because of avoidable harm and adverse outcomes.

With the convergence of clinical care, safety priorities, and economic stability, board members' interest will increase over time and create opportunities for healthcare quality professionals to educate organizational leaders on the importance of attending to patient safety. "Board oversight of quality and patient safety rests on the directors' ability to obtain, process, and interpret information; assess current performance; and set strategic direction using a range of metrics tailored to local circumstances."[78(p754)]

Over 100 consensus standards with a focus on patient safety are endorsed by NQF. The first of the 34 endorsed practices are Leadership Structures and Systems.[79] This safe practice for leadership provides an overview of the leadership structures and systems deemed critical to the organization-wide awareness of patient safety performance gaps, direct accountability of leaders for those gaps, and adequate investment in performance improvement abilities, along with the actions necessary to ensure safe care of every patient served.[74] The four distinct elements within the NQF-endorsed safe practice of Leadership Structures and Systems are outlined below.

Awareness Structures and Systems

Awareness structures and systems provide leaders with continuous information about potential risks, hazards, and performance gaps that may contribute to patient safety issues. These structures and systems include (a) identification of risks and hazards; (b) culture management, feedback, and intervention; (c) direct patient input; and (d) governance board and senior management briefings and meetings.

Accountability Structures and Systems

Accountability structures and systems enable leaders to establish direct accountability to the governing body, senior management, mid-level management, physician leaders, and frontline staff. Included in these structures and systems are (a) the patient safety program, (b) the patient safety officer, (c) direct organization-wide leadership accountability, (d) an interdisciplinary patient safety committee, and (e) external reporting activities.

Structures and Systems-Driving Ability

Structures and systems-driving ability allows leaders to assess the capacity, resources, and competence necessary to implement change in the culture and in patient safety performance. This ability includes (a) patient safety budgets, (b) people systems, (c) quality systems, and (d) technical systems.

Action Structures and Systems

Action structures and systems enable leaders to take direct and appropriate action. These structures and systems include (a) quality and performance improvement programs; (b) regular actions of governance, including confirmation of values, basic teamwork training, and governance board competence in patient safety; (c) regular actions of senior administrative leadership, including commitment of time to patient safety; culture measurement, feedback, and interventions; basic teamwork training and team interventions; and identification and mitigation of risks and hazards; (d) regular actions of unit, service line, departmental and mid-level management leaders; and (e) regular actions with respect to independent medical leaders.[74(pp6–10)]

As leaders think about accountability and action, they can foster and reward improvement for the spread of best practices, knowledge and adoption of value-based interventions and innovations in program design and redesign. Measures of success should align the incentives for the improvement of patient safety. Rogers's work on disseminating innovations is also applicable to the widespread adoption of safety practices.[80] A comprehensive discussion of change and innovation can be found in *Performance and Process Improvement*. Also, see *Organizational Leadership* for more information about leadership, quality improvement, and strategy.

Patient Safety Principles and Practices

Human error is inevitable, even among the most conscientious professionals who are practicing the highest standards of care. Human error happens when "there is general agreement that the individual should have done other than what they did, and in the course of that conduct inadvertently causes or could cause an undesirable outcome, the individual is labeled as having committed an error."[81(p6)] Identification and reporting of human error events are critical to an organization's efforts to continuously improve patient safety and contribute to a robust learning environment. Likewise, healthcare leaders have a duty to recognize the inevitability of human error, design systems that make such error less likely, and avoid punitive reactions to honest errors. Pham et al.[82] offer that IRS can help the organization identify local system hazards, bolster the patient safety culture, and share lessons within and across organizations. Incident reporting, however, should not be the only component of an enterprise-wide patient safety program.

A formal patient safety program is part of system design. The program considers the following:

- Mission, vision, core values, and goals of the organization
- Interrelationships between and among functions, departments and disciplines
- Acknowledging differences in the patient safety mindset
- Silos that might exist for overlapping or misaligned goals and objectives
- Forming cross-departmental teams for collaboration
- Identifying where processes can be streamlined to improve organizational or system effectiveness.

The written program and plan incorporates the patient safety goals and objectives. It describes how efforts are coordinated to support organization-wide assessment, evaluation, and improvement of interrelated processes. Different aspects of the plan can include the following:

- Governance and leadership
- Goals and objectives
- Planning, designing, and redesigning safe processes
- Culture of safety
- Reduction of preventable errors (e.g., identifying and mitigating risks and hazards, adverse events, sentinel events, and peer review processes)
- Adherence to clinical practice guidelines
- Patient, family, and caregiver engagement

- Measurement, monitoring, and evaluating program effectiveness/success
- Transparency and dissemination of results across the organization.

The healthcare quality professional can guide the organization in determining which performance improvement methodology can be adopted proactively and retrospectively. An organization also can look to build the skills of those working on improving patient safety, such as avowing common pitfalls when conducting a root cause analysis (RCA)[83] and developing strong harm reduction actions that are sustainable.

Harm Reduction

The IOM report, *To Err Is Human: Building a Safer Health System*,[21] and its subsequent reports, garnered the attention of providers, payers, and consumers by illustrating the direct relationship between quality of care and patient outcomes. Further, Becher and Chassin[84] pointed out the experience of patient harm as the result of three types of quality issues: underuse, overuse, and misuse of health services. Underuse occurs when patients do not receive beneficial health services. For instance, only 10% of patients who have an addiction problem receive treatment.[85] Overuse occurs when patients undergo treatment or procedures from which they do not benefit (e.g., X-rays performed on patients with back pain are unnecessary). Misuse occurs when patients receive appropriate medical services provided poorly, adding to the risk for preventable complications.

Underuse, overuse, and misuse are considered waste and waste is costly. Berwick and Hackbarth[86] believe the best healthcare reform and cost reduction strategy is to eliminate waste. They identified six categories where considerable costs are represented by waste. Below are the categories and the estimated wasteful spending to the U.S. healthcare system. Total waste cost of the United States was $558 billion to $1,263 billion in 2011. These are examples of waste related to harm reduction:

1. Failures of care delivery: Waste from poor execution or lack of best practice adoption resulting in injuries and poor outcomes ($102 billion to $154 billion).
2. Failures of care coordination: Waste related to fragmented care resulting in complications, readmissions, declines in functional status, and increased dependency of the chronically ill ($25 billion to $45 billion).
3. Overtreatment: Waste from rendering care that is not useful ($158 billion to $226 billion).

Human Factors

Human factors (also called human factors engineering) "is the application of knowledge about human capabilities (physical, sensory, emotional, and intellectual) and limitations to the design and development of tools, devices, systems, environments, and organizations. . . ."[87(p1)] The human factors associated with healthcare personnel and patient safety are complex. Employee attitudes, motivation, physical and psychological health, education, training, and cognitive functioning can influence the likelihood of a medical error.

In healthcare, 85% of errors are the result of systems issues, and 15% are attributable to human factors.[88] According to IHI, "The key to reliable, safe care does not lie in exhorting individuals to be more careful and try harder. It lies in learning about causes of error and designing systems to prevent human error whenever possible."[77(p19)] Causes for human error are important in system design and redesign. Examples of human factors found to contribute to errors include the following:

- Human interaction with machines
- Workload leading to errors and mistakes in providing the best care for patients, when there are not enough staff to handle the workload or work hours are inadequate
- Disruptive behavior of healthcare personnel that undermines a culture of patient safety[89]
- Fatigue and stress leading to less than expected performance.[90(p100)]

Any improvement efforts focused on eliminating errors requires a just culture, detailed analysis of the care delivery process, human factors influencing processes of care, and the resources to bring about sustained system change. Drawing from many other disciplines such as anatomy, physiology, physics, biomechanics, and ergonomics, the IHI defines human factors as "the study of all the factors that make it easier to do the work in the right way"[91(¶1)] The science applied to healthcare fosters these principles in designed work processes:

- Simplify to take steps out of a process.
- Standardize to remove variation and promote predictability and consistency.
- Use forcing functions and constraints that makes it impossible to do a task incorrectly and creates a hard stop that cannot be passed unless actions are changed. Check, restrict, or compel to avoid or perform some action.
- Use redundancies such as double-checking someone's work.
- Avoid reliance on memory by using tools such as checklists.
- Take advantage of habits and patterns to perform consistently (habit) and in a recognizable way (pattern).
- Promote effective team functioning (e.g., teamwork and communication).
- Automate and use technology carefully.[91]

High Reliability

Healthcare organizations and systems are working toward becoming highly reliable. As Gordon et al.[92] pointed out, to become a high-reliability industry healthcare "needs a radical cultural transformation, like the one that has taken place in aviation over the past thirty years. . . . If aviation could do it, health care can too."[92(p7)] Adopting high-reliability principles and practices helps the healthcare organization strive toward a near-zero-defect culture. Reason[45] stated: "Perhaps the most important distinguishing feature of high reliability organizations is their collective preoccupation with the possibility of failure. They expect to make errors and train their workforce to recognize and recover them."[45(p770)]

HROs are "organizations with systems in place that are exceptionally consistent in accomplishing their goals and avoiding catastrophic errors."[93,94(p298)] Five key concepts frame the HRO. They include the following:

1. Sensitivity to operations. Preserving constant awareness and vigilance by leaders and staff about the state of the systems and processes affecting patient care. This awareness is central to noting risks and preventing them.
2. Reluctance to simplify. Simple processes are good, but simplistic explanations for why things work or fail are risky. Avoiding overly simple explanations of failure (unqualified staff, inadequate training, communication failure, etc.) is essential to understand the true reasons patients are placed at risk.
3. Preoccupation with failure. When near misses occur, these are viewed as evidence of systems to improve for reduction of potential harm to patients. Rather than viewing near misses as proof the system has effective safeguards, they are viewed as symptomatic of areas in need of more attention.
4. Deference to expertise. If leaders and supervisors are not willing to listen and respond to the insights of staff who know how processes work and the risks patients face, high reliability in the organization's safety culture may not be possible.
5. Resilience. Leaders and staff need to be trained and prepared to know how to respond when system failures do occur.[95(p1)]

These concepts lead to mindfulness, an important component of reliability, which keep HROs at a high level of vigilance.[95(p7)] Chassin and Loeb[96(p481)] propose organizations use *robust process improvement*, "a combination of Lean, Six Sigma, and change management" as a new set of tools to achieve high reliability and maintain patient safety. These can achieve outcomes such as decreased morbidity and mortality through the application of replicable and scalable patient safety interventions. Many organizations now use the Lean practice of system redesign with a focus on the human factors in their patient safety programs. See *Performance and Process Improvement* for more information on Lean and Six Sigma, and *Organizational Leadership* for more information on change management.

Weick and Sutcliffe[97,98] explain the success of an HRO—by acting mindfully, an HRO organizes itself so the unexpected is noticed and stopped from advancing. Five principles are found to impact HRO performance and responsiveness:

1. Preoccupation with failure. Attention on close calls and near misses ("being lucky vs being good"); focus more on failures rather than successes.
2. Reluctance to simplify interpretations. Solid "root cause" analysis practices.
3. Sensitivity to operations. Situational awareness and carefully designed change management processes.
4. Commitment to resilience. Resources are continually devoted to corrective action plans and training.
5. Deference to expertise. Listen to the experts on the frontlines (e.g., authority follows expertise).

Using these principles, the healthcare quality professional can work with others in the organization to create a mindful infrastructure that prevents harm from happening, reduces the damage produced by unexpected events, and promotes reliable performance.

Marx has been working with high reliability in the context of a just culture for over 20 years and offered that "it is through the lessons of our everyday errors that we can design our work environment."[81(p3)] High reliability is dependent on making good choices and becoming less error prone and more error tolerant. Marx works from a model-based approach to managing risk proactive or anticipatory) instead of an event-driven approach (reactive). The focus on highly reliable outcomes derives from a core set of principles[99] that include the following:

- Zero is not possible.
- There is no such thing as an HRO; there are only organizations that are highly reliable around those things they value.
- Humans are not inherently rule followers—they are threat and hazards avoiders.
- There is a preoccupation with risk. Faulty equipment and fallible human beings can still produce great results.
- Strive to be three human errors away from harm with robust system design.
- It is about system design and choices and managing the right things.
- Doing less is often the better path—adopt smart designs that are often less extensive.

An example of system design and redesign is the Lean Healthcare program developed and deployed by Hagg et al.[100] for different initiatives. The program strategy enabled the robust implementation of quality and performance improvement initiatives including clinical practice bundles. See FIGURE 2-4 for techniques and methodologies used. The program applied Lean and systems engineering methodologies and was structured to sustain improvements in process effectiveness and patient outcomes. The idea is to build sustainable programs as when change is frequent or not sustained, the result is often accompanied by increased staff fatigue, a more stressful work environment, and increased costs.[100(p1)] Different projects were successfully implemented that affected patient safety such as emergency department patient flow, surgical flow, medication delivery process redesign, ICU length of stay reduction (including ventilator-associated pneumonia [VAP]/ glycemic control bundles), central line and methicillin-resistant *Streptococcus aureus* bundles, and patient fall reduction. Mitigating risk by using proven techniques contributes to high reliability—whether it is the behavior of the organization or the outcomes that result from the organization's processes.

Another example of system design for infection prevention and control is the "Journey to Zero" that includes innovative strategies to eradicate HAIs through a process of laying the foundation (sizing the burden), crafting a multipronged

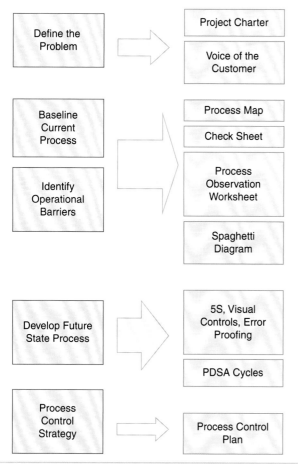

Figure 2-4 Lean healthcare system redesign approach. PDSA, Plan–Do–Study–Act. (From Hagg HW, Workman-Germann J, Flanagan ME, Doebbeling BN. Techniques and methodologies utilized within the Lean Healthcare Program. In: Henriksen K, Battles JB, Keyes MA, Grad ML, eds. *Implementation of Systems Redesign: Approaches to Spread and Sustain Adoption. Advances in Patient Safety: New Directions and Alternative Approaches* (Vol. 2: Culture and Redesign). Rockville, MD: Agency for Healthcare Research and Quality; 2008.)

strategy (establishing frontline awareness and minimizing pathogen opportunity), and ensuring sustainable success and promoting long-term gains.[14(pp18–19)] Hand hygiene is an example of where the principles of high reliability bring promise. To get to zero HAIs, the Joint Commission Center for Transforming Healthcare developed a Hand Hygiene Targeted Solutions Tool to manage change so it can be sustained using principles of leadership, safety culture, and performance improvement.[101] Many organizations use this tool to increase hand hygiene.

Risk Management

In the 1970s, RM was the initial reaction to continually increasing litigation. However, as litigation continued to rise, RM assumed a more proactive role in reducing the incidents of unsafe care. Today, healthcare organizations focus on maintaining good and defined standards of practice to identify hazards posing risks to patients, assess the risks associated with healthcare hazards against the intended benefit, and eliminate or reduce risks to patients.[102] **TABLE 2-6** summarizes how approaches and processes of healthcare risk management (HRM) have evolved.

RM is the process of making and carrying out decisions that will minimize the adverse effects of accidental losses. Whereas the traditional evolution demonstrates a strong focus on clinical HRM, the concept of enterprise risk management is becoming more popular in expanding the focus of risks that affect the entire organization, not just clinical operations. In 2010, Carroll noted that "*Enterprise risk management* (ERM) is a comprehensive business decision-making process instituted and supported by the healthcare organization's board, executive management, and medical staff leadership. ERM recognizes the synergistic effect of risks across the continuum of care, and has as its goals to reduce uncertainty and process variability, promote patient safety and maximize the return on investment through asset preservation, and the recognition of actionable risk opportunities."[103(p585)] The major categories of risk in ERM include the following:

- Strategic: Brand and reputational risks associated with business strategy, changing priorities, and competition;
- Financial: Risks that affect the profitability, cash flow access to capital, or financial ratings;
- Legal and regulatory: Risks associated with licensure, accreditation, product liability, and intellectual property issues;
- Operational: Risks related to the business operation that may result from failed processes, people, or systems;
- Human capital: Risks associated with a tight labor market, including selection, retention, and compensation;
- Technology: Risks associated with machines, equipment, devices, hardware, and software; and

Table 2-6 Evolution of Healthcare Risk Management

Past	Present
Number one goal: protect financial resources and reputation.	Number one goal: improve patient safety and minimize risk of harm to patient through better understanding of systemic factors that limit caregiver's ability to provide safe care.
Paper occurrence form required for reporting.	Variety of methods to report: paper form, electronic form, telephone call, anonymous reporting, person-to-person reporting.
Investigate only the serious occurrences.	Encourage reporting of "near misses," and investigate and discuss the potential root causes for any incident, regardless of severity.
Interview staff one-on-one when there is an adverse incident.	Hold root cause analysis meetings with the entire team of caregivers. Identify human and system factors that contributed to the event.
Information from investigation kept confidential.	Develop corrective action, share with patient safety committee and others in the organization who need to know.
Blame and train.	Perform a criticality analysis and determine the root cause of the "near miss" or the adverse occurrence. Identify human and system factors.
Talk to the patient or patient's family only if necessary and be vague about findings.	Advise physician or other caregiver to speak directly with the patient and/or family. Talk with them about any unexpected outcomes and errors. Share steps taken to make environment safe for next patient.
Work with department involved to develop corrective action.	Work with team and organization's leadership to develop a patient safety improvement plan.
Assume that action is taken to correct the problem that occurred, notice only when it happens again that no action was taken.	Monitor the patient safety improvement plan to determine that changes are initiated and that the changes made a difference.
Keep patients in the dark about risk management and occurrence reporting.	Establish ongoing patient safety education; publish patient safety bulletins that address specific patient safety issues and the organization's approach to managing them; provide opportunity for patients to identify methods of improving patient safety and to share them with administration; disclose errors.

Adapted from Kuhn AM, Youngberg BJ. The need for risk management to evolve to assure a culture of safety, *Qual Saf Health Care*. 2002;11:158–162. Copyright 2002 by Quality and Safety in Health Care, BMJ Publishing Group. Used with permission.

- Hazard: risks related to physical loss of assets, often associated with natural hazards such as earthquakes, wildfire, cyclonic storms, flood, and drought.

In 2014, Carroll furthered the definition of ERM in healthcare as a "comprehensive framework for making RM decisions which maximize value protection and creation by managing risk and uncertainty and their connection to total value."[104(p5)] ERM includes components of culture, strategy, objectives, appetite/tolerance, structure and plans, and oversight:

- Culture: A culture supporting ERM, including programs such as HROs, Crew Resource Management, Just Culture, and Mindfulness.

- Strategy: Management's game plan for strengthening enterprise performance, with an organizational strategy linked to vision, mission, goals and objectives.
- Objectives: Ensuring ERM objectives are SMART—specific, measurable, achievable, realistic, and timely.
- Appetite/Tolerance: Determining the desired level of risk the organization will take vis-à-vis its mission and threshold or qualitative range of risks taken in pursuit of the organization's strategy (i.e., tolerance).
- Structure and Plans: Organization-wide communication and education plans describe key roles and committee structures, employee engagement strategies, techniques to update employees on the progress of ERM initiatives,

key performance indicators (KPIs) and key risk indicators (KRIs), and scenarios highlighting the value of ERM to the organization.
- Oversight: Acknowledging the responsibility of the Governing Body for ERM oversight; leadership ensures the Governing Body is regularly apprised of: progress on risk strategies, status of KPIs and KRIs, emerging risks and recommendations for new projects.[104(pp6–8)]

Risk and Quality

Effective strategies for proactively reducing errors and ensuring patient safety require an integrated and coordinated approach to synthesizing knowledge and experience. Staff members are encouraged to learn about errors and permit internal reporting of information without blame. There are interdependencies and intersections between healthcare quality and RM. Healthcare quality professionals work in tandem with enterprise RM to

- improve the effectiveness and efficiency of the organization's processes and operations through consistent identification of risks (threats) to the enterprise;
- identify, evaluate, and prioritize areas of risk affecting the operations of the organization;
- assess whether the identified risks are caused by internal (controllable) or external (uncontrollable) factors;
- develop and propose comprehensive strategies to minimize risks;
- establish action plans to address problems when identified; and
- maintain a periodic evaluation of feedback to monitor the progress of strategies and actions.

HRM can be defined as an "organized effort to identify, assess, and reduce, where appropriate, risk to patients, visitors, staff and organizational assets."[105(p3)] The goal of HRM in any organization is to protect from financial losses, which may arise because of the risks to which it is exposed. A healthcare risk manager must consider such things as regulatory compliance, safety management, credentialing, client–provider relations, publicity and media coverage, and, most importantly, patient care. In this way, HRM and patient safety are closely aligned.

Key to ERM program management is the risk manager. This position is an important asset to the organization and is typically charged with functions related to risk identification, risk assessment and evaluation, and application of techniques to reduce risks. Duties vary widely by organization, but the basic ERM functions are as follows:

- Risk identification, assessment, planning, mitigation, and evaluation;
- Maintenance and monitoring of effective incident reporting and occurrence screen programs;

- Clinical and administrative responsibilities, such as regulatory compliance, policy review, credentialing, contract review, internal and external reporting, and education;
- Collaboration and communication with environmental safety officer, patient safety officer, and quality officer (although not optimal, in some organizations these are the same position);
- Collaboration with the financial officer on insurance and other risk financing methods; and
- Collaboration and communication with legal representatives for claims management.

The risk manager is often charged with developing and deploying the ERM plan to align patient safety efforts so RM activities are not siloed. It is helpful for risk managers to also have some experience and knowledge in these areas: clinical knowledge because they must review care and provide guidance to clinical providers of care; knowledge of healthcare law and thorough understanding of the legal system because review is necessary of defense counsel work and legal documents; knowledge about the insurance industry because risk managers help make decisions about various insurance coverages, such as hospital professional liability, general liability, and workers' compensation.

Risk Management Plan. A healthcare organization typically has a formal, written plan explaining its ERM philosophy. Often the ERM plan is integrated with the quality and patient safety plan because the processes are interdependent. Important plan elements include purpose and board statement of support of ERM, scope of the program, authority, and confidentiality assertions, data collection and reporting mechanisms (both internal and external) and integration with quality management and program effectiveness reviews. Within the plan, prevention of risk is often managed by

- contract review
- internal and external reporting processes
- education of staff and providers
- policy review to protect the organization
- informed consent.

Possible causes of losses for organizations related to patient safety include criminal acts by employees, patient harm related to inability of contractors to perform services, clinical treatment by qualified or unqualified staff, falls with injury, and medication errors with harm. An important aspect of enterprise RM is management of claims. **TABLE 2-7** lists the types of professional liability sources often considered in determining the validity of a claim.

Table 2-7 Professional Liability Sources

Corporate liability	Based on recognition that the organization owes a duty to the patients it serves
Vicarious liability	Indirect responsibility for the acts of another person; *respondeat superior,* which holds the employer responsible for the wrongful acts of its employees
Ostensible agency	Generally an organization is not liable for injuries sustained by patients because of the actions of an independent contractor. However, the extension of *respondeat superior* to the doctrine of the ostensible agency may extend liability exposure to the organization for acts of nonemployed, independent contractor physicians where no employer–employee relationship exists.
Res ipsa loquitur	Allows a patient to prove his or her case without needing to establish the standard of care in which there is clear and obvious negligence

Risk Assessment

Organizations can establish mechanisms for reviewing potential incidents of risk and safety concern. All members of the workforce are responsible for identifying, reporting, and documenting RM and potential quality-of-care problems that influence patient safety. Variance or incident reporting is an important component of any patient safety program. Healthcare quality professionals assist organizations in developing and maintaining IRS. AHRQ[106] describes four attributes of voluntary patient safety event reporting systems:

1. Institution must have a supportive environment for event reporting to protect the privacy of staff who report occurrences.
2. Reports are received from a broad range of personnel.
3. Summaries of reported events must be disseminated in a timely fashion.
4. A structured mechanism must be in place for reviewing reports and developing action plans.[106(¶2)]

Only a small portion of healthcare errors (10% to 20%) is reported. Of the errors reported, 90% to 95% result in no harm to the patient.[107] A report of the DHHS Office Inspector General[108] found "most incidents of patient harm were not being reported. Hospital staff did not report 86 percent of events to incident reporting systems, partly because of staff misperceptions about what constitutes patient harm. Of the events experienced by Medicare beneficiaries discharged in October 2008, hospital incident reporting systems captured only an estimated 14 percent."[(108pii)]

Fear of disciplinary action continues to affect reporting practices by healthcare personnel.[109] Frequent and routine reporting is more likely in organizations with nonpunitive cultures. The *AHRQ Hospital Survey on Patient Safety Culture* showed only 45% of staff feel their mistakes and event reports are not held against them and mistakes are not kept in their personnel file[110]; this rate has been consistently low since 2012 (see **TABLE 2-8**).

Risk Identification

Risk identification is the first step to determine what risks can affect the achievement of organizational goals. Both formal and informal methods are used, and the risks may be internal or external to the organization. Approaches used include retrospective, concurrent, pre-interventional, and prospective. Approaches in risk identification are aimed to identify the root causes of risks for things that do go wrong (e.g., RCA) and possible modes by which these functions might fail to perform (e.g., FMEA). It may be "easier to identify all the factors that are critical to success, and then work backward to identify the things that can go wrong with each one."[111(p24)]

Once the risks have been identified, the next step is to conduct a risk assessment to quantify the magnitude or severity of the risks, the exposure through possible results, frequency of occurrence, probability of the occurrence, and time to act. Through this analysis, the organization can determine RM techniques that can be applied to the exposures to mitigate loss, select the best RM technique for the situation, prioritize actions, identify resources needed, identify risk control and risk financing methods, implement the techniques, monitor the effectiveness of the technique, and trend and analyze results. **TABLE 2-9** shows domains and measures to be considered for possible clinical risk areas based on the NQF's Consensus Standards for Quality of Hospital Care.

Risk Control

Usually risk control is managed through incident (or variance) reporting, occurrence screening, and claims management. Data that may be useful when trended or analyzed include

- liability and workers' compensation;
- tort claims (duty, breach of duty, causation, and injury);
- malpractice coverage;
- incident reports and occurrence screens;
- review of records using criteria to note variations
  - details of the occurrence,

Table 2-8 Hospital Survey Results on Patient Safety Culture: Potential for Improvement			
Areas with Potential for Improvement (Hospitals)	**2012**	**2014**	**2016**
Nonpunitive Response to Error The extent to which staff feel their mistakes and event reports are not held against them, and that mistakes are not kept in their personnel file.	44%	44%	45%
Handoffs and Transitions The extent to which important patient care information is transferred across hospital units and during shift changes.	45%	47%	48%
Staffing The extent to which there are enough staff to handle the workload, and work hours are appropriate to provide the best care for patients.	56%	55%	54%

Adapted from Agency for Healthcare Research and Quality. *Hospital survey on patient safety culture: 2012 User comparative database report;* 2012. http://www.ahrq.gov/sites/default/files/wysiwyg/professionals/quality-patient-safety/patientsafetyculture/hospital/2012/hospsurv121.pdf. Accessed April 17, 2017; Agency for Healthcare Research and Quality. *Hospital survey on patient safety culture: 2016 User comparative database report;* 2014. http://www.ahrq.gov/sites/default/files/wysiwyg/professionals/quality-patient-safety/patientsafetyculture/hospital/2014/hsops14pt1.pdf. Accessed April 17, 2017; Agency for Healthcare Research and Quality. *Hospital survey on patient safety culture: 2016 User comparative database report;* 2016. http://www.ahrq.gov/sites/default/files/wysiwyg/professionals/quality-patient-safety/patientsafetyculture/hospital/2016/2016_hospitalsops_report_pt1.pdf. Accessed April 17, 2017.

○ records that need more in-depth review,
○ confirmation of the variation or absence of an untoward event,
○ summary of data with trends, and
○ patient complaints.

Disclosure of Errors

Disclosing errors to patients and families is becoming more common practice in healthcare organizations across the country, especially in the aftermath of the Josie King incident in Maryland. Disclosure as an important part of error discovery in contrast to tactics of the past, which sprang from fear and blame.[74] A just culture supports the disclosure of successes and failures. Healthcare quality professionals typically are involved in the investigation of errors and work with quality management, enterprise RM, and legal professionals to determine a course of action. **TABLE 2-10** outlines NQF consensus standards regarding the disclosure of error or injury to consumers.

Conway et al. highlight the "respectful management" of adverse events. The aims of this group's work were to

• encourage and help every organization to develop a clinical crisis management plan before they need to use it;
• provide an approach to integrating this plan into the organizational culture of quality and safety with a focus on patient- and family-centered care and fair and just treatment for staff; and
• provide organizations with a concise, practical resource to inform their efforts when a serious adverse event occurs in the absence of a clinical crisis management plan and/or culture of quality and safety.[112(p4)]

Organizations can look for ways to encourage reporting using innovations such as the "Good Catch Awards" at Johns Hopkins Medicine in Baltimore, MD. This reporting system encourages every clinician to report situations in which patients are at risk and potentially lifesaving actions are warranted.[113]

Patient Safety Tools

Professionals who lead patient safety programs and initiatives know the importance of using the most current evidence-based information to inform design and implementation efforts. Effective tools and strategies for implementation support the advances and improvement understanding of risk factors associated with the different aspects of healthcare affecting the safe delivery of healthcare—health IT, adverse events reporting, risk identification, infection prevention and control, medication safety, physical plant, and environment of care to name a few. Using evidence-based tools can promote patient-centered care and accelerate positive changes in the patient safety culture. For example, Plan–Do–Study–Act may help implement sustainable improvement by using small tests of change. See *Performance and Process Improvement* and *Health Data Analytics* for more information about tools for evaluating and improving quality and safety.

Failure Mode and Effects Analysis

A failure mode and effects analysis (FMEA) can be used to develop safety program activities and provide continuous readiness for external surveys. It is a way for staff to be

Table 2-9 Consensus Standards for Quality of Hospital Care

Domain	Measure
Length of stay and readmission	Risk-adjusted average length of inpatient hospital stay
	Overall inpatient hospital average length of stay (ALOS) and ALOS by diagnosis-related group (DRG) service category
	All-cause readmission index
	30-day all-cause risk standardized readmission rate following heart failure hospitalization
	Severity: standardized ALOS—routine care
	Severity: standardized ALOS—special care
	Severity: standardized ALOS—deliveries
Patient safety, adult	Accidental puncture or laceration
	Death in low-mortality DRGs
	Iatrogenic pneumothorax
	Death among surgical inpatients with serious, treatable complications
	Bilateral cardiac catheterization rate
	Blood cultures performed within 24 hours before or 24 hours after hospital arrival for patients who were transferred or admitted to intensive care unit (ICU) within 24 hours of hospital arrival
	Congestive heart failure mortality
	Hip fracture mortality rate
	Transfusion reaction, age 18 years and older
Patient safety, pediatrics	Accidental puncture or laceration
	Decubitus ulcer
	Iatrogenic pneumothorax in non-neonates
	Transfusion reaction, age under 18 years
Pediatrics	Pediatric ICU (PICU) severity-adjusted length of stay
	PICU unplanned readmission rate
	Review of unplanned PICU readmissions
	Home management plan-of-care document given to patient or caregiver
	Pediatric heart surgery mortality
	Pediatric heart surgery volume
	PICU pain assessment on admission
	PICU periodic pain assessment
	PICU standardized mortality ratio
Surgery and anesthesia	Abdominal aortic aneurysm volume
	Abdominal aortic aneurysm repair mortality rate
	Esophageal resection mortality rate
	Esophageal resection volume
	Incidental appendectomy in the elderly rate
	Pancreatic resection mortality rate
	Pancreatic resection volume
	Postoperative wound dehiscence, age under 18 years
	Postoperative wound dehiscence, age 18 years and older
	Foreign body left after procedure, age under 18 years
	Foreign body left in during procedure, 18 years and older
	Failure to rescue—inhospital mortality
	Failure to rescue—30-day mortality

(continued)

Table 2-9 Consensus Standards for Quality of Hospital Care (*continued*)

Domain	Measure
Venous thromboembolism (VTE)	VTE prophylaxis ICU VTE prophylaxis VTE patients with anticoagulation overlap therapy VTE patients—unfractionated heparin dosages/platelet count monitoring by protocol (or nomogram) VTE discharge instructions Incidence of potentially preventable VTE

Reprinted from National Quality Forum. National Quality Forum Endorses Consensus Standards for Quality of Hospital Care: Patient Safety in Hospitals Focus of 48 NQF-Endorsed Measures; 2012. www.qualityforum.org/Projects/h/Hospital_Care_Performance_(2002)/Hospital_Care__Performance_Evaluation_Framework.aspx. Copyright 2012 by National Quality Forum, with permission.

proactive in their pursuit of quality and safety versus to being reactive; to imagine what could go wrong and correct any risk factors before errors occur. FMEA includes review of the following:

- Steps in the process
- Failure modes (What could go wrong?)
- Failure causes (Why would the failure happen?)
- Failure effects (What would be the consequences of each failure?).[91(¶1)]

FMEA and Healthcare FMEA are fully described in detail in *Performance and Process Improvement*.

Root Cause Analysis

Organizations use RCA to determine the cause of a variation in a process. Human, environmental, equipment, policy, and leadership system factors are explored in the analysis. The OPSC has developed an exceptional RCA Toolkit.[114]

It provides a framework for investigating adverse incidents and can be applied in any healthcare setting.

Organizations developing and maintaining robust healthcare safety programs are committed to the process of ongoing risk identification and prevention. Staff in these organizations are encouraged to identify potential errors and report any "near misses" or "close calls" or "good catches" that occur. Even when an event is not considered "reviewable," the HRO conduct RCAs on these identified risks to prevent similar events in the future.

The National Patient Safety Foundation (NPSF) developed a definitive guide on conducting RCAs.[115] These guidelines have been endorsed by TJC and other public and private patient safety organizations. The guide provides teams with effective techniques to conduct comprehensive systematic reviews to develop strong and sustainable actions to prevent future occurrence. See FIGURE 2-5 for the *NPSF Root Cause Analysis and Action (RCA²) Process*.

RCA is described further in *Performance and Process Improvement* and *Health Data Analytics*.

Table 2-10 Consensus Standards Related to Disclosure of Error or Injury

Safe Practice 7: Disclosure Following serious unanticipated outcomes, including those that are clearly caused by systems failures, the patient and, as appropriate, the family should receive timely, transparent, and clear communication concerning what is known about the event.[74]	• The types of serious unanticipated outcomes addressed by this practice include, at a minimum, sentinel events, serious reportable events, and any other unanticipated outcomes involving harm that require the provision of substantial additional care (such as diagnostic tests, therapeutic interventions, or increased length of stay) or that cause the loss of limb or function lasting seven days or longer. • Organizations must have formal processes in place for disclosing unanticipated outcomes, reporting events to those responsible for patient safety, including external organizations where applicable, and identifying and mitigating risks and hazards. • The governance and administrative leadership should ensure that such information is systematically used for performance improvement by the organization. Policies and procedures should incorporate continuous quality improvement techniques and provide for annual reviews and updates. • Adherence to the practice and participation with the support system is expected and may be considered as part of credentialing.

(*continued*)

Table 2-10 Consensus Standards Related to Disclosure of Error or Injury (*continued*)

Applicable Clinical Care Settings	

Applicable Clinical Care Settings
 	
This practice is applicable to CMS care settings, to include ambulatory, ambulatory surgical center, emergency room, dialysis facility, home care, home health services/agency, hospice, inpatient service/hospital, outpatient hospital, and skilled nursing facility.
	Communication with patients, their families and caregivers, should include or be characterized by the following:
	
	• the "facts"—an explicit statement about what happened that includes an explanation of the implications of the unanticipated outcome for the patient's future health, an explanation of why the event occurred, and information about measures taken for its preventability;
	
	• empathic communication of the "facts," a skill that should be developed and practiced in healthcare organizations;
	
	• an explicit and empathic expression of regret that the outcome was not as expected (e.g., "I am sorry this has happened");
	
	• a commitment to investigate and as possible prevent future occurrences by collecting the facts about the event and providing them to the organization's patient safety leaders, including those in governance positions;
	
	• feedback of the results of the investigation, including whether or not it resulted from an error or systems failure, provided in sufficient detail to support informed decision-making by the patient;
	
	• "timeliness"—the initial conversation with the patient and/or family occurs within 24 hours, whenever possible. Early and subsequent follow-up conversations occur, to maintain the relationship and to provide information as it becomes available;
	
	• an apology from the patient's licensed independent practitioner (LIP) and/or an administrative leader should be offered if the investigation reveals the adverse outcome clearly was caused by unambiguous errors or systems failures;
	
	• emotional support for patients and their families provided by trained caregivers should be provided;
	
	• a disclosure and improvement support system should be established and maintained to provide the following to caregivers and staff that includes
	
	  ○ emotional support for caregivers and administrators involved in such events provided by trained caregivers in the immediate post-event period that may extend for weeks afterward,
	
	  ○ education and skill building regarding the concepts, tools, and resources that produce *optimal* results from this practice, centered on systems improvement rather than blame, and with a special emphasis on creating a just culture,
	
	  ○ 24-hour availability of advisory support to caregivers and staff to facilitate rapid responses to serious unanticipated outcomes, including the provision of "just-in-time" coaching and emotional support, and
	
	  ○ Education of caregivers regarding the importance and technique of disclosure to care teams of error or adverse events as they happen;
	
	• healthcare organizations should implement a procedure to ensure and document that all LIPs are provided with a detailed description of the organization's program for responding to adverse events, including the full disclosure of error(s) that may have caused or contributed to patient harm. This is done with the expectation that the healthcare organizations and/or the LIPs will provide this information to their individual medical malpractice liability carriers in the event that they are provided liability coverage from entities outside of the organization. All new employees should also receive this information;
	
	• a process should be in place to consider providing information to a Patient Safety Organization that would provide a patient safety evaluation program to protect privileged and confidential information; and
	
	• a process should be in place to consider early remediation and the waiving of billing for care services provided during the care episode and for subsequent treatment if the event was due to unambiguous systems failures or human error.

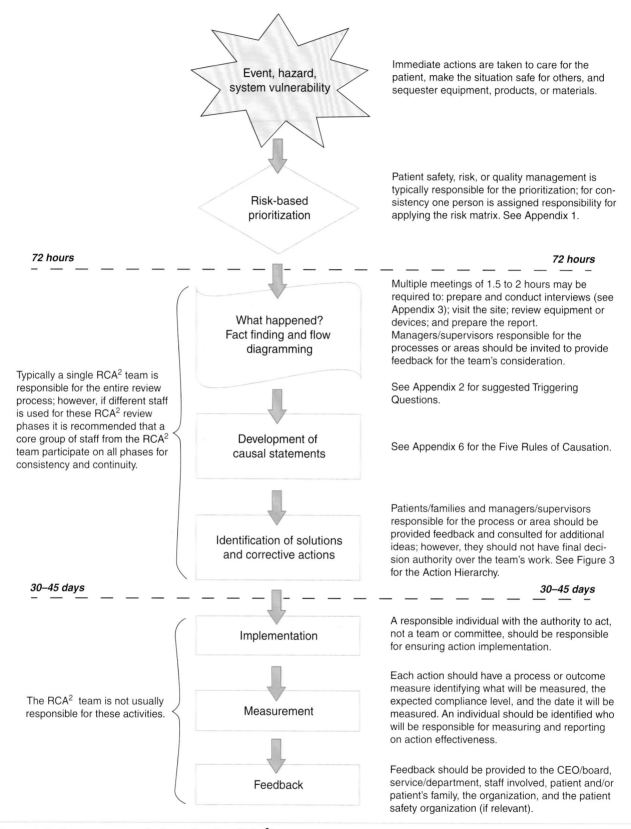

Immediate actions are taken to care for the patient, make the situation safe for others, and sequester equipment, products, or materials.

Event, hazard, system vulnerability

Risk-based prioritization

Patient safety, risk, or quality management is typically responsible for the prioritization; for consistency one person is assigned responsibility for applying the risk matrix. See Appendix 1.

72 hours   *72 hours*

What happened? Fact finding and flow diagramming

Multiple meetings of 1.5 to 2 hours may be required to: prepare and conduct interviews (see Appendix 3); visit the site; review equipment or devices; and prepare the report. Managers/supervisors responsible for the processes or areas should be invited to provide feedback for the team's consideration.

Typically a single RCA^2 team is responsible for the entire review process; however, if different staff is used for these RCA^2 review phases it is recommended that a core group of staff from the RCA^2 team participate on all phases for consistency and continuity.

See Appendix 2 for suggested Triggering Questions.

Development of causal statements

See Appendix 6 for the Five Rules of Causation.

Identification of solutions and corrective actions

Patients/families and managers/supervisors responsible for the process or area should be provided feedback and consulted for additional ideas; however, they should not have final decision authority over the team's work. See Figure 3 for the Action Hierarchy.

30–45 days   *30–45 days*

Implementation

A responsible individual with the authority to act, not a team or committee, should be responsible for ensuring action implementation.

The RCA^2 team is not usually responsible for these activities.

Measurement

Each action should have a process or outcome measure identifying what will be measured, the expected compliance level, and the date it will be measured. An individual should be identified who will be responsible for measuring and reporting on action effectiveness.

Feedback

Feedback should be provided to the CEO/board, service/department, staff involved, patient and/or patient's family, the organization, and the patient safety organization (if relevant).

Figure 2-5 Root cause analysis and action (RCA^2) process. (Reprinted from *RCA²: Root Cause Analyses and Actions to Prevent Harm*. Used with permission of the Institute for Healthcare Improvement (IHI), copyright © 2015.) Appendices referenced in this figure can be found in the original NPSF document.

Red Rules

Another safety practice—Red Rules—is used by highly reliable industries such as aviation and manufacturing, sparking interest for use in healthcare.[116,117] Red Rules are those that must be followed to the letter. The most important aspect of a Red Rule is to empower all workers to speak up when a rule is not being followed and to *stop the line*, regardless of their position in the organization.[118,119]

When properly implemented, Red Rules foster a culture of safety because frontline workers will know they can stop the line when they notice potential hazards. The most important aspect of a Red Rule is its ability to "empower any worker to speak up when the rule is not being followed and to stop the line, regardless of rank or seniority."[119(p2)] ISMP[119] outlines what differentiates a Red Rule from other crucial rules such as policies and procedures:

- It must be possible and desirable for everyone to follow a Red Rule every time in a process under all circumstances (Red Rules do not contain verbiage such as "except when . . ." or "each breach will be assessed for appropriateness").
- Anyone who notices the breach of the Rule has the authority and responsibility to stop further progress of patient care while protecting the patient or healthcare worker from harm.
- Managers and other leaders (including the board of trustees) always support the work stoppage, immediate rectification of the problem, and addressing the underlying reason for breaking the rule.
- People breaching the Red Rule are given an opportunity to support their behavioral choices and are then judged fairly based on the reasons for breaking the rule, regardless of rank and experience.
- There are few Red Rules, and they must be well understood and memorable.[119(¶7)]

Healthcare scenarios for which Red Rules can be beneficial include patient identification (using two identifiers before administering tests of any kind), sponge-count reconciliation, timeouts before an invasive procedure, timely alarm response, and correct labeling of specimens.

Newer to healthcare quality and safety, there is a mixed reception of Red Rules. Red Rules are part of a just culture although the way they are deployed could impact how they are received by affected personnel. There are circumstances where they are experienced as blaming and punitive, which is not aligned with a just culture. The way that Red Rules are deployed may not support trust and transparency. Jones and O'Connor[120] examined four measures of patient safety culture among two groups of hospitals that completed the AHRQ Hospital Survey on Patient Safety Culture and compared hospitals that did or did not implement Red Rules as a patient safety strategy. The four measures were (1) staff perceptions of safety; (2) frequency of events reported; (3) number of events reported; and (4) staff perceptions of no punitive response. The study found that there were no differences in the four measures between those hospitals who used Red Rules and those who did not. The authors did suggest that Red Rules can be effective as part of a comprehensive strategy to improve patient safety when used within a commitment-based management style.

Red Rules can be used as a communication tool to support staff in following safety rules rather than a disciplinary action. If misused or poorly supported, they will not be effective and may even introduce patient risks if systems and processes are not in place to facilitate adherence to the Red Rule.[118]

Safety Checklists

A checklist is an algorithmic, evidence-based listing of actions to be performed with the goal of "no step forgotten." Grounded in human factors engineering, checklists can shape the organizational and systematic thinking and behaviors in healthcare delivery. Checklists are found to

- improve communication,
- strengthen adherence with guidelines,
- improve human factors,
- reduce the incidence of adverse events, and
- decrease mortality and morbidity.[121]

Patient safety checklists "allow complex pathways of care to function with high reliability by giving users the opportunity to pause and take stock of their actions before proceeding to the next step."[122(¶1)] Checklists can be developed for internal processes (surgical checklist) or can be consumer-focused.[123] Surgical checklists are the most commonly used, but other checklists are developed for safe childbirth, trauma care, and Pandemic H1N1[122] and other patient safety events, such as blood clots and central line–associated blood stream infections. Recently, the CDC[124] released its *Checklist for Core Elements of Hospital Antibiotic Stewardship Programs*, which is recommended for facilities to systematically assess the core key elements, actions to ensure optimal antibiotic prescribing, and limiting the overuse and misuse of antibiotics.

Checklists are helpful in preparing, implementing, monitoring, and evaluating workforce and environmental safety. Healthcare services can be directly or indirectly provided to individuals in a variety of settings (e.g., hospitals, clinics, emergency departments, home health, and skilled nursing facilities). There are many health and safety hazards that workers face across the different settings including blood-borne pathogens, potential drug exposures, respiratory hazards, ergonomic hazards, and workplace violence. There are accreditation standards, regulations and state, federal and local laws governing workplace safety. Checklists can support an organization's workforce and environmental safety efforts. FIGURE 2-6 offers an example for blood-borne pathogens in residential care.

The following checklist is designed to assist with determining which OSHA standards apply to your practice/facility and assessing your current state of compliance. It includes the most common hazards found in residential facilities. However, there are a number of other potential safety and health hazards were not addressed. If the following hazards exist in your facility, please refer to OSHA's Compliance Assistance eTool for long-term care facilities (https://www.osha.gov/SLTC/etools/nursinghome/index.html), or contact your state's OSHA Consultation Program for assistance:

- Ergonomic Hazards associated with patient handling;
- Slips, trips, and falls;
- Influenza;
- Tuberculosis;
- Emergency response hazards; and
- Latex allergies.

Completed	In Progress	Not Started	
The facility has workplace policies in place to protect employees from occupational exposure to blood and other potentially infectious materials (OPIM). These policies must include:			
			Practicing universal precautions
			Using safety engineered needles and sharps
			Consideration and documentation of safety engineered sharps on an annual basis, including documented input from non-managerial staff with occupational exposure
			Having sharps containers as close as possible to the immediate area where sharps are used, and routinely inspecting to ensure that they do not become overfilled
			Place sharps containers in shower rooms
			Disposable razors are placed in sharps container once used
			Washing exposed skin following contact, and washing hands after glove removal
			Having eyewash stations located within 10 seconds of where exposure is likely to occur
			Using personal protective equipment (PPE) whenever exposure is possible. PPE should be provided at no cost to the employees, and should be suitably sized and impervious
			Maintaining a sufficient supply of protective equipment necessary for day-to-day operations
			Creating and following a documented housekeeping schedule for cleaning and disinfecting equipment and work surfaces that may become contaminated with blood or OPIM. The schedule should include frequency of activities and the registered disinfectants being used
			Eating, drinking, smoking, applying cosmetics or lip balm, and handling contact lenses are prohibited in work areas where there is a reasonable likelihood of occupational exposure
			Storing food and drinks only in areas where blood or OPIM are not present
			Offering Hepatitis B vaccinations to all employees with exposure to blood or OPIM
			Maintaining vaccination and treatment records or declination forms in the employees' medical file in a secure and locked location.

Figure 2-6 **Controlling hazards in residential care facilities checklist: control of exposure to blood-borne pathogens (29 CFR 1910.1030).** (Reprinted with permission from Occupational Safety & Health Consultation Program, Georgia Technical and Research Institute. Controlling hazards in residential care facilities checklist. *Occup Saf Health Program.* www.oshainfo.gatech.edu. Accessed January 17, 2017. Copyright © 2016 Georgia Tech Research Corporation. All rights reserved.)

The benefit of using checklists was cemented with the publication of the "Keystone Initiative" findings by Pronovost in the *New England Journal of Medicine*. This project focused on the reduction of catheter-related bloodstream infection using a checklist to ensure adherence to infection-control practices—handwashing, using full-barrier precautions during the insertion of central venous catheters, cleaning the skin with chlorhexidine, avoiding the femoral site if possible, and removing unnecessary catheters. This project garnered success by reducing and sustaining rates of catheter-related bloodstream infection that was maintained throughout the 18-month study period.[125]

Gawande[126,127] advanced the thinking about the use of checklists in healthcare. The regimentation offered by checklists can reduce risk and save lives in complex situations. Healthcare is highly specialized. Couple complexity with specialization, the routine might be overlooked and steps skipped in processes. Consistent use and improvement of checklists may offer healthcare providers a tool to focus less of their efforts on the routine and more on the difficult.

There is resistance to the adoption of checklists in healthcare. Based on work by Treadwell, Lucas and Tsou,[128] barriers to implementation can fall into these categories:

1. Confusion regarding how to properly use the checklist, efficient workflow, access to resources, and individual beliefs and attitudes.
2. Workflow problems such as extra time, duplication of safety checks already routinely performed, and access to resources required to fulfill the checklist.
3. Individual attitudes of staff toward the checklist such as resistance to changing habits and interpersonal hierarchy (e.g., operating room).
4. Legal responsibility and RM.

Healthcare quality professionals can bring knowledge about the benefits of checklists as part of the organization's overall quality management system. Examples of sources include ISO9001:2015 and the Baldrige Excellence Framework.

See *Performance and Process Improvement* for more discussion on tools.

Evaluating and Improving Patient Safety

Healthcare quality professionals work collaboratively with others to improve compliance with standards set forth by TJC National Patient Safety Goals (NPSGs), Leapfrog Safe Practices, NQF-endorsed measures, and federal government-vetted measures (e.g., AHRQ, National Health Safety Network). Standards for patient safety practices include recommendations to improve accuracy in patient identification, effectiveness of communication among caregivers, precautions when using high-alert medications, and surgery

safeguards.[129] Proposed solutions to improving patient safety range from making electronic health information readily available to providers and consumers to inviting patients to make decisions collaboratively with their care providers.[28,130]

When thinking about meeting or exceeding standards, part of the healthcare quality professional's work is to identify what interventions to use and their effects—some small things can lead to big and sustainable change. There are important resources to consider, such as systems for collecting reliable and valid data, selecting measures that provide the information for evaluation, and focusing on relevant high-volume problem prone areas such as safe medication practices. As healthcare quality professionals aim to improve safety for the patient, organization, or system of care, they might consider the following for launching routine monitoring and evaluation of activities and specific projects:

- Establishing the plan to evaluate the actual impact on health outcomes, quality of care, and patient safety due to the effort (patient, healthcare personnel, clinical workflow, other relevant indicators);
- Feasibility, usability, and possibilities when identifying the target population and/or problem to be addressed;
- Clearly defining the quantifiable impact of the effort (e.g., number of incidents, rates of occurrence) and who is affected (e.g., patients, clinicians, department, unit);
- Determining appropriate tools to use (e.g., RCA, FMEA, other Lean tools); and
- Identifying mechanisms to share results and efforts resulting in improved safety (e.g., board reports, enterprise-wide communications, patient materials).

As part of developing the patient safety plan, healthcare organizations can conduct a thorough analysis of where patients and healthcare personnel are at risk for errors. In doing so, systems and processes can be hardwired. Actively engage employees in analyzing processes to ensure the organization achieves desired outcomes. Look for the differences in mindsets and close the gap by removing silos. Cross-functional objectives will promote collaboration in developing the plan.

Patient safety plans are often integrated in quality or performance improvement program plans. These are five components of an effective patient safety system:

1. monitoring of progress and maintenance of vigilance,
2. knowledge of the epidemiology of patient safety risks and hazards,
3. development of effective practices and tools,
4. building infrastructure for effective practices, and
5. achieving broader adoption of effective practices.[129(p4)]

Two exemplars shown here are University of California, Los Angeles (UCLA) Health System and Intermountain

Healthcare. The UCLA Health System's Performance Improvement & Patient Safety Plan goals include the following:

- Achieve a patient safety conscious environment throughout the facility.
- Improve the reporting of medical errors by establishing a policy focusing on corrective actions through staff education for those reporting their errors, rather than punitive or disciplinary actions.
- Implement confidential electronic event reporting process that includes documentation of follow-up and reporting processes.
- Expand the implementation of evidence-based practices.
- Monitor hospital-wide indicators for established areas of focus.
- Reduce the number of medication errors.
- Monitor patient safety indicators related to an area's specific "Scope of Service."
- Conduct a proactive risk assessment utilizing the FMEA methodology.
- Monitor and improve areas identified through patient satisfaction surveys.[131(p4)]

Intermountain Healthcare's Quality & Patient Safety Plan goals include the following:

- Attain optimal patient outcomes and patient and family experience.
- Support an engaged and safe workforce.
- Enhance appropriate utilization.
- Minimize risks and hazards of care.
- Develop and share best practices.[132(p6)]

When deploying the plan, various statistical process control and quality improvement tools can be used in patient safety initiatives. Statistical process control techniques and performance improvement tools are applicable to the deployment of patient safety practices throughout a healthcare enterprise. The healthcare quality professional serves an essential role in helping the organization determine if a safety issue in an organization is an infrequent event or endemic. Prioritizing functions should be utilized as part of the safety program.

See *Health Data Analytics* and *Performance and Process Improvement* for more principles, practices and tools.

Health Information

Health IT holds the promise of making healthcare services safer and offers clinical decision support through electronic health records (EHR). If health IT is to work, the healthcare consumer must be at the center of the healthcare system and be empowered with their personal healthcare data. Often these questions are asked. Is health IT easy to use? How quickly does it process information? How functional is it? How can it help me? If health IT is to be effective in the care setting, it needs to be integrated with the patient and clinical workflow and aligned with available resources and the expectations of the end users.

Leadership plays a critical role in the adoption of health IT (EHRs, personal health records, and e-prescribing systems) and ensuring risks associated with heath IT are avoided altogether or mitigated. TJC provides a framework for maintaining a culture of safety vis-à-vis health IT by

1. collective mindfulness focused on identifying, reporting, analyzing, and reducing health IT-related hazardous conditions, close calls, or errors;
2. comprehensive and systematic analysis of each adverse event causing harm to determine if health IT contributed to the event in any way; and
3. shared involvement and responsibility for the safety of health IT among the healthcare organization, clinicians, and vendors/developers.[133(pp2-3)]

EHRs typically include four core components: electronic clinical documentation, results reporting and management, e-prescribing, and clinical decision support. Over time, other functionalities such as barcoding and patient engagement tools were added. Health IT and interoperable systems are requisites for healthcare delivery in the 21st century. In 2012, an IOM report examined the state of the art in system safety and opportunities to build safer systems and concluded as follows:

- Safety is an emergent property of a larger system that accounts for not just the software but also how it is used by clinicians.
- The "sociotechnical system" includes technology (software, hardware), people (clinicians, patients), processes (workflow), organization (capacity, decisions about how health IT is applied, incentives), and the external environment (regulations, public opinion).
- Safer implementation and use of health IT is a complex, dynamic process that requires a shared responsibility between vendors and healthcare organizations.
- Poor user-interface design, poor workflow, and complex data interfaces threaten patient safety.
- Lack of system interoperability is a barrier to improving clinical decisions and patient safety.
- Constant, ongoing commitment to safety—from acquisition to implementation and maintenance—is needed to achieve safer, more effective care.[134(ppS2-S4)]

EHRs have the potential to capture data for purposes of patient safety performance and improvement. However, some say not enough evidence exists to support the link between the EHR and patient safety[135] and may have unintended consequences as follows:

- Workarounds and alarm fatigue such as "delayed response time to alarms, disabled alarms, volumes set to inaudible, parameters limits set to unsafe zones, or alarms paused without a thoughtful consideration of the warning message."[136(pE1)]

- Incorrect patient matching where some or all data retrieved via health information exchange (HIE) relate to a different (and incorrect) patient. Such errors can happen because of flawed matching algorithms used for HIE.
- Data quality issues, such as incomplete patient data, duplicate patient records, or data entry errors, can propagate through HIE, increasing the potential for adverse safety events.
- Loss of data integrity during transmission. For example, if the HIE process alters the meaning of the data or errors in translation that occur between different systems, reflecting differences in vocabularies. If the HIE degrades EHR or other system performance, critical delays in accessing HIE data can result.[137]

TABLE 2-11 provides potential benefits and safety concerns of IT components commonly used in healthcare.

As part of national efforts to improve the use of health IT, the Nationwide Health Information Network (NHIN)

was established. The NHIN is comprised of standards, services, and a trust fabric that enables the secure exchange of health information over the Internet. This critical part of the national health IT agenda is that health information follows the consumer, is available for clinical decision-making, and supports appropriate use of healthcare information beyond direct patient care to public health. A key component of the technology strategy is providing a common platform for HIE across diverse entities, within communities and across the country, helping to achieve the goals of the Health Information Technology for Economic and Clinical Health Act.[138(p4)]

Free, open source software was developed to support local and national efforts to provide HIE. This kind of information exchange is critical for community-wide patient safety efforts as the NHIN will

- improve the coordination of care information among hospitals, laboratories, physician offices, pharmacies, and other providers;

Table 2-11 Potential Benefits and Safety Concerns of Health Information Technology (IT) Components

Computerized Provider Order Entry (CPOE) (e-Prescribing)
An electronic system that allows providers to record, store, retrieve, and modify orders (e.g., prescriptions, diagnostic testing, treatment, and/or radiology/imaging orders)

Potential Benefits	Safety Concerns

- Large increases in legible orders
- Shorter order turnaround times
- Lower relative risk of medication errors
- Higher percentage of patients who attain their treatment goals
	- Increases relative risk of medication errors
	- Increased ordering time
	- New opportunities for errors, such as
	  ○ fragmented displays preventing a coherent view of patients' medications,
	  ○ inflexible ordering formats generating wrong orders,
	  ○ function separation that facilitates double dosing, and
	  ○ incompatible orders
	- Disruptions in workflow

Clinical Decision Support (CDS)
Monitors and alerts clinicians of patient conditions, prescriptions, and treatment to provide evidence-based clinical suggestions to health professionals at the point of care

Potential Benefits	Safety Concerns

- Reductions in
  ○ relative risk of medication errors,
  ○ risk of toxic drug levels,
  ○ time to therapeutic stabilization,
  ○ management errors of resuscitating patients in adult trauma centers, and
  ○ prescriptions of nonpreferred medications
- Can effectively monitor and alert clinicians of adverse conditions
- Improve long-term treatment and increase the likelihood of achieving treatment goals
	- Rate of detecting drug–drug interactions varies widely among different vendors
	- Increases in mortality rate
	- High override rate of computer generated alerts (alert fatigue)

(continued)

Table 2-11 Potential Benefits and Safety Concerns of Health Information Technology (IT) Components (*continued*)

Barcoding

Barcoding can be used to track medications, orders, and other healthcare products. It can also be used to verify patient identification and dosage

Potential Benefits	*Safety Concerns*

• Significant reductions in relative risk of medication errors associated with
   ○ transcription,
   ○ dispensing, and
   ○ administration errors
	• Introduction of workarounds; for example, clinicians can
	   ○ scan medications and patient identification without visually checking to see if the medication, dosing, and patient identification are correct;
	   ○ attach patient identification bar codes to another object instead of the patient; and
	   ○ scan orders and medications of multiple patients at once instead of doing it each time the medication is dispensed.

Patient Engagement Tools

Tools such as patient portals, smartphone applications, e-mail, and interactive kiosks, which enable patients to participate in their healthcare treatment

Potential Benefits	*Safety Concerns*

• Reduction in hospitalization rates in children
• Increases in patients' knowledge of treatment and illnesses
	• Reliability of data entered by
	   ○ patients,
	   ○ families,
	   ○ friends, or
	   ○ unauthorized users.

This table is not intended to be an exhaustive list of all potential benefits and safety concerns associated with health IT. It represents the most common potential benefits and safety concerns. Reprinted from Institute of Medicine, Committee on Patient Safety and Health Information Technology. Health IT and Patient Safety: Building Safer Systems for Better Care; 2012. Copyright 2012 by National Academies Press, with permission.

• ensure appropriate information is available at the time and place of care;

• ensure consumer health information is secure and confidential;

• give consumers new capabilities to manage and control their personal health records, as well as providing access to their health information from EHRs and other sources;

• reduce risks from medical errors and support the delivery of appropriate, evidence-based medical care; and

• lower healthcare costs resulting from inefficiencies, medical errors, and incomplete patient information.[139]

An exemplar of this strategy is the implementation of a Virtual Lifetime Electronic Record (VLER) by the U.S. Department of Veterans Affairs (VA). The VLER program ensures an EHR for each veteran that is accessible, with consent, by public and private sector healthcare providers. The first pilot of this program occurred in San Diego, CA, between the VA, the U.S. Department of Defense, and Kaiser Permanente. VLER has advanced HIEs nationally and the data sharing capability was deployed in 2013.[140] Another more recent example is the Delaware Health Information Network, a public–private partnership that includes all hospitals, skilled nursing facilities and laboratories in the state, 95% of its imaging centers, and 62% of the state's pharmacies.[141]

Healthcare quality professionals work with others in the organization to use health IT to mitigate risks, manage care, and reduce preventable harm. As work is undertaken, consider the available tools to organize and support initiatives. For example, patient identification-related events present risk for patient care. The partnership for Health IT Patient Safety is a multi-stakeholder group working to identify how to optimize health IT for safer care. The partnership currently offers two toolkits—patient identification and cut and paste. The *Health IT Safe Practices: The Safe Use of Health IT for Patient Identification* toolkit offers a framework of eight safety practice recommendations using IDENTIFY—Include, Detect, Evaluate, Normalize, Tailor, Innovate, Follow-up, and Yield.[142] This model is useful when looking at the independent and interacting effects of behaviors and technology. The partnership descriptions for each practice is shown in FIGURE 2-7.

Also, see *Health Data Analytics* for more discussion of health information.

Measurement and Improvement

Continuous measurement and monitoring can yield important insights about the impact of interventions and improvement projects on patient safety. These insights can be leveraged

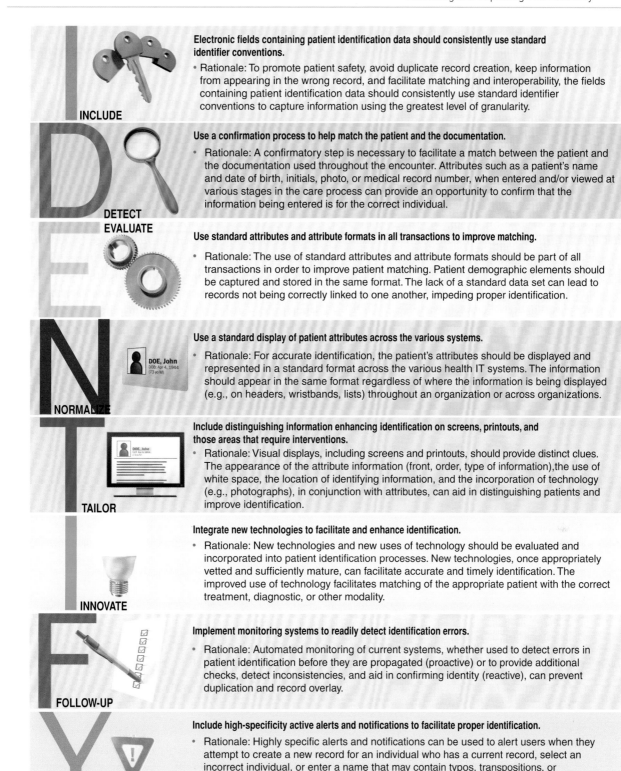

INCLUDE

Electronic fields containing patient identification data should consistently use standard identifier conventions.

- Rationale: To promote patient safety, avoid duplicate record creation, keep information from appearing in the wrong record, and facilitate matching and interoperability, the fields containing patient identification data should consistently use standard identifier conventions to capture information using the greatest level of granularity.

DETECT
EVALUATE

Use a confirmation process to help match the patient and the documentation.

- Rationale: A confirmatory step is necessary to facilitate a match between the patient and the documentation used throughout the encounter. Attributes such as a patient's name and date of birth, initials, photo, or medical record number, when entered and/or viewed at various stages in the care process can provide an opportunity to confirm that the information being entered is for the correct individual.

Use standard attributes and attribute formats in all transactions to improve matching.

- Rationale: The use of standard attributes and attribute formats should be part of all transactions in order to improve patient matching. Patient demographic elements should be captured and stored in the same format. The lack of a standard data set can lead to records not being correctly linked to one another, impeding proper identification.

NORMALIZE

Use a standard display of patient attributes across the various systems.

- Rationale: For accurate identification, the patient's attributes should be displayed and represented in a standard format across the various health IT systems. The information should appear in the same format regardless of where the information is being displayed (e.g., on headers, wristbands, lists) throughout an organization or across organizations.

TAILOR

Include distinguishing information enhancing identification on screens, printouts, and those areas that require interventions.

- Rationale: Visual displays, including screens and printouts, should provide distinct clues. The appearance of the attribute information (front, order, type of information),the use of white space, the location of identifying information, and the incorporation of technology (e.g., photographs), in conjunction with attributes, can aid in distinguishing patients and improve identification.

INNOVATE

Integrate new technologies to facilitate and enhance identification.

- Rationale: New technologies and new uses of technology should be evaluated and incorporated into patient identification processes. New technologies, once appropriately vetted and sufficiently mature, can facilitate accurate and timely identification. The improved use of technology facilitates matching of the appropriate patient with the correct treatment, diagnostic, or other modality.

FOLLOW-UP

Implement monitoring systems to readily detect identification errors.

- Rationale: Automated monitoring of current systems, whether used to detect errors in patient identification before they are propagated (proactive) or to provide additional checks, detect inconsistencies, and aid in confirming identity (reactive), can prevent duplication and record overlay.

YIELD

Include high-specificity active alerts and notifications to facilitate proper identification.

- Rationale: Highly specific alerts and notifications can be used to alert users when they attempt to create a new record for an individual who has a current record, select an incorrect individual, or enter a name that may contain typos, transpositions, or misspellings. Monitoring how alerts are used and providing direct feedback will improve proper identification.

Figure 2-7 Eight safe practices for patient identification. (Reprinted from ECRI Institute for Health IT Patient Safety. Eight safe practice recommendations; 2016. https://www.ecri.org/Resources/HIT/Patient%20ID/Recommendations_Patient_ID_Handout.pdf. p.1. Accessed April 19, 2017. Copyright © 2017 ECRI Institute Partnership for Health IT Patient Safety. www.ecri.org. 5200 Butler Pike, Plymouth Meeting, PA 19462. 610-825-6000.)

into the ongoing, sustainable action plan. Gathering and using real-time data will help the organization improve and protect patients from harm. Selected measures may relate to structure, process, outcomes, resource use, or composite of measure attributes. With the proliferation of reliable and valid safety measures, the healthcare quality professional can examine available measures and determine which will be the most meaningful to the organization's internal and external stakeholders.

There is no one single source for safety measures, so the healthcare quality professional can review available measures for the healthcare setting. The most logical place to start are measures from organizations that require certain measures for payment or accreditation. These measures may have been developed and validated by the sponsoring organization (e.g., NCQA and HEDIS) or are endorsed measures that are used by third-party payers or accreditation agencies (e.g., NQF). The following are possible sources of such measures.

The Joint Commission. TJC, through its accreditation standards and other activities, strives to help organizations achieve zero patient harm. TJC standards require the organization gather and analyze the data generated through standardized monitoring. Results are used to inform the goals and objectives of care, treatment, or services, and the outcomes of care, treatment, or services provided to the population served by aggregating and analyzing the data gathered through the standardized monitoring effort. The agency assists healthcare organizations in collecting and reporting performance improvement and accountability data through ORYX and Core Measure Sets.

The NPSGs are another way that TJC assists healthcare organizations and programs in the United States through accreditation surveys and continuous readiness. Currently, there are safety goals for ambulatory healthcare, behavioral healthcare, critical access hospitals, home care, hospitals, laboratories, nursing care centers, and office-based surgery.[143] **TABLE 2-12** describes examples of the current NPSGs for hospitals.

Table 2-12 **Examples of the National Patient Safety Goals**	
Goal 1. Improve the accuracy of patient identification	
Example	Use at least two patient identifiers to verify a patient's identity upon admission or transfer to another hospital or other care setting and prior to the administration of care.
Goal 2. Improve the effectiveness of communication among caregivers	
Example	Report critical results of tests on a timely basis by defining who should receive the results; who should receive the results when the ordering provider is not available, what results require timely and reliable communication, when the results should be actively reported to the ordering provider with explicit timeframes, how to notify the responsible provider, and how to design, support, and maintain the systems involved (Hanna et al., 2005).
Goal 3. Improve the safety of using medications	
Example	Maintain and communicate accurate patient medication information through medication reconciliation to avoid inadvertent inconsistencies across transitions in care by reviewing the patient's complete medication regimen at the time of care transitions (e.g., admission, transfer, discharge) (AHRQ, 2015).
Goal 7. Reduce the risk of healthcare-associated infections	
Example	Comply with current hand hygiene guidelines (i.e., Centers for Disease Control and Prevention [CDC] or current World Health Organization [WHO] hand hygiene guidelines).
Goal 15. The hospital identifies safety risks inherent in its patient population	
Example	Use a Zero Suicide approach to identify patients at risk for suicide by screening for suicidal thoughts or behaviors at admission or intake and complete a full risk assessment when a patient screens positive.
Universal Protocol for Preventing Wrong Site, Wrong Procedure, and Wrong Person Surgery	
Example	A time-out is performed before the procedure that includes the confirmation of the correct patient, correct side and site, agreement on the procedure to be performed, correct patient position, availability of needed equipment/supplies/implants, and the presence and review of relevant radiologic images (if applicable) (Feldman, 2008).

Adapted from Agency for Healthcare Research and Quality. Patient safety primer: Medication reconciliation; 2015. https://psnet.ahrq.gov/primers/primer/1/medication-reconciliation. Accessed May 17, 2017; Feldman DL. The inside of a time out. Cases & commentaries, WebM&M; 2008. https://psnet.ahrq.gov/webmm/case/177/the-inside-of-a-time-out. Accessed May 17, 2017; Hanna D, Griswold P, Leape LL, Bates DW. Communicating critical test results: safe practice recommendations. *J Qual Patient Saf.* 2005;31(2):68–80; The Joint Commission. National Patient Safety Goals effective January 2017. https://www.jointcommission.org/assets/1/6/NPSG_Chapter_HAP_Jan2017.pdf. Accessed April 27, 2017; World Health Organization. WHO draft guidelines for adverse event reporting and learning systems (Publication No. WHO/EIP/SPO/QPS/05.3); 2007. http://apps.who.int/iris/bitstream/10665/69797/1/WHO-EIP-SPO-QPS-05.3-eng.pdf. Accessed April 27, 2017; Zero Suicide. Zero Suicide Toolkit; 2015. http://zerosuicide.sprc.org/toolkit. Accessed May 17, 2017.

The Leapfrog Group. The Leapfrog Group's safe practices informed the development of 34 NQF-endorsed safety practices. These hospital practices, if implemented, reduce harm in several areas. The practices comprise elements related to leadership, care needs, information transfer and communication, medication management, HAIs, and specific care processes. On the 2016 Leapfrog Hospital Survey, 1,266 hospitals reported on C-sections, 987 reported mortality rates for surgeries, and 1,702 reported their Never Events policy.[144]

National Quality Forum. As a leader in patient safety, NQF is recognized as a voluntary consensus standards-setting organization as defined by the National Technology Transfer and Advancement Act of 1995 and Office of Management and Budget Circular A-119. Since 2002, NQF assembled a portfolio of more than 600 NQF-endorsed measures in use by both the private and public sectors for public reporting and quality improvement. Most notably, NQF accomplished the following:

- 2003: Endorsed a set of 30 practices for universal use in applicable clinical care settings to reduce the risk of harm to consumers.
- 2006: Undertook an update of the original set and endorsed practices with significantly expanded specifications, supporting literature, and guidance for implementation.
- 2009: Endorsed practices were updated to address pediatric imaging, organ donation, caring for caregivers, glycemic control, and falls prevention.

- 2010: Added evidence to the existing practices, and more direction was given to healthcare professionals for implementation and patient and family engagement.[157]

NQF has endorsed over 100 consensus standards with a focus on patient safety.[79] The NQF's consensus-setting efforts support the evaluation of patient safety using standardized performance measurement. The NQF also maintains the Quality Positioning System (QPS), which helps to select measures that might align with monitoring, reporting, and improvement interests.[145] **TABLE 2-13** presents the NQF Patient Safety Portfolio of Measures representing structure, process and outcomes.

Evaluating the Culture of Safety

How does an organization evaluate its progress and success in achieving a culture of safety? Safety culture is generally measured by patients and healthcare providers. Safety culture measures reflect teamwork training, executive walk rounds, and establishing unit-based safety teams. These have been associated with improvements in safety culture measures but have not yet linked to lower error rates. Other methods, such as "rapid response teams and structured communication methods such as SBAR, are being widely implemented to help address cultural issues such as rigid hierarchies and communication problems, but their effect on overall safety culture and error rates remains."[146] SBAR is an acronym for

Table 2-13 Portfolio of Patient Safety Measures

	Process	Outcome/Resource Use	Structure	Composite
Falls	2	4	–	–
Healthcare-associated infections	1	7	–	–
Medication safety	10	–	–	–
Mortality	–	4	–	–
Perioperative safety	–	6	–	–
Pressure ulcers	1	3	–	–
Venous thromboembolism	1	1	–	–
Workforce	–	–	2	1
General	2	5	–	2
TOTAL	17	30	2	3

Situation, Background, Assessment, Recommendation, which is a standardized tool used in healthcare settings to facilitate communication.

Surveys are the most common approach to evaluating the safety climate or safety culture. For the purposes of reporting on NQF Safe Practice 2: Culture Measurement, Feedback, and Intervention, hospitals must conduct a culture of safety survey of their employees within the past 24 months. The units surveyed must account for at least 50% of the aggregated care delivered to patients within the facility, and includes the high patient safety risk units or departments using a nationally recognized tool that has demonstrated validity, consistency, and reliability. When selecting a survey tool for the organization, the healthcare quality professional should consider the following:

- Alignment of survey with setting where survey will be administered.
- Nationally recognized survey that is determined valid and reliable.
- Survey supported by evidence from peer-reviewed literature.
- Respondent burden is minimized.
- Results offer information that is actionable.
- Benchmarking data are available.[147–149]

Validated surveys will have well-detailed methodology to assure a successful survey administration. Healthcare quality professionals should consider using a third-party vendor for the survey administration—the vendor can be a safe intermediary for data collection, ensure anonymity of respondents, and work with the organization to achieve higher response rates. Descriptions of more commonly used assessment and survey tools follow.

The Oro 2.0 High Reliability Organizational Assessment.
TJC Center for Transforming Health Care Oro 2.0 High Reliability Organizational Assessment consists of a series of questions for senior leaders to reflect upon and come to consensus on the organization's current high-reliability status. The Assessment looks at the organization's level of maturity and incorporates multiple domains across 14 areas of performance such as leadership commitment to achieving zero patient harm, how the safety culture is functioning, and the deployment of performance improvement tools. Per the Center, the Oro 2.0 accomplishes the following:

- Serves as a guiding force for transformation.
- Provides crucial information about strengths, opportunities, and potential investment strategies for achieving high performance.
- Can be repeated to assess the organization's progress in its high-reliability journey over time.[150]

All staff at accredited hospitals and critical access hospitals can access ORO 2.0 through the Joint Commission Center for Transforming Healthcare's website, or can be granted access through Joint Commission Connect.

Physician Practice Patient Safety Assessment.
When the IOM published *Crossing the Quality Chasm* in 2001, the extent of preventable medical errors was far reaching.[21] Many initiatives focus on inpatient care and fewer focus on other settings such as ambulatory or nursing home care. The Health Research and Educational Trust (HRET)—in partnership with the AHA, the Institute for Safe Medication Practices (ISMP), and the Medical Group Management Association and its certifying body, the American College of Medical Practice Executives—developed the Physician Practice Patient Safety Assessment (PPPSA) for the medical practice setting.[151] The PPPSA is an interactive self-assessment tool for evaluating medication safety, handoffs and transitions, surgery and invasive procedures, personnel qualifications and competency, practice management and culture, and patient education and communication. Healthcare quality professionals in ambulatory settings can use the PPPSA to

- gain specific ideas to improve patient safety,
- compare data to aggregate results for similar practices,
- enhance team's awareness of patient safety issues,
- heighten provider awareness of characteristics that make a practice safer,
- create a new reference point and baseline to enhance and support patient safety, and
- document successes and track progress.[152]

University of Texas Safety Attitudes Questionnaire.
This Safety Attitudes Questionnaire (SAQ) measures caregiver attitudes about six patient safety-related domains, allows organizations to compare themselves to others, prompt interventions to improve safety attitudes, and measure the effectiveness of these interventions. The SAQ domain scales are teamwork climate, job satisfaction, perceptions of management, safety climate, working conditions, and stress recognition.[148,153] An organization can use the tool to gather baseline data and measure the effectiveness of change and the adoption of patient safety practices.

Patient Safety Climate in Healthcare Organizations.
The Patient Safety Climate in Healthcare Organizations survey is designed to assess the healthcare workforce's perception about the culture of safety in their organization. It assesses different aspects of safety including contributions to safety climate from the hospital, work unit, interpersonal and other. Contributing factors are measured including engagement, resources, emphasis on patient safety, unit support,

unit-level factors (e.g., safety norms, recognition, support, and collective learning). The fear of shame and fear of blame and punishment subscales are considered interpersonal contributions to safety climate. The provision of safe care is also examined.[149,154]

AHRQ Surveys on Patient Safety Culture.

As part of its goal to support a culture of patient safety and quality improvement in the nation's healthcare system, AHRQ developed its patient safety culture assessment tools for healthcare. In 2004, AHRQ developed and distributed a valid and reliable safety culture survey, the Hospital Survey on Patient Safety Culture,[155] to help hospitals, nursing homes, and ambulatory outpatient medical offices evaluate the culture of safety in their institutions. In 2008, AHRQ

released its first benchmarking report based upon an analysis of data from 400 voluntary participating hospitals. Healthcare organizations can use these surveys to track changes in patient safety over time and evaluate the effects of patient safety interventions.[34]

The *Hospital Survey on Patient Safety Culture: 2016 User Comparative Database Report* is a compilation of the most recent survey findings. Based on data provided voluntarily by hospitals, the report provides results hospitals can use as benchmarks to establish a culture of safety in comparison to similar hospitals or hospital units. The survey evaluates patient safety issues, medical errors, and event reporting. It includes 42 items that measure 12 areas, or composites, of patient safety culture. Each of the 12 composites or areas and their definitions are described in **TABLE 2-14**.

Table 2-14 Patient Safety Culture Composites and Definitions

Patient Safety Culture Composite	Definition: *The extent to which . . .*
Communication openness	Staff freely speak up if they see something that may negatively affect a patient and feel free to question those with more authority.
Feedback and communication about error	Staff are informed about errors that happen, given feedback about changes implemented, and discuss ways to prevent errors.
Frequency of events reported	Mistakes of the following types are reported: (1) mistakes caught and corrected before affecting the patient, (2) mistakes with no potential to harm the patient, and (3) mistakes that could harm the patient but do not.
Handoffs and transitions	Important patient care information is transferred across hospital units and during shift changes.
Management support for patient safety	Hospital management provides a work climate that promotes patient safety and shows that patient safety is a top priority.
Nonpunitive response to error	Staff feel their mistakes and event reports are not held against them and that mistakes are not kept in their personnel file.
Organizational learning—continuous improvement	Mistakes have led to positive changes and changes are evaluated for effectiveness.
Overall perceptions of patient safety	Procedures and systems are good at preventing errors, and there is a lack of patient safety problems.
Staffing	There are enough staff to handle the workload, and work hours are appropriate to provide the best care for patients.
Supervisor/manager expectations and actions promoting safety	Supervisors/managers consider staff suggestions for improving patient safety, praise staff for following patient safety procedures, and do not overlook patient safety problems.
Teamwork across units	Hospital units cooperate and coordinate with one another to provide the best care for patients.
Teamwork within units	Staff support each other, treat each other with respect, and work together as a team.

From Agency for Healthcare Research and Quality. *Hospital Survey on Patient Safety Culture: 2016 User comparative database report; 2016:3-4.* http://www.ahrq.gov/sites/default/files/wysiwyg/professionals/quality-patient-safety/patientsafetyculture/hospital/2016/2016_hospitalsops_report_pt1.pdf

In 2016, 680 hospitals submitted survey data, representing 447,584 staff respondents representing medicine, surgery, and other areas. The results reflected progress in teamwork, management expectations around promoting patient safety, and organizational learning. However, continued potential for improvement in most hospitals was found for patient safety practices, particularly nonpunitive response to reporting, hand offs and transitions, and workload. Areas of strength are shown in **TABLE 2-15** and issues presenting the most potential for improvement are shown in Table 2-8.

Validated provider surveys from AHRQ's portfolio of *Patient Safety Culture Surveys* survey instruments include the following:

- Hospital Survey on Patient Safety Culture
- Medical Office Survey on Patient Safety Culture
- Nursing Home Survey on Patient Safety Culture
- Community Pharmacy Survey on Patient Safety Culture
- Ambulatory Surgery Center Survey on Patient Safety Culture.

These surveys ask providers to rate the safety culture in their unit and the whole organization. Annual benchmarking data are available in AHRQ's comprehensive reports.

Monitoring Safe Medication Practices

Even though many treatment procedures involve some risk, by far the most common errors occur with the use of medications. The frequency of medication use in the United States is startling. More than four out of five U.S. adults take at least one medication (prescription or over-the-counter drug, vitamin, mineral, or herbal supplement), and almost one-third take at least five different medications. Further, it is estimated the extra medical costs of treating medication-related injuries amounts to $3.5 billion per year.[156] In healthcare facilities, most errors occur in the prescribing and administration stages of medication therapy. Further, it is estimated that it costs the US $289 billion per year for medication non-adherence.[157]

The patient safety culture has its foundation an atmosphere devoid of blame. An organization uses systematic ways to welcome the reporting of medication errors. Because 85% of errors are the result of system failures and traditionally only 15% are due to human error, the exploration of systems issues is primary to identifying a root cause of error.[88] Both public and private sector organizations that have worked tirelessly to reduce medication errors include the ISMP, ECRI Institute, and the FDA.

Through a consensus process, NQF endorsed the adoption of safe practices related to medication administration (**TABLE 2-16**). Other organizations such as the Leapfrog Group have shown support by their endorsements. To improve patient safety and hold the gains, healthcare organizations conduct a thorough analysis of where and how patients are at risk for potential medical errors and hardwire systems and processes to prevent them. Leadership style and climate have also been found to affect medication practices so the routine administration of culture of safety surveys may prove beneficial to identify opportunities for improvement at the organization and unit levels.[158]

Technology Solutions

Various technological solutions are proposed to enhance patient safety programs. A *patient safety solution* is defined as "any system design or intervention that has demonstrated

Table 2-15 Hospital Survey Results on Patient Safety Culture: Strengths

Areas of Strength (Hospitals)	2012 (%)	2014 (%)	2016 (%)
Teamwork within Units The extent to which staff members support each other, treat each other with respect, and work together as a team.	80	81	82
Supervisor/Manager Expectations and Actions Promoting Patient Safety The extent to which supervisors/managers consider staff suggestions to improve patient safety, praise staff for following patient safety procedures, and do not overlook patient safety problems.	75	76	78
Organizational Learning, Continuous Improvement The extent to which mistakes lead to positive changes and changes are evaluated for effectiveness.	72	73	73

Adapted from Agency for Agency for Healthcare Research and Quality. *Hospital Survey on Patient Safety Culture: 2012 User Comparative Database Report;* 2012. http://www.ahrq.gov/sites/default/files/wysiwyg/professionals/quality-patient-safety/patientsafetyculture/hospital/2012/hospsurv121.pdf. Accessed April 17, 2017; Agency for Healthcare Research and Quality. *Hospital Survey on Patient Safety Culture: 2014 User Comparative Database Report;* 2014. http://www.ahrq.gov/sites/default/files/wysiwyg/professionals/quality-patient-safety/patientsafetyculture/hospital/2014/hsops14pt1.pdf. Accessed April 17, 2017; Agency for Healthcare Research and Quality. *Hospital Survey on Patient Safety Culture: 2016 User Comparative Database Report.* 2016. http://www.ahrq.gov/sites/default/files/wysiwyg/professionals/quality-patient-safety/patientsafetyculture/hospital/2016/2016_hospitalsops_report_pt1.pdf. Accessed April 17, 2017.

Table 2-16 Safe Practices Related to Medication Administration

Safe Practice 13: Order Read-back and Abbreviations	Incorporate within the organization a safe, effective communication strategy, structures, and systems to include the following: • For verbal or telephone orders or for telephonic reporting of critical test results, verify the complete order or test result by having the person who is receiving the information record and "read back" the complete order or test result. • Standardize a list of "Do Not Use" abbreviations, acronyms, symbols, and dose designations that cannot be used throughout the organization.
Safe Practice 16: Safe Adoption of Computerized Prescriber Order Entry	• Implement a computerized prescriber order entry (CPOE) system built upon the requisite foundation of reengineered evidence-based care, an assurance of healthcare organization staff and independent practitioner readiness, and an integrated information technology infrastructure.
Safe Practice 17: Medication Reconciliation	• The healthcare organization must develop, reconcile, and communicate an accurate medication list throughout the continuum of care.
Safe Practice 18: Pharmacist Leadership Structures and Systems	• Pharmacy leaders should have an active role on the administrative leadership team that reflects their authority and accountability for medication management systems performance across the organization.

Reprinted from National Quality Forum. Safe Practices for Better Healthcare—2010 Update: A Consensus Report (abridged version); 2010. Copyright 2010 by National Quality Forum, with permission.

the ability to prevent or mitigate patient harm stemming from the processes of health care."[159(p2)] The premise of these solutions is that if processes are standardized and the potential for medical error is reduced by the automation of processes, errors will be mitigated. Clancy[33] proposed a formula for healthcare improvement comprised of four health IT elements: (1) connect health records, (2) build smart systems, (3) put the patient at the center of care, and (4) put prevention at the center of treatment. This is illustrated in **TABLE 2-17.**

Patient Safety and the Learning Organization

It is imperative that a continuous, dynamic learning healthcare system is achieved. This system is one that "provides the best care at lower cost: (1) managing rapidly increasing complexity; (2) achieving greater value in health care; and (3) capturing opportunities from technology, industry, and policy."[160(p8)] How can this be achieved by a learning organization? The infrastructure of a learning organization embraces lifelong learning as a value and opportunities are continually provided for capacity building, developing core competencies, and seeking patient safety innovations. This includes cultivating good judgment and having the opportunity to use it. A learning organization embraces team learning, shared vision and goals, shared ways of thinking, individual commitment to lifelong learning, and systems thinking.[161] Greater attention is paid to learning that fosters more rapid progress in patient safety, increases organizational capabilities, strengthens a culture of

safety, fixes process problems that contribute to patient harm, and produces higher reliability.[162]

Creating the infrastructure for learning can be accomplished in many ways. As summarized by the ISMP,[163] these are suggested steps for creating an infrastructure for learning that were informed by Conway's work (2008). These include the following:

• Identifying reliable sources of information about errors and risks
• Establishing a systematic way to review external information about errors and risk
• Bringing outside points of view into an organization from the literature or experts
• Leveraging the learning of other organizations that had high-profile errors (e.g., contributing factors, how the error was addressed)
• Integrating learning into existing processes in the organization (e.g., safety committee, board reports, unit-level quality teams).

The healthcare quality professional can work with others in the organization to build a sustainable infrastructure that includes a multifaceted learning and organizational development plan for patient safety that is appropriate for the healthcare setting and is reflective of the development needs of personnel. The plan should be competency-based where individual and team clinical and interpersonal skill development will result in performance excellence for safety processes and outcomes. The plan can be supported by evidence-based publications and materials available from

Table 2-17 Information Technology Commonly Used by Healthcare Professionals

Direct Care Delivery Technology	*Patient Assessment, Monitoring, and Surveillance*
• Barcode medication administration	• Telemetry
• Automated medication cabinets	• Bedside monitoring
• Call systems, including emergency call bell	• Ventilators
• Computerized physician/provider order entry	• Video surveillance
• Clinical results available at point of care	• Pulse oximetry
• Standardized order sets	• Smart pumps
• e-Prescribing	
Indirect Care Delivery Technology	*Remote Patient Monitoring*
• Robotics	• Telemedicine and telehealth
• Radio frequency identification	• Robotics
• Electronic inventory systems	
• Computerized staffing systems	
• Automated customized patient directives and education	
Communication with Healthcare Team Members	*Continuous Learning*
• Electronic medical records	• Distance learning
• Documentation at point of care	• Video conferencing
• Electronic ordering systems	• Online training (Webinars)
• Clinical decision support	
• Communication devices (cell phones, personal digital assistants, interactive voice response systems, paging systems)	
Patient Protective Devices	*Pattern Identification (to learn from errors and systems; influences adverse events)*
• Abduction, Elopement or wandering alarms	• Electronic medical or health record
• Fall alarms	• Workload and staffing data systems
• Alerts or results on handheld devices	• Interdisciplinary charting
• Radio frequency identification	• Laboratory, pathology, and radiology results
	• Automated patient safety-related reports

Adapted from Powell-Cope G, Nelson AL, Patterson ES, Patient care technology and safety. In: Hughes RG, ed., *Patient Safety and Quality: An Evidence-Based Handbook for Nurses* (AHRQ Publication No. 08-0043). Rockville, MD: Agency for Healthcare Research and Quality; 2008:3. https://archive.ahrq.gov/professionals/clinicians-providers/resources/nursing/resources/nurseshdbk/nurseshdbk.pdf. Accessed April 17, 2017. Copyright 2008 by Agency for Healthcare Research and Quality.

national and international organizations who already have developed curricula for teaching patient safety.

In 2017, IHI and Safe & Reliable Healthcare released their white paper that talked about the importance of continuous reflection to assess performance. Learning systems that support reflection work to "identify defects and act on them; they reward proactivity rather than reactivity. Learning and a healthy culture reinforce one another by identifying and resolving clinical, cultural, and operational defects. By effectively applying improvement science, organizations can learn their way into many of the cultural components of the framework."[164] The intersections between culture and learning in this framework are shown in FIGURE 2-8.

Some examples to use in building infrastructure are shown alphabetically below and is by no means exhaustive. These resources are evidence-based and include validated tools for

improving safety practices. All organizations offer professional development and learning programs, some with nominal or no charge to the user.

Agency for Healthcare Quality and Research

AHRQ offers a portfolio of free curriculum tools and toolkits for all healthcare settings.[165] AHRQ tools are practical and research-based. Healthcare professionals in all settings can use these tools to make care safer and improve their communication and teamwork skills. Examples of these tools are provided here:

- Diabetes Planned Visit Notebook
- Advancing Pharmacy Health Literacy Practices Through Quality Improvement

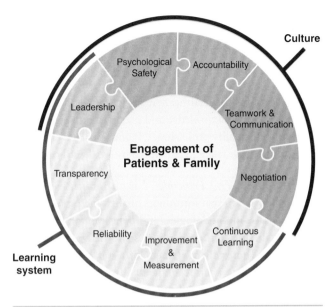

Figure 2-8 Learning system and culture framework.
(Reprinted with permission from Frankel A, Haraden C, Federico F, Lenoci-Edwards J. *A framework for safe, reliable, and effective care*. White Paper. Cambridge, MA: Institute for Healthcare Improvement, 2017. www.IHI.org.)

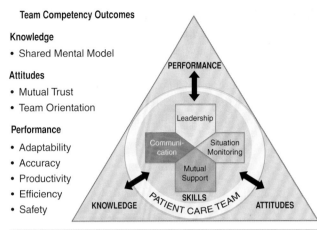

Figure 2-9 TeamSTEPPS 2.0 framework and competencies. (From Agency for Healthcare Research and Quality. Pocket Guide: TeamSTEPPS team strategies & tools to enhance performance and patient safety; 2013. https://www.ahrq.gov/sites/default/files/wysiwyg/professionals/education/curriculum-tools/teamstepps/instructor/essentials/pocketguide.pdf. Accessed April 17, 2017.)

- Staying Healthy Through Education and Prevention (STEP)
- Chronic Care Model
- Central Line-associated Blood Stream Infection (CLABSI) Tools
- Comprehensive Unit-based Safety Program (CUSP) Toolkit
- SHARE Approach.

One of the more widely used programs, Team Strategies and Tools to Enhance Performance and Patient Safety (Team-STEPPS) is a teamwork system developed by AHRQ and the Department of Defense. It is based on team structure and four teachable-learnable skills: communication, leadership, situation monitoring, and mutual support. FIGURE 2-9 shows the framework where there is

> a two-way dynamic interplay between the four skills and the team-related outcomes. Interaction between the outcomes and skills is the basis of a team striving to deliver safe, quality care and support quality improvement. Encircling the four skills is the team structure of the patient care team, which represents not only the patient and direct caregivers, but also those who play a supportive role within the health care delivery system.[166(p4)]

TeamSTEPPS 2.0 serves as the core curriculum for training. It is scientifically rooted in more than 20 years of research and lessons from the application of teamwork principles and system error prevention.[167(¶2)] Using tools such as SBAR, huddles and Two-Challenge Rule, TeamSTEPPS intends

to produce outcomes such as mutual trust, adaptability and shared mentality. TeamSTEPPS provides higher quality, safer patient care by increasing team awareness and clarifying team roles and responsibilities.[167(¶3)]

ECRI Institute

This nonprofit organization is dedicated to bringing applied scientific research to improving patient care using the best medical procedures, devices, drugs, and processes. Resources are offered by clinical specialty, care setting, and role. This member service organization's clients include hospitals, health systems, public and private payers, U.S. federal and state government agencies, health clinics, patients, policymakers, ministries of health, associations, and accrediting agencies worldwide. In 2014, ECRI convened the Partnership for Health IT Patient Safety, which develops and publicly disseminates resources and educational tools that help identify and remediate harm associated with health IT. Another valuable patient safety resource for is the ECRI's Medical Device Safety Reports (MDSR) database. The MDSR is a repository of medical device incident and hazard information independently investigated by ECRI. It offers updated reviews of the types of problems occurring with medical devices and lessons learned over the past three decades.

Institute for Healthcare Improvement

Through its "Open School," the IHI offers quality improvement and patient safety courses based on introductory concepts, intermediate concepts, specialized topics, and project-based learning. Faculty are offered tools for tracking successful completion of online courses for a nominal fee. The courses specifically related to patient safety include: Introduction to Patient Safety; From Error to Harm; Human Factors and Safety; Teamwork and Communication in a Culture of Safety; Responding to Adverse Events; Root Cause and Systems Analysis; Building a Culture of Safety; Partnering to Heal: Teaming Up Against Healthcare-Associated Infections; and Preventing Pressure Ulcers.[168]

Institute for Safe Medication Practices

For over 25 years, the ISMP has been dedicated to learning about medication errors and understanding their system-based causes while promulgating practical recommendations that can help healthcare providers, consumers, and the pharmaceutical industry prevent errors. The ISMP initiatives include *ISMP Medication Safety Alert!* newsletters for healthcare professionals, frequent educational programs, and teleconferences on current medication use issues. The organization develops posters, videos, patient brochures, books and other resources and has valuable medication safety tools such as lists of high-alert drugs and potentially dangerous abbreviations. ISMP is a PSO and provides confidential consulting services to healthcare systems to proactively evaluate medication systems or analyze medication-related sentinel events.[169]

The Joint Commission

TJC accredits organizations across the continuum of care and leverages decades of knowledge and experience to develop and share literature from industry experts and safety scholars from other industries (e.g., nuclear power, air transportation). In addition to developing standards of care, TJC offers conceptual and practical frameworks for patient safety programs, methods, and practices (e.g., safety culture, high reliability, RCA, sentinel events).

In 2008, the Joint Commission Center for Transforming Healthcare was formed to pursue solutions to healthcare's most critical safety and quality problems. Useful resources specific to patient safety are described below:

- Patient Safety Systems. This chapter from the *2017 Comprehensive Accreditation Manual for Hospitals* is intended to help inform and educate hospitals about the importance and structure of an integrated patient safety system. Although the information is drawn from hospital patient safety, there is general discussion of leadership, patient safety culture, effective use of data, and proactive risk assessment to prevent harm.[170]
- Oro 2.0 Resource Library. Provides more than 125 references and tools to help organizations learn about the 14 component areas of performance within the High Reliability Maturity Model.

National Association for Healthcare Quality

The National Association for Healthcare Quality (NAHQ) was founded in 1976 and is solely dedicated to the healthcare quality profession. It is the primary source for healthcare quality education for the healthcare quality professional and has defined the body of knowledge and essential competencies for the healthcare quality professional. Professional development opportunities that relate to patient safety are described below.

HQ Principles. *HQ Principles*[171] is an interactive online certificate program that introduces quality and patient safety fundamentals, methodologies, and concepts for healthcare professionals. The certificate validates knowledge and demonstrates value. Those who can benefit from this program include individuals new to healthcare quality, individuals who have been given added responsibilities or who are looking to refresh their knowledge, and healthcare leaders with teams that need foundational healthcare quality learning opportunities.

HQ Essentials. *HQ Essentials*[172] defines six areas of competence and applies to all healthcare settings across the continuum of care. The six areas are performance improvement and process improvement; population health and care transitions; health data analytics; patient safety; regulatory and accreditation; and quality review and accountability. *HQ Essentials* for patient safety outlines the competency dimensions for safety, which include (1) foster a culture of safety, (2) adopt methods to identify and evaluate risk for harm, and (3) managing and mitigating risk for harm. Within each dimension, descriptors are provided for advances and master proficiency levels. As example, FIGURE 2-10 shows the dimension for mitigating and managing risk for harm. When used as an individual or organizational assessment and development tool, it can provide valuable information to gauge strengths and opportunities and identify where resources can be allocated to support learning, competency development, and capacity building.

National Patient Safety Foundation

The NPSF creates resources for the community to create a world where patients and caregivers are free from harm. As voice for patient safety since 1997, it focuses on patient safety and healthcare workforce safety and disseminates strategies to prevent harm. In March 2017, it announced a merger with IHI. Online learning includes the following:

- Professional Learning Series Webcasts offering continuing education and peer-to-peer collaboration.
- Patient Safety Curriculum: Online courses providing the context, key principles, and competencies associated with the discipline of patient safety and their application in everyday practice.

Dimension 3: Mitigate and Manage Risk for Harm

Provide oversight to the coordination of actions taken to lessen or eliminate a risk, thereby reducing the likelihood of occurrence/recurrence, or prevent and reduce the level of harm should the risk occur/reoccur. This includes a plan for implementing interventional strategies and a process for monitoring progress and effectiveness.

Proficiency Levels and Descriptors

Competency	Proficiency 1: Advanced	Proficiency 2: Master
3.1. Identify the active and inactive conditions within the work environment that contribute to the specific area(s) of risk/defect.	3.1.1a. Demonstrate knowledge of the foundational elements of human, environmental, and organizational factors that can contribute to behaviors or conditions that lead to risk/defect. 3.1.1b. Guide improvement teams in the identification and removal of risk/defect.	3.1.2a. Develop improvements to processes that remove or reduce the defects caused by risky human, environmental, and organizational factors that have the potential to introduce harm into the environment. 3.1.2b. Identify root causes and trends associated with human, environmental, and organizational factors from aggregated safety reports or events.
3.2. Integrate best practices and evidence-based mitigation strategies.	3.2.1a. Use authoritative databases to locate and share evidence-based guidelines or practices for risk or error reduction associated with specific events or conditions. 3.2.1b. Guide improvement teams in the application of newly identified best evidence-based practices to prevent or reduce risk/defect. 3.2.1c. Access evidence-based resources for identifying best practices and mitigation strategies.	3.2.2a. Identify research themes and best practices that can be applied and spread to other areas within the organization to prevent or reduce risk/defect. 3.2.2b. Participate in internal and external work groups to identify and develop best practices for safety improvement initiatives or programs.
3.3. Determine appropriate actions for mitigation or management of identified risks, defects, and root causes.	3.3.1a. Guide improvement teams in selection of actions from a hierarchy of weak, intermediate, and strong actions, while encouraging the usage of stronger actions, whenever possible, within a specific time period. 3.3.1b. Assist with identification of alternative action in cases where the process actions failed to meet the set expectations or when consensus/process reconciliation is needed. 3.3.1c. Monitor proactive interventions applied to high-risk and high-stress environments for reliability improvement.	3.3.2a. Monitor implemented actions and system changes to determine if the actions implemented are reliable, valid, and effective and have not created any unintended consequences within appropriate time expectations. 3.3.2b. Share information on organizational-wide usage of intervention and trends in terms of lessons learned, strengths, time to implement, and effectiveness. 3.3.2c. Encourage leadership efforts to continuously review operations for proactive patient safety improvements.

Figure 2-10   **Patient safety competency dimension for mitigating and managing risk.**

Source: National Association for Healthcare Quality. Patient safety. *HQ essentials: Competencies for the healthcare profession*. Chicago: NAHQ; 2017, p. 17.

- Educational Modules: Educational resources developed by experts in the field offering self-paced learning options and continuing medical education credits.
- Health IT: Educational module that explores the fundamentals of health IT and examines the challenges for information collection, use, and application in health systems.

- Diagnostic Errors: Education for clinicians on strategies for reducing the prevalence of diagnostic errors.
- Patient Blood Management: Although blood has played a central role in clinical practice for decades, the proof of safety and efficacy of blood transfusions remains ill-defined in comparison to other forms of medical and surgical interventions. Safety implications of blood

transfusion are reviewed with an introduction of Patient Blood Management.

World Health Organization

The *Patient Safety Curriculum Guide* presents an interprofessional educational approach for healthcare professionals. The *Guide* offers tools and resources on the following topics:

1. What is patient safety?
2. Why applying human factors is important for patient safety?
3. Understanding systems and the effect of complexity on patient care
4. Being an effective team player
5. Learning from errors to prevent harm
6. Understanding and managing clinical risk
7. Using quality improvement methods to improve care
8. Engaging patients and caregivers
9. Infection prevention and control
10. Patient safety and invasive procedures
11. Improving medication safety.[90(p28)]

See WHO facts related to patient safety in **TABLE 2-18.**

Other Resources

Other patient safety resources that can be useful to healthcare quality professionals include the following:

- The Josie King Foundation offers a patient safety curriculum. Based on the Josie King story, the curriculum includes 16 sessions, developed from a caregiver's viewpoint.[173]
- The NPSF "Getting the Right Diagnosis" checklist helps patients prepare as much information as possible for appointments with healthcare providers.

Table 2-18 Ten Facts on Patient Safety

1. **Patient safety is a serious global public health issue**. There is now growing recognition that patient safety and quality is a critical dimension of universal health coverage. Since the launch of the WHO Patient Safety Programme in 2004, over 140 countries have worked to address the challenges of unsafe care.

2. **One in 10 patients may be harmed while in the hospital**. Estimates show that in developed countries as many as one in 10 patients is harmed while receiving hospital care. The harm can be caused by a range of errors or adverse events.

3. **Hospital infections affect 14 out of every 100 patients admitted.** Of every 100 hospitalized patients at any given time, 7 in developed and 10 in developing countries will acquire healthcare-associated infections (HAIs). Hundreds of millions of patients are affected worldwide each year. Simple and low-cost infection prevention and control measures, such as appropriate hand hygiene, can reduce the frequency of HAIs by more than 50%.

4. **Most people lack access to appropriate medical devices.** There are an estimated 1.5 million different medical devices and over 10,000 types of devices available worldwide. The majority of the world's population is denied adequate access to safe and appropriate medical devices within their health systems. More than half of low- and lower middle-income countries do not have a national health technology policy which could ensure the effective use of resources through proper planning, assessment, acquisition and management of medical devices.

5. **Unsafe injections decreased by 88% from 2000 to 2010**. Key injection safety indicators measured in 2010 show that important progress has been made in the reuse rate of injection devices (5.5% in 2010), while modest gains were made through the reduction of the number of injections per person per year (2.88 in 2010).

6. **Delivery of safe surgery requires a teamwork approach.** An estimated 234 million surgical operations are performed globally every year. Surgical care is associated with a considerable risk of complications. Surgical care errors contribute to a significant burden of disease despite the fact that 50% of complications associated with surgical care are avoidable.

7. **About 20–40% of all health spending is wasted due to poor quality care**. Safety studies show that additional hospitalization, litigation costs, infections acquired in hospitals, disability, lost productivity and medical expenses cost some countries as much as US$19 billion annually. The economic benefits of improving patient safety are therefore compelling.

8. **A poor safety record for healthcare.** Industries with a perceived higher risk such as the aviation and nuclear industries have a much better safety record than healthcare. There is a 1 in 1,000,000 chance of a traveler being harmed while in an aircraft. In comparison, there is a 1 in 300 chance of a patient being harmed during healthcare.

9. **Patient and community engagement and empowerment are key.** People's experience and perspectives are valuable resources for identifying needs, measuring progress and evaluating outcomes.

10. **Hospital partnerships can play a critical role.** Hospital-to-hospital partnerships to improving patient safety and quality of care have been used for technical exchange between health workers for a number of decades. These partnerships provide a channel for bi-directional patient safety learning and the co-development of solutions in rapidly evolving global health systems.

- The Institute for Patient- and Family-Centered Care provides consumers and providers resources, roadmaps and toolkits to foster patient- and family-centered care within the healthcare organization and delivery system.[174]
- Think Cultural Health features information, continuing education opportunities, resources, and more for healthcare professionals to learn about CLAS and its implications for safe and effective healthcare delivery.
- Videos can be helpful learning and teaching aids. Consider these personal stories to complement learning activities:
  - Frontline Innovators: Patient- and Family-Centered Care (AHRQ)
  - Open School Video Library (IHI)
  - The Josie King Story (IHI)
  - My Prepared Patient Story: Jessie Gruman (Center for Advancing Health)
  - Patient and Family-Centered Care: Partnerships for Quality and Safety (AHA)
  - Waiting Room (AHRQ).

Section Summary

Healthcare professionals work diligently to identify and act on opportunities to improve safety. Attention is given to planning, development, implementation, and evaluation, as well as to continuous improvement. In summary, the following tenets are imperative for an effective patient safety program in any healthcare organization:

- Healthcare leaders set the vision, mission, purpose, intention, and direction and provide the resources necessary to adopt evidence-based patient safety practices.
- Error prevention and harm reduction are the shared responsibility of the board, executive leaders, medical leaders, healthcare personnel, and the patient and family. At every intersection, there is an opportunity to take different actions to mitigate risks and reduce harm.
- Organizations create and maintain a fair and just culture by being mindful, taking actions to reduce preventable errors and mitigate risks, and emphasizing learning to support the workforce in eliminating or preventing future errors.
- Patient empowerment and engagement in patient safety will lead to better outcomes and fewer errors.
- Safety program development, implementation, and evaluation considerations include
  - identifying needs and priorities at the organization, department, unit, team, and individual levels;
  - determining how technology can support the program;
  - integrating efforts with RM and infection prevention;
  - monitoring and analyzing close calls, near-misses, and errors;

  - supporting ethical practices in patient safety using fair and just culture principles; and
  - identifying strategies for adoption, spread, and evaluation of evidence-based safety interventions and innovations.

Patient safety gets better through learning and doing using advanced technology, teamwork, and communication approaches that have been proven to mitigate errors, reduce harm and save lives. Healthcare quality professionals can lead and collaborate on these efforts. They possess the unique experience and expertise to advance safety practices in their organizations and the community-at-large. This can be accomplished by bringing knowledge, promising practices, improvement tools, and safety innovations to the healthcare setting.

References

1. Agency for Healthcare Research and Quality. Advancing Patient Safety: A Decade of Evidence, Design and Implementation. AHRQ Publication No. 09(10)-0084; 2009. https://www.ahrq.gov/sites/default/files/publications/files/advancing-patient-safety.pdf. Accessed January 22, 2017.
2. National Quality Forum. *Serious Reportable Events in Healthcare—2011 Update: A Consensus Report.* Washington, DC: Author; 2011.
3. National Priorities Partnership. *Input to the Secretary of Health and Human Services on priorities for the National Quality Strategy.* Washington, DC: National Quality Forum; 2011.
4. Centers for Medicare & Medicaid Services. CMS Quality Strategy 2016. https://www.cms.gov/medicare/quality-initiatives-patient-assessment-instruments/qualityinitiativesgeninfo/downloads/cms-quality-strategy.pdf. Accessed April 19, 2017.
5. U.S. Department of Health & Human Services. Report to Congress: National strategy for quality improvement in health care; 2011. https://www.ahrq.gov/workingforquality/reports/index.html. Accessed April 17, 2017.
6. National Priorities Partnership. *Executive Summary: National Priorities and Goals: Aligning Our Efforts to Transform America's Healthcare.* Washington, DC: National Quality Forum; 2008.
7. Agency for Healthcare Research and Quality. Patient Safety and Quality Improvement Act of 2005. https://www.gpo.gov/fdsys/pkg/PLAW-109publ41/pdf/PLAW-109publ41.pdf. Accessed April 17, 2017.
8. Agency for Healthcare Research and Quality, Office for Civil Rights, & U.S. Department of Health & Human Services. Patient safety and quality improvement; final rule. *Fed Regist.* 2008;73(226):70732–70814.
9. Cartwright-Smith L, Rosenbaum S, Sochacki C. The Patient Safety and Quality Improvement Act regulations: implications for health information access and exchange. *Legal Notes.* 2011;2(2):1–7.
10. Agency for Healthcare Research and Quality. Patient Safety Organization (PSO) Frequently Asked Questions. https://www.pso.ahrq.gov/faq. Accessed April 17, 2017.
11. Halpern MT, Roussel AE, Treiman K, Nerz PA, Hatlie MJ, Sheridan S. Designing Consumer Reporting Systems for Patient Safety Events. Final Report (Prepared by RTI International and Consumers Advancing Patient Safety under Contract No. 290-06-00001-5).

AHRQ Publication No. 11-0060-EF. Rockville, MD: Agency for Healthcare Research and Quality; April 2011.

12. Health Policy Brief. Public Reporting on Quality and Costs. Health Affairs, March 8, 2012. http://healthaffairs.org/healthpolicybriefs/brief_pdfs/healthpolicybrief_65.pdf. Accessed April 19, 2017.

13. Hanlon C, Sheedy K, Kniffin T, Rosenthal J. *2014 Guide to State Adverse Event Reporting Systems*. Washington, DC: National Academy for State Health Policy; 2015. http://www.nashp.org/2014-guide-state-adverse-event-reporting-systems/. Accessed April 17, 2017.

14. The Advisory Board Company. *The Journey to Zero: Innovative Strategies for Minimizing Hospital-Acquired Infections*. Washington, DC: Author; 2008.

15. Centers for Disease Control and Prevention. National Healthcare Safety Network; 2017. https://www.cdc.gov/nhsn/. Accessed April 20, 2017.

16. Kohn LT, Corrigan J, Donaldson MS. *To Err is Human: Building a Safer Health System*. Washington, DC: National Academy Press; 1999.

17. National Committee for Quality Assurance. HEDIS measures; 2017. http://www.ncqa.org/hedis-quality-measurement/hedis-measures. Accessed April 17, 2017.

18. The Leapfrog Group. The Leapfrog Group mission and vision; 2016. http://www.leapfroggroup.org/about/mission-and-vision. Accessed April 17, 2017.

19. Centers for Medicare & Medicaid Services. About the CMS Innovation Center; 2016. https://innovation.cms.gov/About/index.html. Accessed April 17, 2017.

20. Centers for Medicare & Medicaid Services. Partnership for Patients Pledgers. https://partnershipforpatients.cms.gov/partnership-pledge/partnershippledge.html. Accessed July 24, 2017.

21. Institute of Medicine, Committee on Quality of Health Care in America. *Crossing the Quality Chasm: A New Health System for the 21st Century*. Washington, DC: National Academies Press; 2001.

22. Connecticut Center for Patient Safety. Annual report; 2016. http://www.ctcps.org/annual-report.cfm. Accessed April 17, 2017.

23. Oregon Patient Safety Commission. Advancing patient safety in Oregon. Director. http://oregonpatientsafety.org/. Accessed April 17, 2017.

24. Berwick DM, Nolan, TW, Whittington J. The triple aim: care, health, and cost. *Health Affairs*. 2008;27(3):759–769.

25. Sikka R, Morath JM, Leape L. The quadruple aim: care, health, cost, and meaning in work. *BMJ Qual Saf Online*; 2015. http://qualitysafety.bmj.com/content/qhc/24/10/608.full.pdf. Accessed April 17, 2017.

26. Bodenheimer T, Sinsky C. From triple to quadruple aim: care of the patient requires care of the provider. *Ann Family Med*. 2014;12(6):573–576.

27. American Hospital Association, Committee on Research and Committee on Performance Improvement. *Care and Payment Models to Achieve the Triple Aim*. Chicago, IL: American Hospital Association; January 2016.

28. Centers for Medicare & Medicaid Services. Better care, smarter spending, healthier people: improving our health care delivery system; 2015. https://www.cms.gov/Newsroom/MediaRelease Database/Fact-sheets/2015-Fact-sheets-items/2015-01-26.html. Accessed April 17, 2017.

29. Patient-Centered Outcomes Research Institute. What we do; 2014. http://www.pcori.org/about-us. Accessed April 17, 2017.

30. Patient-Centered Outcomes Research Institute. National Priorities and research agenda; 2014. http://www.pcori.org/research-results/research-we-support/national-priorities-and-research-agenda. Accessed April 17, 2017.

31. Hughes RG. Tools and strategies for quality improvement and patient safety. In: Hughes RG, ed. *Patient Safety and Quality: An Evidence-Based Handbook for Nurses*. Rockville, MD: Agency for Healthcare Research and Quality (US); 2008. https://www.ncbi.nlm.nih.gov/books/NBK2682/. Accessed April 17, 2017.

32. Aspden P, Corrigan J, Wolcott J, Erickson SM, editors. *Patient Safety: Achieving a New Standard for Care*. Washington, DC: National Academies Press; 2004.

33. Clancy CM, Farquhar MB, Sharp BA. Patient safety in nursing practice. *J Nurs Care Qual*. 2005;20(3):193–197.

34. Agency for Healthcare Research and Quality Patient Safety Network. Glossary; 2008. http://psnet.ahrq.gov/glossary.aspx#R. Accessed April 17, 2017.

35. Emanuel L, Berwick D, Conway J, et al. What exactly is patient safety? In: Henriksen K, Battles J B, Keyes MA, Grady ML, eds. *Advances in Patient Safety: New Directions and Alternative Approaches*. Rockville, MD: Agency for Healthcare Research and Quality; 2008.

36. Angood P, Colchamiro E, Lyzenga A, Marinelarena M. *Meeting of the National Quality Forum Patient Safety Team*. Washington, DC. Unpublished; August 2009.

37. World Health Organization. Patient Safety. www.who.int/patientsafety/en. Accessed April 17, 2017.

38. Kabcenell A, Nolan TW, Martin LA, Gill Y. *The Pursuing Perfection Initiative: Lessons on Transforming Health Care*. IHI Innovation Series white paper. Cambridge, MA: Institute for Healthcare Improvement; 2010.

39. May EL. The power of zero: Steps toward high reliability healthcare. *Healthcare Executive*. 2013;28(3):16–22.

40. National Patient Safety Foundation Lucien Leape Institute. *Transforming Healthcare: A Compendium of Reports from the NPSF's Lucien Leape Institute*; 2016. http://www.npsf.org/page/reportcompendium. Accessed April 17, 2017.

41. Dunham RB, Pierce JL. *Management*. Glenview, IL: Scott Foresman and Company; 1989.

42. Botwinick L, Bisognano M, Haraden C. *Leadership Guide to Patient Safety*. IHI Innovation Series white paper. Cambridge, MA: Institute for Healthcare Improvement; 2006. www.ihi.org

43. The Joint Commission. Sentinel event data summary. Joint Commission Online; 2017. https://www.jointcommission.org/sentinel_event_statistics_quarterly/. Accessed April 17, 2017.

44. Reason J. Achieving a safety culture: theory and practice. *Br Med J*. 1998;12(3):293–306.

45. Reason J. Human error: models and management. *Br Med J*. 2000;320:768–770.

46. Quality Interagency Coordination Task Force. Doing What Counts for Patient Safety: Federal Actions to Reduce Medical Errors and Their Impact; 2000. https://archive.ahrq.gov/quic/report/errors6.pdf. Accessed April 16, 2017.

47. Agency for Healthcare Research and Quality Patient Safety Network. Adverse Events, near misses and errors; July 2016. https://psnet.ahrq.gov/primers/primer/34/adverse-events-near-misses-and-errors. Accessed April 16, 2017.

48. The Joint Commission. Sentinel event policy and procedure. https://www.jointcommission.org/sentinel_event_policy_and_procedures/. Accessed April 17, 2017.

49. Institute for Safe Medication Practices. *Patient Safety: Achieve a New Standard for Care*. Washington DC: National Academies Press; 2004.

50. Barnard D, Dumkee M, Bains B, Gallivan B. Implementing a Good Catch Program in an integrated health system. *Healthcare Qual*. 2006;9: Spec No. 22-27.

51. Kaplan HS, Fastman B. Organization of reporting data for sense making and system improvement. *Qual Safe Health Care.* 2003;12 (Supple 2: ii68-72).

52. Marks CM, Kasda E, Paine L, Wu AW. "That was a close call": Endorsing a broad definition of near misses in health care. *J Qual Pat Saf* / Joint Commission Resources. 2013;39(10):475–479.

53. Institute of Medicine. *Patient Safety: Achieving a New Standard of Care.* Washington, DC: National Academies Press; 2004.

54. California Patient Safety Action Coalition. CAPSAC Fair and just culture; 2016. http://www.capsac.org/our-approach-to-safety/fair-and-just-culture/

55. Outcome Engenuity. What does our model of accountability look like? https://www.outcome-eng.com/getting-to-know-just-culture/. Accessed April 17, 2017.

56. Josie King Foundation. About; 2016. www.josieking.org/about. Accessed April 24, 2017.

57. The Patient Safety Group. About us; 2016. https://www.patient safetygroup.org/about/about.cfm. Accessed April 17, 2017.

58. Agency for Healthcare Research and Quality. The SHARE approach–Achieving patient-centered care with shared decision making: A brief for administrators and practitioners; 2014. http://www.ahrq.gov/professionals/education/curriculum-tools/shareddecision making/tools/tool-9/index.html. Retrieved April 17, 2017.

59. Hibbard JH, Greene J. What the evidence shows about patient activation: better health outcomes and care experiences; fewer data on costs. *Health Affairs.* 2013;32(20):207–214. doi:10.1377/hlthaff.2012.1061

60. The Joint Commission. Facts about Speak Up™; 2012. www.jointcommission.org/facts_about_speak_up_initiatives. Accessed April 17, 2017.

61. OpenNotes. What is OpenNotes? http://www.opennotes.org/about-opennotes/. Accessed April 17, 2017.

62. OpenNotes. (n.d.). OpenNotes patient safety initiative. Retrieved April 17, 2017 from http://www.opennotes.org/research/opennotes-patient-safety-initiative/

63. Frampton SB, Guastello S, Hoy L, Naylor M, Sheridan S, Johnston-Fleece M. *Harnessing Evidence and Experience to Change Culture: A Guiding Framework for Patient and Family Engaged Care.* Discussion paper. Washington, DC: National Academy of Medicine; 2015. https://nam.edu/wp-content/uploads/2017/01/Harnessing-Evidence-and-Experience-to-Change-Culture-A-Guiding-Framework-for-Patient-and-Family-Engaged-Care.pdf. Accessed April 17, 2017

64. Institute of Medicine. What healthcare consumers need to know about racial and ethnic disparities in healthcare; 2002. http://www.nationalacademies.org/hmd/~/media/Files/Report%20Files/2003/Unequal-Treatment-Confronting-Racial-and-Ethnic-Disparities-in-Health-Care/Disparitieshcproviders8pgFINAL.pdf. Accessed April 17, 2017.

65. Cross TL, Bazron BJ, Dennis KW, Isaacs MR. *Towards a Culturally Competent System of Care.* National Institute of Mental Health, Child and Adolescent Services Program (CASSP). Washington, DC: Technical Assistance Center, Georgetown University Child Development Center; 1989.

66. The Joint Commission. Overcoming the challenges of providing care to LEP patients. *Quick Saf.* 2015;13:1-4.

67. Divi C, Koss RG, Schmaltz SP, Loeb JM. Language proficiency and adverse events in US hospitals: a pilot study. *Int J Qual Health Care.* 2007;19:60–67.

68. The Joint Commission. Patient safety. *Joint Commission Online.* April 29, 2015. http://www.jointcommission.org/assets/1/23/jconline_April_29_15.pdf. Accessed April 23, 2017.

69. World Health Organization. Social Determinants of Health. http://www.who.int/social_determinants/en/. Accessed April 17, 2017.

70. U.S. Department of Health & Human Services, Office of Minority Health. National standards for culturally and linguistically appropriate services in health and health care: a blueprint for advancing and sustaining CLAS policy and procedure; 2013. The case of the enhanced national CLAS standards. https://www.thinkculturalhealth.hhs.gov/pdfs/EnhancedCLASStandardsBlueprint.pdf. Accessed April 17, 2017.

71. Saha S, Beach MK, Cooper LA. Patient centeredness, cultural competence and healthcare quality. *J Natl Med Assoc.* 2008;100(11):1275–1285.

72. U.S. Department of Health & Human Services, Office of Minority Health. National Standards for Culturally and Linguistically Appropriate Services in Health Care: FINAL REPORT; 2001. https://minorityhealth.hhs.gov/assets/pdf/checked/finalreport.pdf. Accessed February 22, 2017.

73. Shojania KG, Duncan BW, McDonald KM, Wachter RM. Making health care safer: A clinical analysis of patient safety practices. Evidence Report/Technology Assessment No. 43; 2001. https://archive.ahrq.gov/clinic/ptsafety/pdf/ptsafety.pdf. Accessed April 17, 2017.

74. National Quality Forum. *Safe Practices for Better Healthcare—2010 Update: A Consensus Report* (abridged version). Washington, DC: Author; 2010.

75. Moody's Global Credit Research. *Clinical Quality Initiatives Have Positive Long-Term Impact on Not-For-Profit Hospital Bond Ratings.* New York: Moody's Investor Services; 2008.

76. Moody's Investors Services. Healthcare Quarterly; 2017. April 17, 2017. Moody's.Com.

77. Institute for Healthcare Improvement. 2008 Progress Report: Quality rules! How far have we come? http://www.ihi.org/about/Documents/2008_IHIProgressReport.pdf. Accessed April 17, 2017.

78. Millar R, Mannion R, Freeman T, Davies HTO. Hospital board oversight of quality and patient safety: a narrative review and synthesis of recent empirical research. *Milbank Quart.* 2013;91(4):738–770.

79. National Quality Forum. Patient safety 2016: Final report; 2017. http://www.qualityforum.org/Publications/2017/03/Patient_Safety_Final_Report.aspx. Accessed April 17, 2017.

80. Rogers EM. *Diffusion of Innovations* (5th ed.). New York: Free Press; 2003.

81. Marx D. Patient safety and the "Just Culture": A primer for health care executives; 2001. http://www.chpso.org/sites/main/files/file-attachments/marx_primer.pdf. Accessed April 17, 2017.

82. Pham JC, Thierry G, Pronovost PJ. What to do with healthcare Incident Reporting Systems. *J Public Health Res.* 2013;2:e27. https://www.ncbi.nlm.nih.gov/pmc/articles/PMC4147750/pdf/jphr-2013-3-e27.pdf. Accessed April 20, 2017.

83. Institute for Safe Medication Practices. Building patient safety skills: Common pitfalls when conducting a root cause analysis. *ISMP Medication Safety Alert!* 2011;9(3):1–4.

84. Becher EC, Chassin MR. Improving the quality of health care: Who will lead? *Health Affairs.* 2001;20(5):164–179. doi:10.1377/hlthaff.20.5.164

85. Center for Behavioral Health Statistics and Quality. *2015 National Survey on Drug Use and Health: Detailed tables.* Rockville, MD: Substance Abuse and Mental Health Services Administration; 2016.

86. Berwick DM, Hackbarth AD. Eliminating waste in US health care. *JAMA.* 2012;307(14):1513–1516. doi:10.1001/jama.2012.362

87. Association for the Advancement of Medical Instrumentation. ANSI/AAMI HE75, 2009 R (2013): *Human Factors Engineering—Design of Medical Devices.* Arlington, VA: AAMI; 2013.

88. Deming WE. *Out of the Crisis.* Cambridge, MA: MIT Press; 2000.

89. The Advisory Board. *Managing Disruptive Behavior: Creating a Healthy Workplace Culture.* Washington, DC: Author; 2010.

90. World Health Organization. *Patient Safety Curriculum Guide: Multi-Professional Edition.* Geneva, Switzerland: Author; 2011.

91. Institute for Healthcare Improvement. IHI Open School: Patient Safety 102: Human factors and safety; 2016. http://www.ihi.org/education/ihiopenschool/Courses/Documents/SummaryDocuments/PS%20102%20SummaryFINAL.pdf. Accessed April 17, 2017.

92. Gordon S, Mendenhall P, O'Connor BB. *Beyond the Checklist: What Else Health Care Can Learn from Aviation Teamwork and Safety.* Ithaca, NY: Cornell University ILR; 2013.

93. Agency for Healthcare Research and Quality. Patient safety primer: Safety Culture (last updated July 2016); 2016. https://psnet.ahrq.gov/primers/primer/5/safety-culture. Accessed April 17, 2017.

94. McKeon LM, Oswaks JD, Cunningham PD. Safeguarding patients: complexity science, high reliability organizations, and implications for team training in healthcare. *Clin Nurse Specialist.* 2006;20(6):298–304.

95. Hines S, Luna K, Lofthus J, Marquardt M, Stemokas D. *Becoming a High Reliability Organization: Operational Advice for Hospital Leaders.* AHRQ Publication No. 08-0022. Rockville, MD: Agency for Healthcare Research and Quality; 2008.

96. Chassin MR, Loeb JM. High-reliability health care: getting there from here. *Milbank Quart.* 2013;91(3):459–490.

97. Weick KE, Sutcliffe KM. *Managing the Unexpected—Assuring High Performance in an Age of Complexity.* San Francisco, CA: Jossey-Bass; 2001.

98. Weick KE, Sutcliffe K. *Managing the Unexpected: Resilient Performance in the Age of Uncertainty.* 2nd ed. San Francisco, CA: John Wiley &Sons, Inc.; 2007.

99. Outcome Engenuity. The model for engineering better outcomes; 2017. https://www.outcome-eng.com/the-model-for-high-reliability-organizations/. Accessed April 16, 2017.

100. Hagg HW, Workman-Germann J, Flanagan ME, Doebbeling BN. Implementation of Systems Redesign: Approaches to Spread and Sustain Adoption in book: Advances in Patient Safety: New Directions and Alternative Approaches (Vol. 2: Culture and Redesign), Publisher: Agency for Healthcare Research and Quality (US); 2008, Editors: Kerm Henriksen, James B Battles, Margaret A Keyes, Mary L Grad.

101. Joint Commission Center on Transforming Healthcare. Get to zero HAIs! Hand Hygiene Targeted Solutions Tool® implementation guide for health care organizations; 2014. http://www.centerfortransforminghealthcare.org/assets/4/6/HH_TST_Implementation_Guide.pdf. Accessed April 20, 2017.

102. National Patient Safety Agency. A commitment to patient safety; 2012. www.nrls.npsa.nhs.uk. Accessed April 17, 2017.

103. Carroll R, editor. *Risk Management Handbook for Healthcare Organizations* (student ed.). San Francisco: Jossey-Bass; 2010.

104. Carroll R. *Enterprise Risk Management: A Framework for Success.* Chicago: American Society for Health Risk Management; 2014:5.

105. Kavaler F, Spiegel A. *Risk Management in Health Care Institutions: A Strategic Approach.* Sudbury, MA: Jones & Bartlett; 1997.

106. Agency for Healthcare Research and Quality (AHRQ). Patient safety primer: Voluntary patient safety event reporting (incident reporting); 2014. https://psnet.ahrq.gov/primers/primer/13/voluntary-patient-safety-event-reporting-incident-reporting. Accessed April 17, 2017.

107. Griffin FA, Resar RK. *IHI Global Trigger Tool for Measuring Adverse Events.* IHI Innovation Series white paper. Cambridge, MA: Institute for Healthcare Improvement; 2007.

108. U.S. Department of Health & Human Services, Office of Inspector General. Hospital incident reporting systems do not capture most patient harm; 2012. https://oig.hhs.gov/oei/reports/oei-06-09-00091.pdf. Accessed April 17, 2017.

109. AbuAlRub RF, Al-Akour NA, Alatari NH. Perceptions of reporting practices and barriers to reporting incidents among registered nurses and physicians in accredited and nonaccredited Jordanian hospitals. *J Clin Nursing.* 2015;24(19-20):2973–2982.

110. Agency for Healthcare Research and Quality. *Hospital Survey on Patient Safety Culture: 2016 User Comparative Database Report.* 2016. http://www.ahrq.gov/sites/default/files/wysiwyg/professionals/quality-patient-safety/patientsafetyculture/hospital/2016/2016_hospitalsops_report_pt1.pdf. Accessed April 17, 2017.

111. National Academy of Sciences. *The Owner's Role in Project Risk Management.* Washington, DC: Author; 2005.

112. Conway J, Federico F, Stewart K, Campbell M. *Respectful Management of Serious Clinical Adverse Events* (2nd ed.). IHI Innovation Series white paper. Cambridge, MA: Institute for Healthcare Improvement; 2011.

113. Herzer KR, Mirrer M, Xie Y, et al. Patient safety reporting systems: sustained quality improvement using a multidisciplinary team and "good catch": awards. *Jt Comm J Qual Saf.* 2012;38(8):339–347.

114. Oregon Patient Safety Commission. Introduction: Root cause analysis toolkit; 2016. https://oregonpatientsafety.org/resource-center/opsc-resources/root-cause-analysis-toolkit/432. Accessed April 17, 2017.

115. National Patient Safety Foundation. RCA² Improving root cause analyses and actions to prevent harm; 2016. (Version 2) http://www.npsf.org/?page=RCA2. Accessed April 17, 2017.

116. Griffith S. An examination of red rules in a just culture; 2008. https://www.ismp.org/newsletters/acutecare/articles/20080424.asp. Accessed April 16, 2017.

117. Scharf WR, Red rules: an error-reduction strategy in the culture of safety. *Focus Patient Saf.* 2007;10(1):1–2.

118. Grissinger M. Some red rules shouldn't rule in hospitals. *Pharm Ther.* Jan 2012;37(1):4–5.

119. Institute for Safe Medication Practices–Acute Care. Some red rules shouldn't rule in hospitals. *ISMP Medication Safety Alert!* 2008;13(8): 1–3.

120. Jones LK, O'Connor SJ. The use of red rules in patient safety culture. *Univ J Manage.* 2016;4(3), 130–139.

121. Thomassen O, Storesund A, Softeland E, Brattebo G. The effects of safety checklists in medicine: a systematic review. *Acta Anaesthesiol Scand.* 2013;58(1):5–18. doi:10.1111/aas.12207

122. World Health Organization. Patient safety checklists. http://www.who.int/patientsafety/implementation/checklists/en/. Accessed April 17, 2017.

123. National Patient Safety Foundation. Checklist for getting the right diagnosis; 2014. https://c.ymcdn.com/sites/npsf.site-ym.com/resource/collection/930A0426-5BAC-4827-AF94-1CE-1624CBE67/Checklist-for-Getting-the-Right-Diagnosis.pdf. Accessed April 17, 2017.

124. Centers for Disease Control and Prevention. Checklist for Core Elements of Hospital Antibiotic Stewardship Programs; 2017. https://www.cdc.gov/getsmart/healthcare/implementation/checklist.html. Accessed April 13, 2017.

125. Pronovost P, Needham D, Berenholtz S, et al. An intervention to decrease catheter-related bloodstream infections in the ICU. *N Engl J Med.* 2006;355:2725–2732. doi:10.1056/NEJMoa061115

126. Gawande A. The checklist. *Ann Med.* 2007. http://www.newyorker.com/magazine/2007/12/10/the-checklist. Accessed April 17, 2017.

127. Gawande A. *The Checklist Manifesto: How to Get Things Right.* New York: Metropolitan Books; 2009.

128. Treadwell JR, Lucas S, Tsou AY. Surgical checklists: a systematic review of impacts and implementation. *BMJ Qual Saf.* 2014;3: 299–318.

129. Farley DO, Morton SE, Damberg CL, et al. *Assessment of the AHRQ Patient Safety Initiatives: Moving from Research to Practice. Evaluation Report II* (2003–2004). Santa Monica, CA: RAND Corporation; 2007.

130. Pelletier LR, Stichler JF. Action brief: Patient engagement and activation: A health care reform imperative and improvement opportunity for nursing. *Nursing Outlook.* 2013;61(1):51–54. doi:10.1016/j.outlook.2012.11.003

131. University of California, Los Angeles. UCLA Health System performance improvement & patient safety plan; 2017. https:// quality.mednet.ucla.edu/file/1546079/PerformanceImprovement-Plan.pdf. Accessed April 19, 2017.

132. Intermountain Healthcare. Quality & patient safety plan; 2014. https://intermountainhealthcare.org/-/media/files/facilities/uvrmc/quality-plan.pdf?la=en. Accessed April 19, 2107.

133. The Joint Commission. Sentinel event alert; 2015. Issue 54: Safe use of health information technology. http://www.jointcommission.org/assets/1/18/SEA_54.pdf. Accessed April 17, 2017.

134. Institute of Medicine, Committee on Patient Safety and Health Information Technology. *Health IT and Patient Safety: Building Safer Systems for Better Care.* Washington, DC: National Academies Press; 2012.

135. Parente ST, McCullough JS. Health information technology and patient safety: evidence from panel data. *Health Affairs.* 2009;28(2):357–360. doi:10.1377/hlthaff.28.2.357

136. Sowan AK, Reed CC. A complex phenomenon in complex adaptive health care systems—alarm fatigue. *JAMA Pediatr.* 2017. Published online April 10, 2017. http://jamanetwork.com/journals/jamapediatrics/fullarticle/2614070. Accessed April 17, 2017.

137. Graber ML, Johnston D, Bailey R. *Report of the Evidence on Health IT Safety and Interventions.* Research Triangle Park, NC: RTI International; 2016.

138. Nationwide Health Information Network (NHIN). Exchange Architecture Overview (Draft 0.9); 2012. https://www.healthit.gov/sites/default/files/nhin-architecture-overview-draft-20100421-1.pdf. Accessed April 17, 2017.

139. U.S. Department of Health & Human Services, Office of the National Coordinator. Get the facts about the Nationwide Health Information Network, Direct Project, and CONNECT software; 2010. https://www.healthit.gov/sites/default/files/pdf/fact-sheets/get-the-facts-about-nationwide-hit-direct-project-and-connect.pdf. Accessed April 17, 2017.

140. Byrne CM, Mercincavage LM, Bouhaddou O, et al. The Department of Veterans Affairs/VA implementation of the Virtual Lifetime Electronic Record (VLER): findings and lessons learned from health information exchanges at 12 sites. *Int J Med Inf.* 2014;83(8):537-547. doi:10.1016/ijmedinf.2014.04.005

141. Morrissey J. How to surmount health care's interoperability challenge. *Hospitals & Health Networks*; 2016. http://www.hhnmag.com/articles/7188-how-to-surmount-health-cares-interoperability-challenge. Accessed April 17, 2017.

142. ECRI Institute for Health IT Patient Safety. Health IT safe practices: toolkit for the safe use of health IT for patient identification. https://www.ecri.org/Resources/HIT/Patient%20ID/Patient_Identification_Toolkit_final.pdf. Accessed April 19, 2017.

143. The Joint Commission. National patient safety goals effective January 2017; 2017. https://www.jointcommission.org/standards_information/npsgs.aspx

144. The Leapfrog Group. Home; 2016. http://www.leapfroggroup.org/. Accessed April 17, 2017.

145. National Quality Forum. Field guide to NQF resources: What is the best way to pick measures to use; 2013. http://www.qualityforum.org/Field_Guide/. Accessed April 16, 2017.

146. Agency for Healthcare Research and Quality. Patient safety culture surveys; 2016. http://www.ahrq.gov/professionals/quality-patient-safety/patientsafetyculture/index.html. Accessed April 17, 2017.

147. The Leapfrog Group. Guidelines for a Culture of Safety Survey; 2016. http://www.leapfroggroup.org/sites/default/files/Files/Guidelines_CultureSurvey_updated08032016_0_0.pdf. Accessed April 17, 2017.

148. Sexton JB, Helmreich RL, Neilands TB, et al. The safety attitudes questionnaire: psychometric properties, benchmarking data, and emerging research. *BMC Health Serv Res.* 2006;6(1):44. doi:10.1186/1472-6963-6-44

149. Singer SJ, Meterko M, Baker L, Gaba G, Falwell A, Rosen A. Workforce perceptions of hospital safety culture: development and validation of the Patient Safety Climate in Healthcare Organizations survey. *Health Services Res.* 2007;42(5): 1999–2021.

150. Joint Commission Center for Transforming Healthcare. Facts about Oro™ 2.0 High Reliability Organizational Assessment; 2017. http://www.centerfortransforminghealthcare.org/assets/4/6/Oro_Fact_Sheet.pdf. Accessed April 18, 2017.

151. Health Research and Educational Trust. About the Physician Practice Patient Safety Assessment (PPPSA); 2006. www.mgma.com/pppsa. Accessed April 17, 2017.

152. Medical Group Management Association. About the Physician Practice Patient Safety Assessment (PPPSA); 2016. http://www.mgma.com/practice-resources/tools/patient-safety-tools-for-physician-practices/about-the-physician-practice-patient-safety-assessment-(pppsa). Accessed April 17, 2017.

153. Thomas EJ, Sexton JB, Helmreich RL. Discrepant attitudes about teamwork among critical care nurses and physicians. *Crit Care Med.* 2003;31(3):956–959. doi:10.1097/01.CCM.0000056183.89175.76

154. Singer SJ, Meterko M, Baker L, Gaba D, Falwell A, Rosen A. Patient safety climate in healthcare organizations (PSCHO). Measurement instrument database for the social sciences; 2012. http://www.midss.org/sites/default/files/pscho_survey_2006.pdf. Accessed April 17, 2017.

155. Agency for Healthcare Research and Quality. *Hospital Survey on Patient Safety Culture: 2008 Comparative Database Report* (AHRQ Publication No. 08-0039). Rockville, MD: Author; 2008.

156. Aspden P, Wolcott J, Bootman JL, Cronenwett LR. *Preventing Medication Errors.* Washington, DC: National Academies Press; 2006.

157. The Advisory Board. 5 ways to improve medication adherence–health care's $289 billion problem. https://www.advisory.com/daily-briefing/2017/04/19/medication-adherence. Accessed April 26, 2017.

158. Faraq A, Tullai-McGuinness S, Anthony MK, Burant C. Do leadership style, unit climate, and safety climate contribute to safe medication practices? *J Nurs Administration.* Jan 2017;47(1): 8–15.

159. The Joint Commission, Joint Commission International, World Health Organization. Patient safety solutions preamble; 2007. http://www.who.int/patientsafety/solutions/patientsafety/Preamble.pdf. Accessed April 17, 2017.

160. Institute of Medicine. *Best Care at Lower Cost: The Path to Continuously Learning Health Care in America*. Washington, DC: National Academies of Sciences, Engineering and Medicine; 2012.

161. Senge PM. *The Fifth Discipline: The Art and Practice of the Learning Organization* (2nd ed). New York: Doubleday; 2006.

162. Edwards MT. An organizational learning framework for patient safety. *Am J Med Qual*. 2016;32(2):148–155.

163. Institute for Safe Medication Practices. Using information from external errors to signal a "clear and present danger." *Patient Saf Qual Healthcare*. 2017;14(2):32–34.

164. Frankel A, Haraden C, Federico F, Lenoci-Edwards J. *A Framework for Safe, Reliable, and Effective Care*. White Paper. Cambridge, MA: Institute for Healthcare Improvement and Safe & Reliable Healthcare; 2017:6–7.

165. Agency for Healthcare Research and Quality Patient Safety Network. Training catalog. https://psnet.ahrq.gov/pset. Accessed April 17, 2017.

166. Agency for Healthcare Research and Quality. Pocket Guide: TeamSTEPPS team strategies & tools to enhance performance and patient safety; 2013. https://www.ahrq.gov/sites/default/files/wysiwyg/professionals/education/curriculum-tools/teamstepps/instructor/essentials/pocketguide.pdf. Accessed April 17, 2017.

167. Agency for Healthcare Research and Quality. About TeamSTEPPS; 2016. https://www.ahrq.gov/teamstepps/about-teamstepps/index.html. Accessed April 17, 2017.

168. Institute for Healthcare Improvement. IHI Open School online course; 2016. http://app.ihi.org/lmsspa/#/6cb1c614-884b-43ef-9abd-d90849f183d4. Accessed April 17, 2017.

169. Institute for Safe Medication Practices. Learn about us: the institute for safe medication practices. http://www.ismp.org/about/ismp-decade.pdf. Accessed April 16, 2017.

170. The Joint Commission. Patient safety systems; 2017. https://www.jointcommission.org/assets/1/18/CAMH_04a_PS.pdf. Accessed April 16, 2017.

171. National Association for Healthcare Quality. HQ Principles: Build your quality toolbox. http://nahq.org/education/hq-principles. Accessed April 15, 2017.

172. National Association for Healthcare Quality. *HQ Essentials: Competencies for the Healthcare Profession*. Chicago: NAHQ; 2017.

173. Kaprielian VS, Sullivan DT. Josie's story: A patient safety curriculum; 2009. http://josieking.org/jkf-tools/josies-story-a-patient-safety-curriculum/. Accessed April 17, 2017.

174. Institute for Patient and Family-Centered Care. IPFCC; 2016. http://www.ipfcc.org/about/index.html. Accessed April 17, 2017.

Suggested Readings

Alan J, Card JW, Clarkson PJ. Successful risk assessment may not always lead to successful risk control: a systematic literature review of risk control after root cause analysis. *J Healthcare Risk Manage*. 2012;31(3):6–12. doi:10.1002/jhrm.20090

Card AJ, Ward JR, Clarkson PJ. Beyond FMEA: the structured what-if technique (SWIFT). *J Healthcare Risk Manage*. 2012;31(4):23. doi:10.1002/jhrm.20101

Chuk A, Maloney R, Gawron J, Skinner C. Utilizing electronic health record information to optimize medication infusion devices: a manual data integration approach. *J Healthcare Qual*. 2016;38(6):370–378. doi: 10.1111/jhq.12073

Dixon JL, Stagg HW, Wehbe-Janek H, Jo C, Culp W, Jr, Shake JG. A standard handoff improves cardiac surgical patient transfer: operating room to intensive care unit. *J Healthcare Qual*. January/February 2015;37(1):22–32.

Donaldson N, Aydin C, Fridman M, Foley M. Improving medication administration safety: using naïve observation to assess practice and guide improvements in process and outcomes. *J Healthcare Qual*. 2014;36(6):58–68.

Frankel A, Haraden C, Federico F, Lenoci-Edwards J. *A Framework for Safe, Reliable, and Effective Care*. White Paper. Cambridge, MA: Institute for Healthcare Improvement and Safe & Reliable Healthcare; 2017.

Gleason KM, Brake H, Agramonte V, Perfetti C. *Medications at Transitions and Clinical Handoffs (MATCH) Toolkit for Medication Reconciliation* (prepared by the Island Peer Review Organization, Inc., under Contract No. HHSA2902009000 13C; AHRQ Publication No. 11(12)-0059). Rockville, MD: Agency for Healthcare Research and Quality; 2011.

Haraden C, Leitch J. Scotland's successful national approach to improving patient safety in acute care. *Health Affairs*. 2011;30(4):4755–4763. doi:10.1377/hlthaff.2011.0144

Hefner JL, McAlearney AS, Mansfield J, Knupp AM, Moffatt-Bruce SD. A falls wheel in a large academic medical center: an intervention to reduce patient falls with harm. *J Healthcare Qual*. November/December 2015;37(6):374–380.

Hong AL, Sawyer MD, Shore A, et al. On behalf of the On the CUSP: Stop BSI Program. Decreasing central-line-associated bloodstream infections in Connecticut intensive care units. *J Healthcare Qual*. 2013;35(5):78–87.

Huerta TR, Walker C, Murray KR, et al. Patient safety errors: leveraging health information technology to facilitate patient reporting. *J Healthcare Qual*. 2016;38(1):17-23.

Hurtado MP, Swift EK, Corrigan JM, eds. *Envisioning the National Health Care Quality Report*. Washington, DC: National Academies Press; 2001. Retrieved from www.nap.edu/catalog.php?record_id=10073

Institute of Medicine, Committee on Enhancing Federal Healthcare Quality Programs. *Leadership by example: Coordinating government roles in improving health care quality*. In: Corrigan JM, Eden J, Smith BM, eds. Washington, DC: National Academies Press; 2001. www.nap.edu/catalog.php?record_id=10537. Accessed April 17, 2017.

Leape L. Full disclosure and apology—an idea whose time has come. *Physician Executive*. 2006;32(2):16–18.

Lyren A, Brilli R, Bird M, Lashutka N, Muething S. Ohio Children's Hospitals' Solutions for Patient Safety: a framework for pediatric patient safety improvement. *J Healthcare Qual*. 2016;38(4):213–222. doi: 10.1111/jhq.12058

Maurer M, Dardess P, Carman KL, Frazier K, Smeeding L. Guide to patient and family engagement: Environmental scan report; 2012. https://www.ahrq.gov/sites/default/files/wysiwyg/research/findings/final-reports/ptfamilyscan/ptfamilyscan.pdf. Accessed April 17, 2017.

Michael M, Schaffer SD, Egan PL, Little BB, Pritchard PS. Improving wait times and patient satisfaction in primary care. *J Healthcare Qual*. 2013;35(2):50–60.

Mitchell SE, Martin J, Holmes S, et al. How hospitals reengineer their discharge processes to reduce readmissions. *J Healthcare Qual*. 2016;38(2):116–126.

Morse RB, Pollack MM. Root cause analyses performed in a children's hospital: events, action plan strength, and implementation rates. *J Healthcare Qual*. 2012;34:55–61. doi:10.1111/j.1945-1474.2011.00140.x

Pelletier LR. Quality and safety. In: Huber DL, ed. *Leadership and Nursing Care Management*. 6th ed. Philadelphia: W. B. Saunders; 2017.

Reason J. Human error: models and management. *Br Med J*. 2000;320:768–770. doi:10.1136/bmj.320.7237.768

Reason J. *Human Error*. Cambridge, UK: Cambridge University Press; 1990.

Schuller KA, Lin S, Gamm LD, Edwardson N. Discharge phone calls: a technique to improve patient care during the transition from hospital to home. *J Healthcare Qual*. 2015;37(3):163–172.

Stolldorf DP, Mion LC, Jones CB. A survey of hospitals that participated in a statewide collaborative to implement and sustain rapid response teams. *J Healthcare Qual*. 2016;38(4):202–212.

Thomas MJW, Schultz TJ, Hannaford N, Runciman WB. Failures in transition: learning from incidents relating to clinical handover in acute care. *J Healthcare Qual*. 2013;35(3):49–56.

Trompeter JM, McMillan AN, Rager ML, Fox JR. Medication discrepancies during transitions of care: a comparison study. *J Healthcare Qual*. 2015;37(6):325–332.

Tupper JB, Gray CE, Pearson KB, Coburn AFL. Safety of rural nursing home-to-emergency department transfers: improving communication and patient information sharing across settings. *J Healthcare Qual*. 2015;37(1):55–65.

Wachter R, Sehgal N, Ranji S, Shojania K, Cucina R. AHRQ patient safety network: patient safety primers; n.d. https://psnet.ahrq.gov/primers. Accessed April 17, 2017.

Wagner B, Meirowitz N, Shah J, et al. Comprehensive perinatal safety initiative to reduce adverse obstetric events. *J Healthcare Qual*. 2012;34(1):6–15. doi:10.1111/j.1945-1474.2011.00134.x

Wasserman M, Renfrew MR, Green AR. Identifying and preventing medical errors in patients with limited English proficiency: key findings and tools for the field. *J Healthcare Qual*. 2014;36(3):5–16.

Weick KE, Sutcliffe KM. *Managing the Unexpected: Resilient Performance in an Age of Uncertainty*. 2nd ed. (MP3-CD Edition). Audible Studios on Brilliance Audio.

Yoon RS, Alaia MJ, Hutzler LH, Bosco JA III. Near misses analysis to prevent wrong-site surgery. *J Healthcare Qual*. 2015;37(2):126–132. doi: 10.1111/jhq.12037

Zrelak PA, Utter GH, Tancredi DJ, et al. How accurate is the AHRQ patient safety indicator for hospital-acquired pressure ulcer in a national sample of records? *J Healthcare Qual*. 2015;37(5):287–297. doi: 10.1111/jhq.12052

Online Resources

Agency for Healthcare Research and Quality (AHRQ)

- **Advances in Patient Safety**
  https://www.ahrq.gov/professionals/quality-patient-safety/patient-safety-resources/resources/advances-in-patient-safety/

- **Advancing Patient Safety: A Decade of Evidence, Design and Implementation**
  https://www.ahrq.gov/sites/default/files/publications/files/advancing-patient-safety.pdf

- **CAHPS Ambulatory Care Improvement Guide**
  https://www.ahrq.gov/cahps/quality-improvement/improvement-guide/improvement-guide.html

- **Education and Training for Health Professionals**
  https://www.ahrq.gov/professionals/education/index.html

- **Improving Patient Safety in Nursing Homes**
  https://www.ahrq.gov/sites/default/files/wysiwyg/professionals/quality-patient-safety/patientsafetyculture/nursing-home/resources/nhimpptsaf.pdf

- **National Guideline Clearinghouse**
  www.guideline.gov

- **Oral, Linguistic, and Culturally Competent Services: Guides for Managed Care Plans**
  https://www.ahrq.gov/professionals/systems/primary-care/cultural-competence-mco/index.html

- **Patient Safety Measure Tools and Resources**
  https://www.ahrq.gov/professionals/quality-patient-safety/patient-safety-resources/index.html

- **Patient Safety and Quality: An Evidence-Based Handbook for Nurses**
  https://archive.ahrq.gov/professionals/clinicians-providers/resources/nursing/resources/nurseshdbk/

- **Quality and Patient Safety**
  https://www.ahrq.gov/qual/pips/issues.htm

- **TeamSTEPPS**
  http://teamstepps.ahrq.gov.

- **Web M&M (Morbidity & Mortality Rounds on the web)**
  https://www.ahrq.gov/cpi/about/otherwebsites/webmm.ahrq.gov/index.html

American Board of Internal Medicine Foundation—Choosing Wisely
  www.choosingwisely.org

American Hospital Association

- **Hospitals Against Violence**
  http://www.aha.org/advocacy-issues/violence/index.shtml

- **Hospitals in Pursuit of Excellence**
  www.hpoe.org

- **A Leadership Resource for Patient and Family Engagement Strategies**
  http://www.hpoe.org/resources/hpoehretaha-guides/1407

- **Patient and Family Resource Compendium**
  http://www.hpoe.org/resources/hpoehretaha-guides/2735

American Society for Healthcare Risk Management
  http://www.ashrm.org/

American Society of Health-System Pharmacists: Patient Safety Resource Center
  http://www.ashp.org/patientsafety

Patient and Family Engagement in Healthcare

- **A Roadmap for Patient + Family Engagement in Healthcare**
  http://patientfamilyengagement.org/

Canadian Patient Safety Institute
  http://www.patientsafetyinstitute.ca/en/pages/default.aspx

Center for Advancing Health
  http://www.cfah.org/

Centers for Disease Control and Prevention

- **Guidelines for the Prevention of Intravascular Catheter-Related Infections**
  http://www.cdc.gov/mmwr/preview/mmwrhtml/rr5110a1.htm

- **Medication Safety Program**
  www.cdc.gov/medicationsafety

- **National Healthcare Safety Network**
  https://www.cdc.gov/nhsn/

- **NHSN Patient Safety Component Manual**
  https://www.cdc.gov/nhsn/pdfs/pscmanual/pcsmanual_current.pdf

- Ten Things You Can Do to Be a Safe Patient

    http://www.cdc.gov/HAI/patientSafety/patient-safety.html

Centers for Medicare & Medicaid Services

- **A Practical Guide to Implementing the National CLAS Standards: For Racial, Ethnic and Linguistic Minorities, People with Disabilities and Sexual and Gender Minorities**

    https://www.cms.gov/About-CMS/Agency-Information/OMH/Downloads/CLAS-Toolkit-12-7-16.pdf

- **Partnership for Patients**

    https://partnershipforpatients.cms.gov/about-the-partnership/aboutthepartnershipforpatients.html

The Cochrane Collaboration

    http://www.cochrane.org

Cynosure Health

    http://www.cynosurehealth.org/

ECRI Institute

    http://www.ecri.org

Food & Drug Administration, Medical Devices

    https://www.fda.gov/MedicalDevices/Safety/

- **Drugs**

    https://www.fda.gov/Drugs/default.htm

- **MedWatch**

    www.fda.gov/medwatch/index.html

Health and Medicine Division of the National Academies (formerly Institute of Medicine)

    http://www.nationalacademies.org/hmd/

The Health Foundation

- **The Measurement and Monitoring of Safety**

    http://www.health.org.uk/publication/measurement-and-monitoring-safety

- **Health Research & Education Trust**

    http://www.hret-hen.org/

- **HRET Disparities Toolkit: A toolkit for collecting race, ethnicity, and primary language from patients**

    http://www.hretdisparities.org/

Institute for Healthcare Improvement (IHI)

- **Open School for Health Professions**

    http://app.ihi.org/lms/home.aspx

- **Safety Briefings**

    http://www.ihi.org/Engage/Memberships/Passport/Documents/SafetyBriefings.pdf

- **Improvement Map**

- **High-Alert Medication Safety**

    http://www.ihi.org/topics/highalertmedicationsafety/pages/default.aspx

- **Medication Administration**

    http://www.ihi.org/resources/Pages/Changes/ImproveCoreProcessesforAdministering Medications.aspx

Institute for Safe Medication Practices

    www.ismp.org

The Joint Commission

- **The Essential Role of Leadership in Developing a Safety Culture**

    https://www.jointcommission.org/assets/1/18/SEA_57_Safety_Culture_Leadership_0317.pdf

- **Patient Safety Systems**

    https://www.jointcommission.org/assets/1/18/CAMH_04a_PS.pdf

- **Sentinel Events**

    www.jointcommission.org/sentinel_event.aspx

Joint Commission Center for Transforming Healthcare

    http://www.centerfortransforminghealthcare.org/hro_portal_main.aspx

The Joint Commission International—International Center for Patient Safety

    www.jointcommissioninternational.org

Josie King Foundation

    www.josieking.org

The Just Culture Community

    www.outcome-eng.com

The Leapfrog Group

    www.leapfroggroup.org

National Academies Press

    www.nap.edu

National Association for Healthcare Quality

- **Call to Action: Safeguarding the Integrity of Healthcare Quality and Safety Systems**

    http://www.nahq.org/uploads/NAHQ_call_to_action_FINAL.pdf

- **HQ Essentials: Patient Safety**

    http://nahq.org/education/hq-essentials

National Coordinating Council for Medication Error Reporting and Prevention

    www.nccmerp.org

National Network of Libraries of Medicine

    https://nnlm.gov/

National Patient Safety Foundation

    www.npsf.org

Free from Harm

    http://www.npsf.org/?page=freefromharm

Outcome Engenuity

    https://www.outcome-eng.com/

Occupational Health & Safety Administration—U.S. Department of Labor

- **Healthcare**

    https://www.osha.gov/SLTC/healthcarefacilities/index.html

- **Sustainability**

    https://www.osha.gov/sustainability/

Partnership for Patients, Leadership

    https://partnershipforpatients.cms.gov/p4p_resources/tsp-leadership/toolleadership.html

The Patient Safety Group

    www.patientsafetygroup.org/about/about.cfm

Quality and Safety Education for Nurses

    www.qsen.org

Safe & Reliable Healthcare

    https://www.safeandreliablecare.com/

U.S. Department of Health & Human Services, Office of Minority Health

- **Think Cultural Health**

    https://www.thinkculturalhealth.hhs.gov/about

United States Pharmacopeial Convention: USP and Healthcare Professionals

www.usp.org/usp-healthcare-professionals

University of Texas Safety Climate Survey

https://med.uth.edu/chqs/surveys/safety-attitudes-and-safety-climate-questionnaire/

VA National Center for Patient Safety (NCPS)

http://www.patientsafety.va.gov/

World Health Organization

- **Patient Safety**
  www.who.int/patientsafety/en
- **Infection Prevention and Control**
  http://www.who.int/gpsc/en/

Section 3

Performance and Process Improvement

Susan V. White

Abstract

Through understanding performance and process improvement principles, healthcare quality professionals can apply evidence-based techniques to ensure quality and safety in their healthcare organizations. This section provides an overview of the historical development of performance and process improvement as well as the key principles and practices for performance improvement (PI) in healthcare quality and safety. The tenets of quality and safety must first be established through strategic planning to better align the activities with the organization's mission, vision, values, goals, and objectives. Important to an organization's success is the establishment of priorities for quality and PI activities, translating strategic goals into quality outcomes, and aligning organizational culture and structure to support quality. A formal quality and PI program with a defined scope and infrastructure is required to evaluate projects and performance toward desired goals. Fundamentals of a quality and PI program are described including tools and methods for use by healthcare quality professionals. An overview of teams and their roles and responsibilities is provided (e.g., team effectiveness, process champions, and process owners). Approaches to sharing successes and evaluating external award opportunities are also reviewed.

Learning Objectives

1. Understand historical perspectives on healthcare quality and appreciate the contributions of the quality pioneers and visionaries.
2. Describe strategic planning and management considering current and evolving healthcare performance and process improvement approaches.

3. Create a quality and PI plan that establishes priorities for quality, safety, and PI activities, develop action plans and projects, and provide training on performance and process improvement, program development, and evaluation.

4. Establish methods for evidence-based practice (EBP) guidelines, critical pathways, and effective team building.

5. Identify opportunities for rewards, awards, and recognition for healthcare organizations and understand different ways to share organizational and personal successes (e.g., presentations, storyboards, and publications).

The Evolution of Healthcare Quality

There are individuals in the history of quality and PI who were influential in shaping current performance and process improvement approaches and techniques. Early pioneers viewed process as a sequence of activities and communications that fulfilled a service need for a client or customer and improving a process to yield quality outcomes.[1] These early pioneers are briefly presented with their major contributions to the development of quality and performance management.

Quality Pioneers

Walter Shewhart. In the 1920s, Walter Shewhart, a statistician at Bell Telephone Laboratories, developed the Shewhart Cycle, best known as plan–do–check–act (PDCA). This four-step process is designed to continuously improve quality (FIG. 3-1). The PDCA steps include the following:

Plan.   Question the capacity or capability of a process. Pose theories on how to improve the process and predict measurable outcomes.

Do.   Make changes on an experimental, pilot basis.

Check.   Measure outcomes compared to predicted outcomes.

Act.   Implement the changes on a broad scale.[1]

Later, Deming adapted the PDCA cycle as the plan–do–study–act (PDSA) cycle; therefore, it also is referred to as the Deming Cycle, or the Deming Wheel. Both PDCA and PDSA are used as improvement models. Shewhart is also credited with his work on statistical process control (SPC) charts.

W. Edwards Deming. W. Edwards Deming is probably the most famous of the industrial quality gurus. A statistician with doctorates in mathematics and physics, he ultimately became the "philosopher of quality" and the learning organization. The story of post–World War II America's rejection of Deming's quality exhortations—and of his subsequent dealings with a receptive Japan—led to his being referred to as the "father of the third wave of the industrial revolution."[2(p2)] In the 1950s, Deming visited the Western Electric Hawthorne Plant in Chicago while the Harvard University study regarding motivation of workers was in progress (hence the term "Hawthorne Effect" was coined from this work). Following this experience, he proposed replacing traditional management techniques with a statistically controlled management process to determine when—and when not—to intervene in a process.

SPC techniques allow management to determine a range of random variation that always occurs in a process. SPC describes two types of causes of variation: common cause and special cause. Common-cause problems are rooted in basic processes and systems. Special-cause problems stem from isolated occurrences that are outside the system. SPC is discussed in *Health Data Analytics* and further explains how to understand control limits and define common- and special-cause variation. Deming said that 85% of the problems detected are process or system related, whereas 15% are traceable to individuals; this is known as the "85/15

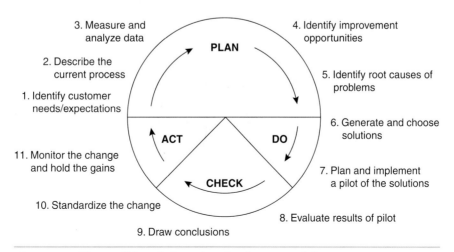

Figure 3-1 The traditional plan–do–check–act model.

theory."[3] Deming's management philosophy is based on his 14 points for businesses that seek to be competitive:

1. Create a constancy of purpose toward quality improvement (QI).
2. Adopt a philosophy that expects good products and services.
3. Cease dependence on mass inspection, and build quality into the product or service.
4. Do not award business solely on price tag.
5. Improve constantly the system of production and service.
6. Institute on-the-job training.
7. Institute leadership with an arm to help people and machines do better jobs.
8. Drive out fear.
9. Break down barriers between departments.
10. Eliminate slogans, exhortations, and targets.
11. Eliminate number quotas and management by objective and substitute leadership.
12. Remove barriers to pride of workmanship.
13. Institute education and self-improvement.
14. Take action to accomplish the transformation.[3,4]

Joseph Juran. Juran's background was in engineering and law. He followed Deming to Japan after World War II, emphasizing the key role of top organizational leadership and the importance "to lean on each other to help the other succeed."[5(p1)] In *Juran on Leadership for Quality*,[6] Juran states that quality is "product performance that results in customer satisfaction; freedom from product deficiencies which avoid customer dissatisfaction."[6(pp16,31)] This concept is known as fitness for use and is explained in Juran's Trilogy. Juran stated that the cost of quality accounting means there is a break-even point of less than 100%. Beyond a certain point, the cost of providing quality exceeds the value of the incremental improvement in quality. Juran's Trilogy is analogous to certain familiar financial processes. Quality planning is equal to budgeting, quality control (sometimes called measurement) is comparable to cost control, and quality and PI relate to cost reduction and margin improvement.[1]

Philip H. Crosby. In the 1970s and 1980s, Crosby developed an important concept known as *the cost of [poor] quality*. His work documented that high quality (what he terms "conformance to expectations") is less costly than the waste and rework that characterizes poor-quality processes. Five stages of management maturity are identified by Crosby in his book, *Quality Is Free*.[7] Crosby's underlying philosophy is "Do it right the first time." The stages are

1. uncertainty (when an organization is characterized by the statement, "We don't know why we have quality problems"),

2. awakening,
3. enlightenment,
4. wisdom, and
5. certainty (reserved for organizations in which top management proclaims, "We know why we don't have quality problems." The mature company is equipped to initiate a QI program[8]).

Crosby also identified 14 steps to improve quality and move a company toward "certainty," including the following:

Step 1. Management is committed to QI.

Step 2. A QI team is formed to oversee actions.

Step 3. Quality measurement is undertaken appropriate to the activities undergoing improvement.

Step 4. Quality cost is evaluated, using estimates as necessary.

Step 5. Quality awareness is promoted through various methods and supervisor involvement.

Step 6. Corrective actions are generated in response to steps 3 and 4.

Step 7. Zero-defects planning is tailored to the company and its products.

Step 8. Supervisory training is undertaken at all management levels.

Step 9. A zero-defects day is held to celebrate a new performance standard.

Step 10. Goals are set for individuals and groups.

Step 11. Error cause(s) is removed by management after notification.

Step 12. Goals are met and recognized.

Step 13. The quality council's experiences, problems, and ideas are shared.

Step 14. The process is repeated (the pursuit of quality is never-ending).

Kaoru Ishikawa. Ishikawa was one of Deming's early Japanese hosts and inventor of the cause-and-effect, or fishbone, diagram and is credited with using the term *total quality control* to imply not just the operational but also the total organizational commitment (marketing, finance, research) needed to fully actualize all components of the modern quality-committed organization. He along with Deming, Juran, and Crosby contributed to the development of *total quality management*.[9]

Healthcare Quality in the 21st Century

A timeline for the healthcare quality movement, which began in the 19th century and continues into the 21st century, is described herein and in FIGURE 3-2.

1863	Florence Nightingale, a nurse, calls for a systematic review of patient care.
1910	Codman proposes an end-result system of hospital standardization and Flexner publishes report calling for American medical schools to enact standards for teaching and research of the medical profession.
1918	The American College of Surgeons develops minimum standards for hospitals and conducts its first survey.
1950	Donabedian formulates a theoretical framework for patient care evaluation (structure, process, outcomes).
1951	Joint Commission on Accreditation of Hospitals founded by Codman introducing quality assurance standards for hospitals (later to become the Joint Commission on Accreditation of Healthcare Organizations and then The Joint Commission).
1960	Japan focuses on becoming a world quality leader; adopts the Deming management philosophy.
1970	Juran and Crosby build on Shewhart and Deming's work; Plan–Do–Check–Act/Plan–Do–Study–Act cycles emerge.
1980	Berwick, Batalden, and James apply quality improvement (QI) methods to healthcare.
1996	Health Insurance Portability and Accountability Act of 1996 (HIPAA) enacted.
1999	Institute of Medicine releases the report, *To Err Is Human*.
2000	Six Sigma, Lean Enterprise, rapid-cycle improvements, safety, and pay for performance begin to have an impact on healthcare quality.
2001	The Committee on Quality of Health Care in America released *Crossing the Quality Chasm* for fundamental change to close the quality gap in the American healthcare system.
2002	Medicare begins a series of quality measurement and reporting initiatives starting with nursing homes, followed by home healthcare, and eventually hospitals and physicians.
2009	American Recovery and Reinvestment Act signed into law that included the Health Information Technology for Economic and Clinical Health Act (HITECH).
2010	The Patient Protection and Affordable Care Act signed into law.
2011	U.S. Department of Health & Human Services releases the *National Quality Strategy* and present three aims to guide efforts to improve quality—Better Care, Healthy People/Healthy Communities, and Affordable Care.
2013	Institute of Medicine (IOM) releases report, *Best Care at Lower Costs: The Path to Continuously Learning Health Care in America*, looking at inefficiencies, an overwhelming amount of data, and other economic and quality barriers hinder progress in improving health and what is needed to achieve continuous improvement and better quality care at a lower cost.

Figure 3-2 **Quality movement timeline.**

The First Era: Nightingale, Codman, and the American College of Surgeons

In 1863, Florence Nightingale noted that patients seemed to fare better in some London hospitals than in others. As a nurse, she was the first to call for systematic inquiry into the nature of care processes that could be related to outcome variability. Although there is little evidence that Nightingale's quality vision came to fruition during her lifetime, Boston surgeon Ernest Codman's early 20th-century efforts had a more formal impact. Codman, who also observed variability in patient outcomes among several hospitals, called for a systematic evaluation process with a view toward improving care.[10] Although his efforts met considerable resistance, Codman's ideas were embodied in the founding of the American College of Surgeons in 1913. This body of work set about the task of establishing quality standards. In 1917, the College established a five-part "minimum standard," and the Hospital Standardization Program was born.[11] These were the early beginnings for hospital accreditation based on standards. The program was based on Codman's end-result system of standardization in which hospitals would track every patient treated for long enough to determine if the treatment was effective. When treatment was found to be ineffective, the hospital would attempt to determine how such similar cases could be treated with success in the future. Codman is best known for his focus on outcomes.

The Second Era: Donabedian and The Joint Commission's Monitoring and Evaluation Process

Accreditation standards evolved slowly throughout the 1950s and early 1960s. At the academic level, the University of Michigan's Dr. Avedis Donabedian examined existing research, formulating a theoretical framework for patient care evaluation.[12] He is best recognized for his "structure, process, outcomes" model of quality evaluation (FIG. 3-3).

This model suggests the importance of relating healthcare structures (qualifications of practitioners and facilities and technology available to them) and processes (activities involved in prevention, diagnosis, and treatment) to outcomes (how patients fare because of their care). In the past, Joint Commission standards mainly reflected the structure and process elements of this model. Surveyors, who reviewed the structures and processes, assessed hospital plans and technology, qualifications of clinicians and administrators, and organizational structures against the annually updated requirements contained in the *Comprehensive Accreditation Manual for Hospitals*. Specialized standards for behavioral health and other services were also developed. Surveyors inferred process from documentation and discussion. They reviewed minutes and interviewed clinical and administrative leaders to ascertain whether designated individuals were following procedures and compliant with quality evaluation processes.

As a matter of policy and practical considerations, accreditation standards did not address patient outcomes directly. First, there were problems with the way "quality" was measured. Second, no professional consensus existed on systematic measures of patient outcomes. Finally, uniform and comparable clinical databases were nonexistent. The problems of measuring and interpreting patient outcomes precluded their practical use in accreditation. Consequently, the accreditation process was necessarily built on an implicit assumption that if proper structures and processes were in place, good outcomes were likely to follow. As measurement systems matured, the evaluation of patient outcomes became

Structure	Process	Outcomes
Professionals	Leadership	Clinical
Facilities	Management	Functional
Technologies	Interaction	Experience
Resources	Diagnosis	Engagement
Organizations	Therapy	

Figure 3-3 **Donabedian's framework.**

a strong focus for accreditation processes as well as the organizational review of different aspects of care, treatment, and services. Current accreditation processes are discussed in detail in *Organizational Leadership*.

The Third Era: Berwick, Batalden, and James "Discover" Deming, Juran, and "Japan, Inc."

The names of Drs. Donald Berwick, Paul Batalden, and Brent James are eminent in the field of healthcare quality and performance management. Like many of their colleagues, these physicians were dissatisfied with traditional healthcare quality assurance (QA) practices. These pioneering physicians, however, went beyond a mere critique of existing QA. Both Berwick and Batalden researched the industrial methods publicized by the Japanese experience. Arising from this research, Berwick's article describing healthcare QA as based upon the "Theory of the Bad Apples" became a classic.[13] Among his many contributions, Batalden translated Deming's famous 14 points[7] into a healthcare context.[14] In 1987, these two physicians played key roles in linking with The Juran Institute and a variety of industrial quality consultants to create the National Demonstration Project on Quality Improvement in Health Care. This multiyear project and its original 21 forward-looking healthcare organizations conclusively demonstrated the applicability of PI processes to healthcare.[15]

James, of the Intermountain Health System, was also a pioneer in applying QI processes directly to patients and clinical outcomes. The success of James and his team measured not only improved results in a single hospital but also across the entire multihospital system.[16,17]

In 1991, Berwick established the Institute for Healthcare Improvement (IHI), a not-for-profit organization that began driving improvements in healthcare. It accomplished this by supporting national projects focused on the six aims—safety, effectiveness, patient centeredness, timeliness, efficiency, and equity.[18] Collaboratives are one approach involving many organizations trying to affect the same issue and using rapid-cycle improvement efforts to implement change. A major benefit of this approach is that the collaborating organizations share their experiences and improvements spread quickly. Projects initiated include improvements in patient safety, chronic care, critical care, and end-of-life care. Berwick was appointed administrator of the Centers for Medicare & Medicaid Services (CMS) in 2010 and served for 18 months in President Obama's administration. While in office, Berwick inculcated the "Triple Aim" into health policy: improving the patient care experience, improving population health, and reducing health costs. Dr. Berwick was also responsible for initiating major changes under the new health reform legislation.[19]

With more and more experience, the list of visionary leaders, both clinical and managerial, continues to grow as evidenced by recent literature and presentations in public forums. Many healthcare organizations are taking the learnings from these leaders as well as newer methodologies and are advancing the science and experience of healthcare quality to serve as role models for others. For example, Virginia Mason led many lean initiatives by modeling the Toyota methods, and Catalysis (formerly ThedaCare Center for Healthcare Value) is sharing its lean journey.

The Fourth Era: Patient Is Front and Center of Quality and Safety with Growth of Advocacy, Engagement, and Activation

Healthcare reform stresses an imperative to engage families in their own care. Enhancing patient-centered care that results in empowerment, engagement, and activation is everyone's job. Patients and their families need to understand their role and responsibilities related to quality and safety. Patient-centered communication is shown to improve clinical outcomes and more patient-centric technology tools are available, which have been found to be most useful in managing chronic disease.[20,21]

Patient advocacy includes addressing the rights and responsibilities of patients and involving them in shared decision making, obtaining informed consent for treatment, and disclosing unanticipated outcomes. An advocate or ombudsman is often available to manage inquiries, requests, complaints, and grievances, with a process to document and track reported issues to resolution. An ethical framework is often applied with ethics consultation to respond to issues that may create conflict with the rights of the patient and the organization or others. A patient's bill of rights was first adopted by the American Hospital Association (AHA) in 1973 and revised in 1992 (FIG. 3-4). More recently, the AHA published *The Patient Care Partnership* replacing the Rights with a plain-language brochure.[22] The protection of the patient rights may include a variety of concerns, such as abuse, neglect, and exploitation; decision-making ability and use of surrogates or durable power of attorney; advance directives or living wills; and treatment without fear of retaliation.

I. Information Disclosure

You have the right to receive accurate and easily understood information about your health plan, healthcare professionals, and healthcare facilities. If you speak another language, have a physical or mental disability, or just don't understand something, assistance will be provided so you can make informed healthcare decisions.

II. Choice of Providers and Plans

You have the right to a choice of healthcare providers that is sufficient to provide you with access to appropriate, high-quality healthcare.

III. Access to Emergency Services

If you have severe pain, an injury, or sudden illness that convinces you that your health is in serious jeopardy, you have the right to receive screening and stabilization emergency services whenever and wherever needed, without prior authorization or financial penalty.

IV. Participation in Treatment Decisions

You have the right to know all your treatment options and to participate in decisions about your care. Parents, guardians, family members, or other individuals that you designate can represent you if you cannot make your own decisions.

V. Respect and Nondiscrimination

You have the right to considerate, respectful, and nondiscriminatory care from your doctors, health plan representatives, and other healthcare providers.

VI. Confidentiality of Health Information

You have the right to talk in confidence with healthcare providers and to have your healthcare information protected. You also have the right to review and copy your own medical record and request that your physician amend your record if it is not accurate, relevant, or complete.

VII. Complaints and Appeals

You have the right to a fair, fast, and objective review of any complaint you have against your health plan, doctors, hospitals, or other healthcare personnel. This includes complaints about waiting times, operating hours, the conduct of healthcare personnel, and the adequacy of healthcare facilities.

(continued)

VIII. Consumer Responsibilities

Greater individual involvement by consumers in their care increases the likelihood of achieving the best outcomes and helps support a quality improvement, cost-conscious environment. Such responsibilities include the following:

 I. Take responsibility for maximizing healthy habits, such as exercising, not smoking, and eating a healthy diet.
 II. Become involved in specific healthcare decisions.
 III. Work collaboratively with healthcare providers in developing and carrying out agreed-upon treatment plans.
 IV. Disclose relevant information and clearly communicate your wants and needs.
 V. Use your health plan's internal complaint and appeal processes to address concerns that may arise.
 VI. Avoid knowingly spreading disease.
 VII. Recognize the reality of risks and limits of the science of medical care and the human fallibility of the healthcare professional.
 VIII. Be aware of a healthcare provider's obligation to be reasonably efficient and equitable in providing care to other patients and the community.
 IX. Become knowledgeable about your health plan coverage and health plan options (when available) including all covered benefits, limitations, and exclusions, rules regarding use of network providers, coverage and referral rules, appropriate processes to secure additional information, and the process to appeal coverage decisions.
 X. Show respect for other patients and health workers.
 XI. Make a good-faith effort to meet financial obligations.
 XII. Abide by administrative and operational procedures of health plans, healthcare providers, and Government health benefit programs.
 XIII. Report wrongdoing and fraud to appropriate resources or legal authorities.

Figure 3-4 **Patients' bill of rights and responsibilities.** (From Agency for Healthcare Research and Quality, President's Advisory Commission on Consumer Protection and Quality in Health Care Industry. Consumer Bill of Rights. Agency for Healthcare Research and Quality; 1998. https://archive.ahrq.gov/hcqual/cborr/. Accessed May 1, 2017.)

Engagement is defined as "actions an individual must make to obtain the greatest benefit from the healthcare services available to them."[23(p2)] Engaging patients produces better health outcomes.[24–26] In this context, patient engagement involves an active process of synthesizing health information, recommendations of healthcare professionals, and personal beliefs and preferences to manage one's illness. Advocacy, engagement, and activation—all offer opportunities for improved healthcare quality and safety in the 21st century. See *Patient Safety* for more discussion of engagement and activation.

Leadership and Performance Improvement

The development of meaningful governance in quality and safety requires assessment of the governing body's knowledge of PI. This is a key role of quality professionals responsible for organizing and coordinating quality management and PI activities for the organization and its medical staff. Healthcare quality professionals can promote the commitment to quality of the governing body and organizational leadership by providing useful information in a format easily understood by members who may lack familiarity with healthcare terminology and procedures.

Fundamental Principles of Leadership

Leadership is the ability to influence an individual or group toward achievement of goals.[27] Leadership and management are not identical. *Leadership* is determining the correct direction or path, whereas *management* is doing the correct things to stay on that path. Kotter[28] notes that management is about coping with complexity through planning and budgeting; setting goals; organizing, staffing, and creating a structure to foster goal attainment; setting up mechanisms for monitoring; and controlling results. In contrast, leaders are responsible for coping with change by developing a vision for change and aligning the subsystems of the organization. Both strong leadership and management are necessary for high performance. Some people are great leaders but poor managers and vice versa; in some cases, a person may be successful in both roles.

Leadership Framework

There are many frameworks for leadership. As is true with the system framework, often it is less important to choose a framework than simply having one to guide behavior. Deming[4] believed that managers were responsible for optimizing the system. Practices of exemplary leaders were explored by Kouzes and Posner,[29] who identified five important general practices: inspire a shared vision, challenge the system, enable others to act, model the way, and encourage the heart. These principles are generic and therefore applicable to any type of organization. These five practices are one way of describing leadership.

1. **Inspire a Shared Vision.** For any change to be successful, leaders must provide a vision for quality and influence people to share that vision. This means getting people

to accept and believe in the core values underlying PI by developing a strong culture.

2. **Challenge the System.** Challenging the system means acting as a change agent for that vision. It also means recognizing good ideas and demonstrating a willingness to stretch and grow to improve the quality of care. This, too, involves adoption of core values as a learning organization.

3. **Enable Others to Act.** The third leadership practice is enabling others to act by sharing decision-making and power. Along with sharing power, enabling involves having an appropriate structural design and resources to support quality and safety initiatives.

4. **Model the Way.** Much behavior is learned through role modeling. Effective leaders must model desired behaviors as actions speak louder than words.

5. **Encourage the Heart.** The last practice is critical. Change is difficult, even if it is done for the right reasons. Encouraging the heart means recognizing contributions employees make and celebrating the core values and victories. The most important point of any reward system is to reward the desired behaviors.

Leaders use these five practices to keep subsystems aligned. However, leaders must first engage people to support a common vision of quality. One way this occurs is through a strong supportive culture of quality and safety. See *Organizational Leadership* for more information on leadership and culture, and their impact on performance and process improvement.

The Governing Body

The organization's governing body or board of directors bears ultimate responsibility for setting policy, financial and strategic direction, and the quality of care and service provided by all its practitioners. Together with the organization's management and medical staff leaders, the governing body sets priorities for QI activities.

The AHA outlined Principles of Accountability for Hospitals and Healthcare Organizations, with specific directives for governing board and leadership.[30] These government and leadership directives are described in **TABLE 3-1**. A new document was published in 2015 with a joint American Hospital Association/American Medical Association (AHA/AMA) statement in *Integrated Leadership for Hospitals and Health Systems: Principles for Success*,[31] which addresses integrated leadership and includes six principles:

1. Physician and hospital leaders who share values and expectations; aligned incentives; goals across the board with appropriate means of measuring them; responsibility for financial, cost and quality targets; accountable service line teams; strategic planning; and a focus on engaging patients as partners.

2. A structure incorporating all disciplines and supporting collaborative decision-making between doctors and hospital executives, with physicians maintaining their clinical autonomy.

Table 3-1 American Hospital Association's (AHA) Principles of Accountability for Hospitals and Healthcare Organizations: Governance/Leadership

Mission and Vision. The organization's governing body and leadership should articulate clearly defined mission and vision statements. With these statements as a foundation, the organization's leadership should develop an action plan with specific goals, time frames for accomplishment, and linked measures of performance for a regular assessment of achievement, with oversight by the governing body. As part of this development process, the organization's governing body and leadership should seek input from relevant stakeholders concerning their needs and interests relative to the organization. The plan and the results should be widely communicated to all individuals who are employed by or affiliated with the organization.

Executive Management Oversight. The organization's governing body is responsible for the oversight of the organization's leadership performance and should periodically evaluate that performance relative to the organization's achievement of its stated strategic goals. As part of the process of evaluating the organization's leadership, the governing body should periodically and systematically assess its own performance relative to defined goals and measures of performance.

Quality Oversight. The organization's governing body and leadership, in conjunction with the clinical staff, are responsible for developing and implementing, in a comprehensive manner, systems and procedures for safeguarding and enhancing the quality of patient care and services. The governing body and leadership, in conjunction with the clinical staff, are also responsible for actively monitoring and immediately acting upon, where appropriate, the results derived from those systems and procedures such that patient and staff safety is ensured or improvements in patient care occur.

Financial Stability. The organization's governing body is responsible for ensuring the financial well-being of the organization and, in conjunction with the organization's leadership, for overseeing the appropriate and most optimal allocation of financial and physical resources for the improvement of patient care. The organization's mission and duty to improve patient care and community health must not be obstructed by (and must take precedence over) the financial interests of individuals or groups employed by or affiliated with the organization.

Reprinted from American Hospital Association. *Accountability—The Pathway to Restoring Public Trust and Confidence for Hospitals and Other Health Care Organizations*, November 11–12, 1999:8, Chicago, IL: AHA; 1999, with permission.

3. Hospital and clinical leadership is integrated at all levels of the health system, and includes nursing and other caregivers, participating in all key management decisions.

4. The partnership between both sides is collaborative, participatory and built on trust, as Combes emphasized. Interdependence and a thrust toward achieving the Triple Aim is "crucial to alignment and engagement," according to the report.

5. Transparency of both clinical and business information, across the entire enterprise, is also crucial.

6. Finally, integrated leadership requires an information technology (IT) system that allows clinicians to capture and report quality and performance data of all participants, with leadership holding its workforce accountable for those measurements.[31]

For practical purposes, day-to-day leadership is the responsibility of the CEO and senior management (collectively known as the C-Suite), elected or appointed members of the medical staff (e.g., chairs), and administrative and clinical staff (e.g., practitioners, quality and PI staff).

Organizational Strategy and Performance Management

The following discussion on performance management centers on the organizational level in the context of meeting the organization's strategic goals and objectives. *Performance management* is defined as "a forward-looking process used to set goals and regularly check progress toward achieving those goals. In practice, an organization sets goals, looks at the actual data for its performance measures, and acts on results to improve the performance toward its goals."[32(p1)] The goal of a performance management system is to make certain that the vision of the organization is being met by defining and measuring outcomes reflected in that vision.

Although there are a variety of quality and PI programs, including the Baldrige Performance Excellence Program and the European Foundation for Quality Management, many government agencies and Fortune 1000 companies use the balanced scorecard (BSC) as an approach to performance management. BSCs are completely compatible with other quality performance programs but go beyond such programs by embedding quality and PI in the strategic framework of the organization.[33]

The BSC was developed by Norton and Kaplan in the early 1990s. The basic idea is that performance measures provide a comprehensive view of organizational performance and not be overly dependent on a few choice indicators. Unlike other performance models, the BSC helps organizations better link long-term strategy with short-term activities.[34]

The BSC approach views the organization from four different perspectives or categories: financial ("How do we look to providers of financial resources?"), customer ("How do our customers see us?"), internal business processes ("At what must we excel?"), and learning and growth ("Can we continue to improve and create value for customers?"). Answers to these questions influence the nature of the strategic goals and objectives that are set and, ultimately, what performance measures are used. The critical aspect of performance indicators is that they must reflect the organization's strategic goals and objectives.

There are likely to be several strategic objectives corresponding to each of the four perspectives. Each of these objectives has at least one measure with vetted measurement properties (e.g., reliability, validity, qualitative data, quantitative data) and can be collected through a variety of means (e.g., surveys, focus groups, patient chart reviews). Health Resources & Services Administration suggests that development and use of different types of measures (i.e., structure, process, outcomes) in each of the categories is an important "balanced" approach.[32]

The foundation for an organization's strategic success begins with its people, who must be willing to learn and grow. To meet the changing needs of customers, they must, for example, learn new technology and acquire new skills to take on new responsibilities. The strategic goal "Develop a state-of-the-art program for breast cancer detection and treatment" could consider measures such as

- structure: quantity of imaging equipment;
- process: number of patients diagnosed with imaging technology; and
- outcome: higher percentage of early diagnoses, due to use of imaging technology.

It is necessary to monitor and improve key processes so that employees can convert learning and growth into products and services or quality outcomes. "Be recognized as one of the top healthcare providers in the community" could be another strategic goal. Measures might include

- structure: resources available for care delivery (e.g., nurse–patient ratio);
- process: care (how patients are diagnosed and treated); and
- outcomes: results of care (e.g., satisfaction, length and quality of life, turnover rates).

Just as different organizational levels and units develop goals and objectives based on corporate strategy, different levels and units also can use the BSC or similar dashboard approach. The use of a scorecard or dashboard to reflect an organization's key strategic goals or priorities or "pillars" is still in active use but terms often morph over time. A review of these concepts can be noted by reviewing Baldrige healthcare recipients in which results are focused on patient safety and quality as key perspectives, not just the traditional BSC perspectives.

Note: for the same strategic goal (e.g., be recognized as one of the top healthcare providers in the community) there are several measures of performance across different perspectives.

Structure for Performance and Process Improvement

Every organization should have an organization-wide plan for PI. The plan defines examples of key activities or core processes and quality control methods for each service. There are numerous federal, state, and local-level regulations and accreditation standards that govern quality monitoring, evaluation, and reporting. This is especially true for diagnostic services such as pathology and laboratory services, radiology, nuclear medicine, and pharmacy. Content experts in these services lead the identification of regulations or other requirements and the specific quality control processes and measures that must be maintained. The requirements may include provisions for employee exposure monitoring, including issuance of individual radiology badges or devices. Quality and performance management personnel are often involved in the direct monitoring within services or the aggregation of data or reports from different services in the organization. The unit or service level is considered a microsystem, and it is at this level that change happens and improvements generally occur. The service-level plan includes

- identifying populations served;
- describing services provided;
- PI priorities at the service level, aligned with the organization's goals and strategic plan;
- identifying any requirements related to PI, quality control, and quality monitoring (e.g., accreditation standards, regulations, device monitoring, quality control);
- selecting valid and reliable metrics for the service;
- developing a monitoring plan (e.g., sample, frequency, reporting);
- developing a plan for evaluating performance; and
- identifying methods for improving the performance.

A standard format can make the development of plans or quality monitoring across multiple services and sites more efficient and effective for tracking, trending, and reporting. The service-level plan should support the organization-wide plan which identifies the framework for all services, organization-level priorities and goals, resources, and metrics. Discussion of the different aspects to consider in the planning process for PI follows.

Setting Priorities

The road to quality healthcare begins with strategic planning to guide the organization in focusing on the most important aspects or priorities. Priorities for performance and process improvement activities are based on several standard approaches. The first approach is that the priorities are aligned with the organization's strategic direction to maximize resources for improvement, and the second is a criteria-based approach considering risk, volume, problem proneness, patient safety, cost, customer satisfaction, and other criteria established specifically by the organization. The pillars identified by Studer are also often used as the categories of improvement priorities: Quality, People, Finance, Service, Growth and Community.[35] In some organizations, safety has recently been added to the pillars of excellence model.

A framework for leadership of improvement is the first step in turning the strategic plan into an operational plan for improvement. In this framework, leaders apply the mission, vision, values, and strategic plan to set direction. This framework is built on a foundational leadership team to support improvement capability. The three components of *will to prepare for change*, *ideas to generate new ways of performing*, and *execution of change* contribute to a leadership system for improvement. Models depicting the framework and how the framework operates in an integrated system are shown in FIGURES 3-5 and 3-6.

Prioritizing evaluates key processes against key business drivers to identify the most important processes to improve and measure in evaluating performance. Applying priorities determines the initiation of an improvement action, based on the analysis of data collection. The goals and drivers of the system are depicted in FIGURE 3-7. Leaders identify a priority list of processes or services for improvement.[36] Healthcare quality professionals facilitate development of priorities by

- establishing criteria for priority assessment (e.g., volume, risk, problem proneness);
- using data on past performance to assess gaps (internal performance);
- using external drivers for consideration (new regulations, standards);
- providing information to leaders with a basis for recommendations;
- using tools to create a matrix for priorities for decision making,
- involving key stakeholders for input; and
- identifying internal and external requirements that influence priorities.

In addition, healthcare quality professionals and their teams use the described criteria to prioritize performance and process improvement activities based on the quantitative and qualitative data available to them. By using past performance, aligned with the criteria and strategic initiatives, the team can determine the priorities for action. A plan is often written by healthcare quality professionals and approved by the clinical leaders to ensure success of the activities, especially in allocating adequate resources for the effort.

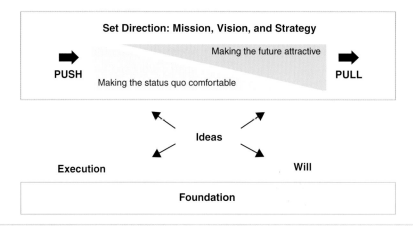

Figure 3-5 Framework for leading improvement. (Reprinted from Reinertsen JL, Bisognano M, Pugh MD. *Seven Leadership Leverage Points for Organization-Level Improvement in Health Care.* 2nd ed. Cambridge, MA: Institute for Healthcare Improvement; 2011, with permission.)

The initiatives having the most opportunity for improvement are often tackled first. Usually, the initiatives selected focus on core clinical processes, high-risk processes, high-risk patients and populations, high-risk medications, or high-risk actions or interventions. The level of risk is based on the potential consequences of injury or harm to patients. In an acute care hospital setting, a high-risk process might be blood transfusions, while in long-term care it might be fall prevention, and within an office practice, it might be ensuring

timely immunizations. Healthcare quality professionals need to identify those processes for specific settings.

Another aspect in assessing level of risk is the frequency with which the process or procedure is performed. For example, responding to a case of sepsis or malignant hyperthermia would be considered high risk for the patient, and if the staff does not manage this scenario often, they may not respond as a highly effective team. Therefore, it may be a priority to perform drills to ensure that staff is competent. Managing

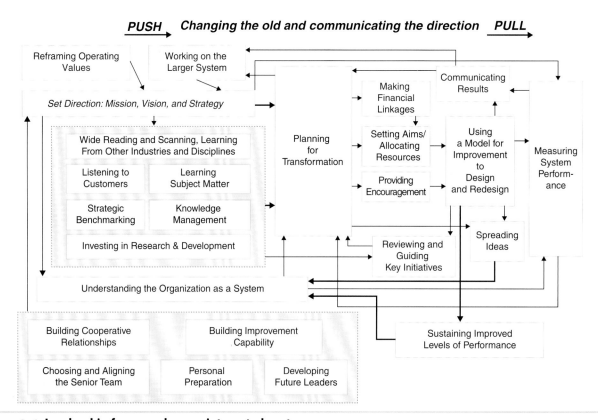

Figure 3-6 Leadership framework as an integrated system. (Reprinted from Institute for Healthcare Improvement. Building a system of leadership for improvement. In: *A Framework for Leadership for Improvement.* Cambridge, MA: IHI; 2006:4, with permission. www.knowledge.scot.nhs.uk/media/CLT/ResourceUploads/4012931/IHILeadershipFramework_FEB2006versionFINAL.pdf.)

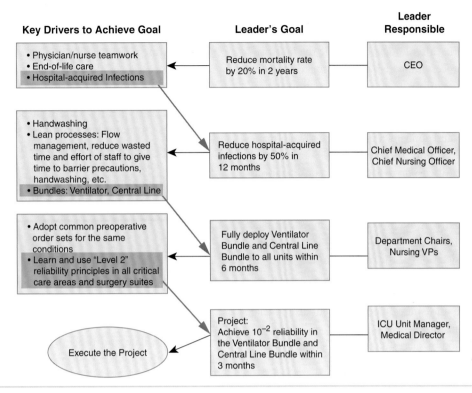

Figure 3-7 Cascading series of goals and drivers for improvement. (Reprinted from Reinertsen JL, Bisognano M, Pugh MD. *Seven Leadership Leverage Points for Organization-Level Improvement in Health Care.* 2nd ed. Cambridge, MA: Institute for Healthcare Improvement; 2011:14, with permission.)

high-risk patients and processes significantly affect morbidity and mortality. Examples of high-risk processes include

- core processes: admission, transfer, discharge, transitions, coordination of care, other handoffs;
- high-risk processes: medication delivery or administration, surgery, resuscitation;
- high-risk patients: patients with reduced renal function, immunocompromised patients, neonates, patients in critical care units, suicidal patients, dementia patients at risk for wandering;
- high-risk medications: heparin (and oral anticoagulants), insulin, chemotherapy, opiates, neuromuscular blocking agents, psychotropics; and
- high-risk actions and interventions: blood and blood product transfusions, use of restraints, extracorporeal circulation, moderate sedation.[37]

After priorities are established, specific initiatives or activities are undertaken. Key steps to implementing PI activities to ensure success of the PI priorities follow:

1. Ensure leadership support and commitment for the PI initiative.
2. Assess priority and feasibility of initiative based on risk, resources, leadership support, and organizational strategies.
3. Identify the aim of the initiative and include the topic, process, or problem to be improved (provide a good rationale).
4. Convene an interdisciplinary team of content and process experts with all key disciplines as participants (involve all the right stakeholders with a champion for change).
5. Use tools and techniques to analyze processes, best practices, research, and consensus-based evidence for the desired change.
6. Develop the change to be implemented and add timelines and accountability for the project.
7. Identify the measures to demonstrate that the change resulted in improvement; set performance goals.
8. Educate staff on the desired change.
9. Implement and test the change via the redesigned processes.
10. Collect, analyze, and evaluate data on the redesigned process.
11. Make additional changes based on findings and disseminate to all areas.
12. Report and display results to reward staff for improvements.
13. Continue to monitor performance to ensure that the change is sustained.
14. Compare performance internally and externally.
15. Celebrate successes internally and externally.[37,38]

When choosing between improvement activities, use a prioritization matrix (FIG. 3-8) to assist in evaluating the items against specific criteria. After leaders determine the improvement priorities for process improvement, they make decisions about the need to organize a team. A prioritization matrix organizes tasks, issues, or actions and prioritizes them based on agreed-upon criteria. The tool is helpful in identifying criteria for specific priorities and applying a rating scale to help make decisions for the selection of specific activities. This matrix applies options under discussion to the priority considerations of the organization. The tool combines the tree diagram and the L-shaped matrix diagram, displaying the best possible effect. The prioritization matrix is often used before more complex matrices are needed. This matrix applies options under discussion to the priority considerations of the organization.

A project selection matrix ranks and compares potential project areas for implementation. Ranking criteria may include organizational and strategic goals, potential financial impact to the organization, effect on patient and employee satisfaction, likelihood of success, and completion within a specified time frame (see FIG. 3-9).

Action Plan and Project Development

Once priorities are identified, an action plan puts them into motion. A standard format includes

- who (accountability),
- what (specific actions or steps to be followed),
- when (time frame),
- status (progress made and ongoing monitoring), and
- completion (closure or closing the loop).

Projects vary greatly, ranging from improving a defined process to complete redesign or even designing a new process or system. Although the scope varies, the key format remains constant. The level of detail, number of steps, and length of time to complete will vary greatly. FIGURE 3-10 shows the framework for execution of plans for a PI project.[39]

Planning and Evaluation of Improvement Projects and Activities

Healthcare quality professionals often guide the planning and evaluation for projects and activities. The first step is to understand data and tools to construct an overall plan and specifically the data collection plan. This includes the following steps:

1. Determine who, what, when, where, how, and why.
2. Structure the design.
3. Choose and develop a sampling method.
4. Determine learning needs and conduct training.

	High Risk	High Volume	Problem Prone	Cost	Customer Satisfaction	Regulatory	Total
Infection Rates	3	2	2	3	1	3	14
Surgical Complications	2	1	2	3	1	3	12
Emergency Department Time to Treatment	1	3	1	1	3	0	9
Falls with Injuries	2	1	1	2	2	2	10
Medication Safety	3	3	3	2	1	2	14

How to construct

1. Create an L-shaped matrix with identified areas on one side and evaluation criteria on the other side.
2. Prioritize and assign weights to the list of criteria that will be used in the prioritization. Define a scoring mechanism such as 1–3 or 1–5. In the example 1–3 is used with 1 = least important and 3 = most important.
3. Prioritize the list of options based on each criterion. Usually, key leaders come to agreement on the ratings.
4. Prioritize and select the items across all the criteria. Use the total scores to order the items from high to low.

When to use

When problems are identified and options must be narrowed down, when options have strong interrelationships, and when all options to be done but prioritization or sequencing is required

Figure 3-8 **Prioritization matrix: clinical improvement priorities.**

	Low Cost	High Strategic Priority	Meets Accreditation Standards	MD Concern	Staff Concern	Total
Repair roof	3	4	2	3	4	16
Purchase new X-ray machine	5	2	0	1	5	13
Develop skilled nursing unit	4	1	0	2	2	9
Develop better communications with home health	2	3	1	4	3	13
Develop staff newsletter	1	5	3	5	1	15

How to construct

1. Create a L-shaped matrix with identified areas on one side and evaluation criteria on the other side.
2. Prioritize and assign weights to the list of criteria that will be used in the prioritization. Define a scoring mechanism such as 1–3 or 1–5. In the example, 1–5 is used with 1 = least important and 5 = most important.
3. Prioritize the list of options based on each criterion. Usually, key leaders come to agreement on the ratings.
4. Prioritize and select the item(s) across all the criteria. Use the total scores to order the items from high to low.

When to use

- When issues are identified and options must be narrowed down
- When options have strong interrelationships
- When options all need to be done, but prioritization or sequencing is needed

Figure 3-9 Prioritization matrix: decision example.

5. Delegate responsibilities.
6. Facilitate coordination.
7. Forecast budget.
8. Conduct pilots or tests of change.

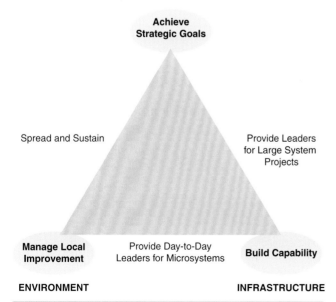

Figure 3-10 Framework for execution. (Reprinted from Reinertsen JL, Bisognano M, Pugh MD. *Seven Leadership Leverage Points for Organization-Level Improvement in Health Care*. 2nd ed. Cambridge, MA: Institute for Healthcare Improvement; 2011:5, with permission.)

A clear understanding of data and tools to assist in problem identification and solutions is needed to facilitate planning and evaluating improvement projects. An overview of data and data management is provided with some of the more common tools used in these processes later in this section.

Evaluation and Selection of EBP Guidelines

Evidence-based medicine (EBM) is the "conscientious, explicit, and judicious use of current best evidence in making decisions about the care of individual patients."[40(p71)] Because multiple disciplines are involved in healthcare delivery, however, the term *evidence-based practice* (EBP) is more appropriate than EBM from a healthcare quality perspective. Clinicians not only base their care on the experimental evidence but also consider experiential evidence, physiologic principles, patient and professional values, and system features in their decision making.[41] This allows individualized application and dissemination of aggregate research evidence.[41,42]

EBP promotes patient safety through the provision of effective and efficient healthcare, resulting in less variation in care and fewer unnecessary or nontherapeutic interventions.[43] EBP and outcomes measurement are iterative; one facilitates the other.[44] EBP complements the principles of continuous quality improvement (CQI). Outcome evaluation at the individual and aggregate level is an essential step in evaluating the impact of EBP.

Evidence-based quality management is based on two types of research: clinical research and health services research. Clinical research evaluates the impact of interventions on patient outcomes. Outcome measures may include clinical outcomes, functional outcomes, and patient satisfaction. This type of research assists healthcare quality professionals in determining clinical evidence-based best practices. Health services research evaluates the health system at the micro and macro levels. Results from this type of research guide healthcare quality professionals in improving work processes and systems of care.

To facilitate research-based practice—that is, to promote research use—healthcare quality professionals must collaborate with organizational leaders to promote a culture of excellence. Healthcare providers must be motivated to provide the best possible care and to use the best system processes based on the evidence in the research literature or on data obtained in their own organizations; they must want to strive for excellence. A key strategy is to keep all discussions based on improving the patient's experience and outcomes and keep personality conflicts out of the conversation, based on previously established ground rules. Research use is a key aspect of the CQI process and critical to obtaining healthcare quality as defined by the Institute of Medicine (IOM).

The rating of evidence for EBP is often based on the U.S. Preventive Services Task Force (USPSTF) levels of evidence and grading system. The USPSTF, created in 1984, is a group of independent experts in prevention and EBM that makes evidence-based recommendations about clinical preventive services. Evidence for practice can be classified by certain levels or strength of the evidence. The USPSTF also defined levels of certainty about net benefit (see **TABLE 3-2**). The USPSTF levels of evidence are often used to rate the evidence so that practitioners can make wise decisions about care and treatment options with some degree of certainty about outcomes. Strong evidence is transformed into practice and then measured in standardized formats. For example, there is strong evidence that timely administration of aspirin in acute myocardial infarction (AMI) decreases mortality. This practice was implemented widely, as in the Joint Commission Core Measure for AMI. As organizations achieved sustained performance, this measure was dropped. Over time as evidence is strengthened, measures will continue to evolve and organizations such as the Joint Commission and CMS and

Table 3-2 Levels of Certainty about Net Benefit

Level of Certainty	Description
High	The available evidence usually includes consistent results from well-designed, well-conducted studies in representative primary care populations. These studies assess the effects of the preventive service on health outcomes. This conclusion is therefore unlikely to be strongly affected by the results of future studies.
Moderate	The available evidence is sufficient to determine the effects of the preventive service on health outcomes, but confidence in the estimate is constrained by factors such as: • the number, size, or quality of individual studies, • inconsistency of findings across individual studies, • limited generalizability of findings to routine primary care practice, and • lack of coherence in the chain of evidence. As more information becomes available, the magnitude or direction of the observed effect could change, and this change may be large enough to alter the conclusion.
Low	The available evidence is insufficient to assess effects on health outcomes. Evidence is insufficient because of: • the limited number or size of studies, • important flaws in study design or methods, • inconsistency of findings across individual studies, • gaps in the chain of evidence, • findings not generalizable to routine primary care practice, and • lack of information on important health outcomes. More information may allow estimation of effects on health outcomes.

Note: The U.S. Preventive Services Task Force (USPSTF) defines certainty as "likelihood that the USPSTF assessment of the net benefit of a preventive service is correct." The net benefit is defined as benefit minus harm of the preventive service as implemented in a general primary care population. The USPSTF assigns a certainty level based on the nature of the overall evidence available to assess the net benefit of a preventive service.
From U.S. Preventive Services Task Force. *Update on Methods: Estimating Certainty and Magnitude of Net Benefit*. January 2017. https://www.uspreventiveservicestaskforce.org/Page/Name/update-on-methods-estimating-certainty-and-magnitude-of-net-benefit.

others will modify requirements. The newest transition is to an electronic capture and submission of measures known as electronic Clinical Quality Measures. Organizations make practices operational by using clinical pathways, standard order sets, plans of care, and ongoing measurement processes.

Common sources for EBP guidelines and national measures are as follows:

- Agency for Healthcare Research and Quality (AHRQ) (e.g., National Clinical Guideline),
- Cochrane (e.g., clinical evidence comparisons),
- Specialty professional associations and societies (e.g., American Cardiology Association),
- The Leapfrog Group (e.g., hospital-based measures), and
- National Quality Forum (NQF) (e.g., 29 Serious Reportable "Never" Events, Nurse Sensitive Measures, Ambulatory Sensitive Measures, Long-Term Care Measures, and Hospital Measures).

The USPSTF updated its definitions of the grades it assigns to recommendations and now includes suggestions for practice associated with each grade (**TABLE 3-3**). These definitions apply to USPSTF recommendations voted on after July 2012.

Clinical Guidelines and Pathways

Clinical guidelines are consensus statements developed to assist in clinical management decisions, and clinical pathways are tools to manage quality outcomes and cost of care based on clinical guidelines and current evidence. Clinical pathways are document-based tools that provide a link between the best available evidence and clinical practice. Clinical pathways, also known as care pathways, critical pathways, integrated care pathways, or care maps, are one tool used to manage the quality in healthcare concerning the standardization of care processes. A variety of terms are used for this tool. For simplicity, the term *clinical pathway* is used here.

Clinical pathways support EBP and clinical guidelines in a time-oriented plan. The use of pathways or guidelines reduces variation of clinical practice to optimize patient outcomes. The concept was introduced in 1985 by Zander and Bower at the New England Medical Center in Boston. They were early nursing pioneers in applying process management thinking and techniques to improve patient care.[45] Clinical pathways operationalize evidence into daily practice for patient care. They are intended to create an integrated comprehensive approach or plan to the patient's care rather than individual professions functioning independently. Interdisciplinary communication, collaboration, and teamwork are enhanced by working from one pathway, and continuity and care coordination are achieved for the patient.

The pathway shapes expectations or outcomes of care as the patient progresses, based on what is the best practice for most patients most of the time. The pathway is written in a manner to ensure that actions or interventions are completed at designated points with the expected outcome. They are designed to support clinical management, clinical and nonclinical resource management, audit management, and

Table 3-3	U.S. Preventive Services Task Force (USPSTF) Grade Definitions (After July 2012)	
Grade	**Definition**	**Suggestions for Practice**
A	The USPSTF recommends the service. There is high certainty that the net benefit is substantial.	Offer or provide this service.
B	The USPSTF recommends the service. There is high certainty that the net benefit is moderate or there is moderate certainty that the net benefit is moderate to substantial.	Offer or provide this service.
C	The USPSTF recommends selectively offering or providing this service to individual patients based on professional judgment and patient preferences. There is at least moderate certainty that the net benefit is small.	Offer or provide this service for selected patients depending on individual circumstances.
D	The USPSTF recommends against the service. There is moderate or high certainty that the service has no net benefit or that the harms outweigh the benefits.	Discourage the use of this service.
I Statement	The USPSTF concludes that the current evidence is insufficient to assess the balance of benefits and harms of the service. Evidence is lacking, of poor quality, or conflicting, and the balance of benefits and harms cannot be determined.	Read the clinical considerations section of USPSTF Recommendation Statement: If the service is offered, patients should understand the uncertainty about the balance of benefits and harms.

From U.S. Preventive Services Task Force. *Grade Definitions*. June 2016. https://www.uspreventiveservicestaskforce.org/Page/Name/grade-definitions.

financial management. Often, the improved clinical outcomes are intended to support cost-effective use of resources such as length of stay, diagnostic tests, and pharmaceutical management. Because there are differences in the responses for the same condition or treatment, individual variances must be captured, documented, and addressed. This continuous monitoring and data evaluation component is essential to pathway improvement through continual revision of pathways. It is expected that over time variation decreases through standardization, costs decrease, and the value of care improves.

Although standardization is important to the pathways, they are not intended to be overly prescriptive and still allow personalized care. However, one critique of pathways is that not all variation in patient care is negative, and standardized care or "cookbook medicine" would be a detriment to patient care and clinician autonomy. Individual patient factors may contribute to variation that cannot be controlled by the system. Pathways tend to address processes in the ideal or uncomplicated patient and may not address problems in most patients. It is important to identify which patients are appropriate for the pathway. In general, pathways are more applicable to patients with uncomplicated illnesses undergoing procedures or surgery. Complex cases with multiple co-morbidities may be more difficult to fit into a standard pathway.

The standardized approach is designed to empower patients such that each patient knows the plan and his or her expected outcome at each phase of recovery (e.g., on postoperative day 2, the hip replacement patient is expected to ambulate a defined number of steps or feet and void without a urinary catheter). Standardization also helps reduce clinical risk by ensuring that for specific conditions there are no lapses in care to be provided, and if outcomes are not met there is an immediate assessment of the reason. When differences or unwanted variances do occur, they are noted and accommodations made in the plan of care to ensure safety and effectiveness. Some common areas addressed by clinical pathways include orthopedic surgery such as hips, knees, and shoulders. Surgical care is more conducive to clinical pathways than medical conditions, where more differences in the patient's condition are more likely to occur.

Clinical pathways facilitate the development of standardized physician order sets, interventions for the patient, and documentation of the patient's condition, and they are often used in the following situations:

- prevalent pathology in the care setting (e.g., pain);
- pathology with a significant risk for patients (e.g., venous thromboembolism), high cost for the hospital (e.g., total hip joint replacement), or well-defined permitting homogeneous care (e.g., laminectomy, transurethral prostate resection);
- predictable clinical course (e.g., total knee or hip replacement);

- possibility of obtaining professional agreement (e.g., coronary angioplasty);
- existence of recommendations of good practices or expert opinion (e.g., diabetes);
- multidisciplinary implementation (e.g., joint replacement); and
- relatively mature guidelines (e.g., stroke).[46]

Although based on current evidence or clinical guidelines, the clinical pathway details the process of care for the specific condition and, in noting any variances, highlights inefficiencies. Twenty-seven studies involving 11,398 participants were included in a meta-analysis of clinical pathway effectiveness.[47] Twenty studies compared stand-alone clinical pathways to usual care. These studies indicated a reduction in inhospital complications and improved documentation. There was no evidence of differences in readmission to hospital or inhospital mortality. Length of stay was the most commonly employed outcome measure with most studies reporting significant reductions. A decrease in hospital costs or charges was also observed. Seven studies compared clinical pathways as part of a multifaceted intervention with usual care. No evidence of differences was found between intervention and control groups.

There are both strengths and limitations of the pathway process that an organization must consider in its development and use of the tool. The development of a clinical pathway includes the following steps:

1. Select the topic. The topic concentrates on high-volume, high-cost diagnoses and procedures; higher mortality; longer length of stay; or greater number of outcome variations. Surgical procedures are more suitable for pathways because of the predictable course of events that occur during the hospitalization.
2. Select a multidisciplinary team, including representatives from all groups that would be affected by the pathway. Without physician support of the pathway, it is unlikely to be successful and achieve any of the stated goals.
3. Evaluate and map the current process of care for the condition or procedure to identify current variation and create an idealized process.
4. Evaluate the current evidence in the literature. In the absence of best practices, comparison with other organizations, or benchmarking, is the best method to use.
5. Determine the clinical pathway form. This may be a hardcopy checklist placed in the patient's medical record or at bedside or an electronic tool capable of tracking variances.
6. Educate all users on how to use the tool and implement it. It is critical to define roles within the pathway for it to be successful.
7. Document and analyze variances that do not meet the expectation of the pathway. Identification of factors that

contribute to variance and interventions to improve those factors are the key features of process improvement. Often, a case manager or other utilization management staff member collects data on use of the pathway and variances. These data must then be analyzed and processes improved to achieve cost savings, quality and safety.

A clinical practice guideline (CPG) is defined in a very structured manner by the Institute of Medicine as a "statement that includes recommendations that intend to optimize patient care. They are informed by a systematic review of evidence and an assessment of the benefits and harms of alternative care options."[48(pp25–26)] A medical guideline (also called a clinical guideline, clinical protocol, or CPG) is a document with the aim of guiding decisions and criteria regarding diagnosis, management, and treatment in specific areas of healthcare. Following a guideline is never mandatory.

The National Guideline Clearinghouse™ (NGC) is a publicly available database of evidence-based CPGs and related documents.[49] It provides Internet users with free online access to guidelines. The NGC is updated weekly as evidence is acknowledged and subject matter experts review guidelines for practice. The key components of the NGC include

- structured, standardized abstracts (summaries) about each guideline and its development;
- a utility for comparing attributes of two or more guidelines in a side-by-side comparison;
- syntheses of guidelines covering similar topics, highlighting areas of similarity and difference;
- links to full-text guidelines, where available, and/or ordering information for print copies; and
- annotated bibliographies on guideline development methodology, structure, implementation, and evaluation.

Guidelines are organized by clinical specialty areas such as Cardiology, Critical Care, Emergency Medicine, Geriatrics, Infectious Diseases, Pediatrics, Physical Medicine and Rehabilitation and Psychiatry. An example of a CPG from the nursing specialty is Prevention of Falls (acute care) and includes recommendations, scope, methodology, evidence, benefits/harms, qualifying statements, implementation, IOM/ NQF report categories, identifying information and any disclaimers. Users of the CPG can check the site periodically as evidence is updated to ensure practice is following the most current evidence.

Another tool to apply evidence into practice to improve healthcare quality is the concept of "bundles."[50] The IHI developed the concept of the bundle in 2001, and it is now commonly used for selected conditions. The original initiative was a joint development of the IHI and the Voluntary Hospitals of America (VHA), focused on improving critical care and increasing reliability of processes and thereby improve outcomes. (*Note that in 2015 the VHA and University

HealthSystem Consortium merged as Vizient, Inc.). A bundle is defined as "a small set of evidence-based interventions for a defined patient segment/population and care setting that, when implemented together, result in significantly better outcomes than when implemented individually."[50(pp1–2)] There are guidelines to the bundle design that include the following:

- The bundle has three to five interventions (elements), with strong clinician agreement.
- Each bundle element is relatively independent.
- The bundle is used with a defined patient population in one location.
- The multidisciplinary care team develops the bundle.
- Bundle elements are descriptive rather than prescriptive, which allows for local customization and use of clinical judgment.[50(p5)]

The first two bundles included ventilator-associated events and central line-associated bloodstream infections (CLABSI). Through ongoing testing and application of the bundles in clinical practice, modifications were made to the original elements and new bundles developed such as the sepsis bundle and perinatal care bundle. "The use of bundles of care interventions as an approach to improving the reliability of care received by patients and preventing certain serious clinical outcomes has been demonstrated successfully for nearly 10 years, with a growing body of published results."[50(pp2–5)]

When assessing processes of bundle use and outcomes, an "all or none" measurement is used to ensure reliability in providing care that offers the best evidence to prevent adverse events and improve outcomes. Often healthcare quality professionals are directly involved in data collection or reporting of bundle compliance as well as the outcomes of care such as ventilator-associated events or CLABSI—key measures of harm to patients.

Performance and Process Improvement Approaches

Definitions and requirements for quality and PI in healthcare evolved over the past decades. In the early 1950s, quality care reviews were conducted exclusively by individual physicians using an unstructured and subjective process that relied on the practitioner's knowledge and experiences. Between 1950 and 1960, the responsibility for quality of care expanded beyond the physician to include both the hospital and the board of directors. Two significant legal decisions marked this transition period:

- *Bing v. Thunig* (1957). In this case, the New York Court of Appeals ruled that the doctrine of charitable immunity no longer applied to hospitals; hospitals are liable for patient injuries sustained through negligence of employees.

- *Darling v. Charleston Community Memorial Hospital* (1965). In this important corporate negligence case, the court ruled that the hospital had a legal responsibility to protect a patient from harm by others by overseeing the quality of patient care.

These cases shifted the thinking about accountability for safety and quality of care delivered by hospitals and set into motion the beginning of quality reviews. This progressed over time into current PI models. There are a variety of PI models and they each have value and usefulness depending on the type of problem, scope, and solution needed. The process for determining which PI model or models to use in an organization requires an analysis of the organization and its track record of success with current and previous models. How will the model be communicated across the organization? Are all staff members expected to know how to use it? Which model or models are a good fit with the culture and the current strategies that are working?

Healthcare quality professionals may be asked to provide a review and analysis of the PI methodology currently in use and compare it with alternative options. As more sophisticated tools and methods become available, the quality professionals must keep pace and serves an important role in the final selection(s) of what tools to use in which situations—the best tool for the right situation at the right time.

Retrospective Audits

A shift from physician review to medical audits occurred in 1955. Medical audits included a systematic procedure using objective, valid criteria with an orientation on outcomes. In 1966, there was a major change whereby the Joint Commission on Accreditation of Hospitals (as it was called then; now The Joint Commission or TJC) focused on optimal, not minimal, standards of care. In 1975, the Joint Commission on Accreditation of Hospitals (JCAH) published the quality of professional services standards, requiring hospitals to demonstrate optimal care using valid and reliable measures. Although *optimal* was never defined, this new focus led to one-time audits of care, known as performance evaluation programs audits. While audits have historical roots, they are still a method often used depending on the type of information to be validated.

Quality Assurance

Audits soon led to a preoccupation with meeting audit number requirements. Thus, in 1980 the JCAH, now known as TJC, developed the first QA standards requiring a problem-focused approach to measuring quality. This approach required organizations to identify and monitor problem

areas. The combined strengths of criteria-based audits and the epidemiologic approach used in infection control in the 1980s resulted in a new focus on systematic monitoring and evaluation in 1985. From this, a 10-step process for quality and PI evolved in 1986 requiring organizations to evaluate important aspects of care and then use the results to identify opportunities for improvement.

Reengineering and System Redesign

In the 1990s, reengineering was one of the major initiatives in hospitals. Most of these efforts were focused on workforce redesign. There was typically a focus on restructuring or redesigning systems and departments into more efficient processes. For example, hospitals experimented with creating new positions that combined work from several different areas. A focus on cross-functional capabilities led to the dissolution of departmental silos. A "patient service associate" or "technical associate" would deliver meals, clean patient rooms, stock supplies, and provide patient transportation. Many hospitals thought that reengineering would increase profit margins and create financial stability. The problem was that reengineering often became associated with mergers, acquisitions, downsizing, and layoffs. When this happened, employee morale declined and productivity suffered. Because of these negative connotations, reengineering fell out of vogue and was replaced by other improvement models and initiatives. The newer approach is to consider adopting the Lean Enterprise method to increase financial stability by eliminating waste.

The key components and tools of a Lean Enterprise include identifying value (value stream mapping and voice of customer), eliminating waste, establishing flow, enabling pull (instead of push) systems, and pursuing perfection. The Six Sigma method includes a five-step process: Define, Measure, Analyze, Improve, and Control (DMAIC). See **TABLE 3-4** for the process and key questions for the healthcare quality professional to consider during each step in the DMAIC process. Lean Enterprise and Six Sigma are often complementary tools. Lean Enterprise focuses on dramatically improving flow in the value stream and eliminating waste to improve efficiency and speed. Six Sigma methodology focuses on eliminating defects and reducing variation in processes to improve effectiveness.

The Health Insurance Portability and Accountability Act of 1996 (HIPAA) established the national Health Care Fraud and Abuse Control Program (HCFAC) under the joint direction of the Attorney General and the Secretary of the U.S. Department of Health & Human Services (HHS). In the latest HCFAC report,[51] the following successes were noted for healthcare fraud and abuse during FY 2016:

- The Federal Government won or negotiated over $2.5 billion in healthcare fraud judgments and settlements.

Table 3-4 The DMAIC Methodology

Phase	Key Questions	Common Tools
Define	• What is the problem? • Why are we working on this project? • Who is going to be working on this project? • What resources do we need to complete this project? What is the scope? • By when must the project be completed? • Who is the customer? • Who are key stakeholders? • What key metrics are important? • What does the current process look like?	Project Charter SIPOC Voice of the Customer Run Chart Process/Flow Map
Measure	• How can we measure the process or performance? • What data sources are available, and what is the data collection method? • What is our current or baseline performance of the process? What data display (graphs) is useful? • What does our customer define as a defect? • How can we stratify data or measure defects? • What benefits do we hope to achieve through solving this problem?	Control Charts Pareto Histogram Other Analysis
Analyze	• Why is there a gap between current performance and customer expectations? • What are the root causes of variability in our processes and have they been verified? • What root causes are the highest priority to focus efforts? • Where is waste in the process and what type of waste?	Process Map Value Stream Map Risk Analysis Cause-and-Effect Diagram (Fishbone/Ishikawa Diagram)
Improve	• What are potential solutions to the root causes? • What solutions have been verified and are the highest priority? • How will we track implementation? • Are there any anticipated barriers to improvement? • How can we best translate the details into standard work expectations? • What will the redesigned process look like and how will it be tested, measured, and validated? • Does the redesigned process reduce waste or variation?	Brainstorming Risk Analysis Standard Work Mistake Proofing Visual Workplace Tools
Control	• How will the improved process be sustained? • Who will be responsible for maintaining/monitoring the improvements and measures? • How will we communicate the new process expectations? • How will we eliminate deviations from standard work and prevent backsliding? • How will we share best practices and lessons learned? • What were the benefits realized from the project?	Control Plan Control Charts Dashboard Standard Operating Procedures and Policy Revision Checklist/Audits

- Investigations conducted by the HHS Office of Inspector General (HHS-OIG) resulted in 765 criminal actions against individuals or entities that engaged in crimes related to Medicare and Medicaid.
- There were 690 civil actions, which included false claims and unjust-enrichment lawsuits filed in federal district court.
- HHS-OIG also excluded 3,635 individuals and entities from participation in Medicare, Medicaid, and other federal healthcare programs. Among these were exclusions based on criminal convictions for crimes related to

  ○ Medicare and Medicaid (1,362),
  ○ other healthcare programs (262),
  ○ patient abuse or neglect (299), and
  ○ result of licensure revocations (1,448).

The HCFAC is in its twentieth year of operation and continues to use a collaborative approach to "identify and prosecute the most egregious instances of healthcare fraud, to prevent future fraud and abuse, and to protect program beneficiaries."[51(p1)]

Rapid-Cycle Improvement

The IHI developed the "collaborative" approach, termed the "Breakthrough Series," to bring about rapid-cycle improvements. Fundamental to the collaborative approach is the acceptance of a model and the establishment of an infrastructure through which collaborating organizations can identify and prioritize aims for improvement and gain access to methods, tools, and materials to conduct sophisticated, evidence-based activities that they could not successfully conduct on their own. The key elements of success are enlisting a broad range of partners, using EBP to improve quality of care, and developing toolkits that contain essential information and resources to manage change.

At the core of the collaborative approach is the PDCA cycle that builds on incremental improvements. The real benefits to organizations that participate in the Breakthrough Series are that they can learn from other organizations' successes and failures. Another key principle in the IHI approach is the concept of spread. IHI proposed that successful small-scale improvement efforts initially affect an individual organization and spread later to the industry (i.e., other hospitals) and eventually to the entire national healthcare system. The spread is fostered through learning sessions in which organizations share their experiences. The IHI approach also can be adapted to a single organization (the work begins in a few units or teams and then is spread to other units and, eventually, to the entire organization). See FIGURE 3-11, which illustrates how the multiple improvement cycles in a collaborative occur.[52] Participation in a collaborative is one

approach that organizations may choose for improvement in a specific area. The IHI is one organization that offers national 10 to 12 month collaboratives such as Reducing Falls and Falls with Injuries; Transforming Care at the Bedside (TCAB); Health Disparities; Primary Care Teams to Meet Patients' Medical and Behavioral Needs; Perinatal Improvement in Community; IHI Triple Aim Improvement Community; and Improving Outcomes for High-Risk and Critically Ill Patients.

Six Sigma

Six Sigma is a business management strategy, originally developed by Motorola. This rigorous methodology, used in many different industry sectors, uses data and statistical analyses to measure and improve performance through the reduction of variation. Quality is improved by eliminating errors in production and service-related processes. Six Sigma is based on the concept of the normal distribution or curve and the belief that there is a point, six standard deviations from the mean, where there should be almost zero defects. Therefore, error rates do not exceed 3.4 defects per million opportunities. Six Sigma can be characterized as obtaining the right measures (or metrics) of quality, using rigorous statistical methods, and possessing a customer-focused and data-driven philosophy.

In 1998, Chassin concluded "We can learn a good deal from industries that are working toward the Six Sigma goal. Let's try it in healthcare and see how close we can get."[53(p587)] Over the past several years, this approach took hold in many hospitals and health systems. With cost, quality, and regulatory pressures continuing to increase within the healthcare industry, Six Sigma gained more attention from hospitals and health systems seeking a better approach to achieving

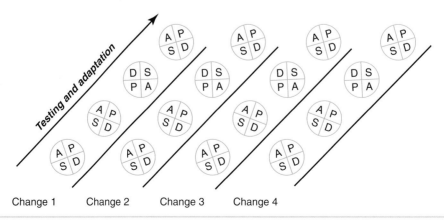

Figure 3-11 **Process for testing multiple cycles of change as used in a collaborative.** (Reprinted from Institute for Healthcare Improvement. *How to Improve: Science of Improvement: Testing Multiple Changes.* Cambridge, MA: IHI; 2017, with permission. http://www.ihi.org/resources/Pages/HowtoImprove/ScienceofImprovementTestingMultipleChanges.aspx.)

long-term results. This approach to improving quality can be used to address many of the challenges facing healthcare, including resource utilization, patient safety, appropriate use of technology, and increasing market share. Six Sigma efforts typically include a methodology that addresses variation and goes by the acronym "DMAIC" (define, measure, analyze, improve, and control).

A Six Sigma project can address process redesign, a problem that needs to be solved, a change that needs to be instituted, or a process that needs to be monitored. Six Sigma projects are managed by Black Belts, who oversee the project. Black Belts are members of the organization who are extensively trained in Six Sigma methods. Black Belts also must be experienced in statistical analysis and interested in teaching others. Projects normally are carried out by Yellow and Green Belts. Yellow and Green Belts are organization frontline members who are knowledgeable about Six Sigma methods but who received less training than Black Belts. For major projects an organization also assigns a senior manager or executive to act as a sponsor. Six Sigma shows success in reducing emergency room wait times, lost charges for billing in financial services, delinquent medical records, diagnostic result turnaround times, account receivable days, patients' length of stay, and medication errors.[54]

Lean Enterprise

The Japanese automotive industry initiated the concept of lean manufacturing, whereby great importance is given to reducing waste and focusing on those activities that add value for the customer. Interest in applying similar principles in service industry environments, including healthcare, is continuing to grow. Lean enterprise includes five basic principles:

1. Specify value from the end customer's perspective.
2. Identify all steps in the value stream for each service, eliminating the non-value-added steps.
3. Make the value-adding steps flow without interruption to the customer.
4. Implement a pull system based on customer demand.
5. As value is specified, value streams are identified, non-value-added steps are removed, and flow and pull are introduced, go back to the first step and continue until a state of perfection is received.[55]

A key focus in a lean enterprise is to eliminate waste in eight key areas: defects, overproduction, waiting, non-utilized talent, transportation, inventory, motion, and extra processing.[56] An explanation of wastes found in healthcare (with examples in each category and the common strategy to address the waste) is given in **TABLE 3-5**. One of the major distinctions of the lean

Table 3-5 Types of Waste in Lean Production Systems

Type of Waste	Description	Lean Strategy to Eliminate Waste
Transportation	Moving material or information	One-piece flow Avoid batching
Inventory (overproduction)	Having more material than you need	Standard work 6S tool
Motion	Moving people to access or process material or information	Standard work Quick changeover Work cell
Waiting	People waiting for material or information, or material or information waiting to be processed	Quick changeover One-piece flow Avoid batching
Overproduction	Creating too much material or information	Standard work One-piece flow Avoid batching
Overprocessing	Processing more than necessary to achieve the desired output	Standard work Mistake proofing is the use of process or design features to prevent errors or the negative impact of errors.
Defects (necessitating rework)	Errors or mistakes necessitating rework to correct the problem	Standard work Mistake proofing

approach versus traditional QI is its emphasis on investigating new ways of getting things done and making the changes in a short period. The basic idea is to identify new procedures that are designed to be more effective than existing systems, ultimately resulting in eliminating waste. QI has typically used the incremental change model, but lean enterprise is more concerned with speed and total redesign. A key element of success is the commitment and involvement of frontline workers and staff in the change process. The typical project includes cross-functional teams with training in lean principles and tools.

Organizations often implement lean methods before considering Six Sigma, because waste should be eliminated prior to fine-tuning the system to deliver excellence. The newer approach is a combination of both Lean and Six Sigma as there is value in reducing waste, speeding up the process, and reducing variation. Naik et al.[57] applied lean principles to their emergency department, which improved overall length of stay, time of arrival to triage completion, time of arrival to being seen by a provider, and increased provider productivity. Significant improvements in workflow were realized.

Of note, the Lean philosophy encompasses the concept of True North. "True North" is a key concept in Lean process improvement that emerged from Toyota and connotes the compass needle for Lean transformation. True North works like a compass, providing a guide to take an organization from the current condition to where they want to be. It might be viewed as a purpose of the organization, and the foundation of a strategic plan. Later other approaches are explained that determine the organization's direction and important metrics, pillars, dashboard metrics, or key success factors.

The use of Lean and Six Sigma constitute what The Joint Commission refer to as *robust process improvement* which supports organizations to be highly reliable.[58]

Performance Monitoring and Evaluation

Performance monitoring is an important component of a quality, safety, and performance management program. Areas for monitoring and evaluation are identified in accreditation standards, local, state and federal regulatory requirements, and organizational demands. Generally, these areas are high risk or problem prone. When quality or safety issues are identified, they may be subject to review or audit. General criteria to be considered for a review or audit include the following:

- Was the intervention used?
- Was it performed properly using specific criteria?
- Was it performed safely?
- Was there any adverse effect or outcome to the patient?
- Was staff competent to perform the intervention?
- Was it effective (this may include cost effectiveness)?
- Was there a better alternative to the intervention?

Areas most commonly monitored are presented and the general criteria are applied to demonstrate specific monitoring and evaluation processes. Examples are provided that may be applied in a variety of settings but may not apply to all settings based on populations served and the specific services and functions within a setting. Healthcare quality professionals work in a variety of settings and will need to determine the key functions within the setting and apply the concepts of prioritization, EBP for the setting/population, and applicable performance monitoring tools.

Not every setting and every type of monitoring process can be discussed in detail. As healthcare quality professionals determine how to apply monitoring resources, they should understand their setting. For example, the hospital setting provides care for the highest risk and most acute patients with the most intense and costly resources (e.g., severity of illness and intensity of services). Depending on the size and complexity of the services offered, this may range from acute trauma, cardiothoracic and neurosurgical care to basic surgery in a rural setting, and initiatives may focus on TCAB, bundles for preventing infections, and core measures. This setting is the costliest, but is episodic and not the primary site for most healthcare. Long-term care services may include short-term rehabilitation, long-term care, and dementia or memory care. While this setting can be costly long term, it serves a specific population. The clinical office is the primary locus of care for most persons. The physician office practice for primary care focuses on preventive measures such as the National Committee for Quality Assurance's (NCQA) Healthcare Effectiveness Data and Information Set (HEDIS), which is aimed at better health and wellness. While a specialty office practice will address unique measures associated with the specialty and address management of specific conditions such as heart failure or diabetes. While monitoring quality performance for care in each setting varies, there are common methods and all have seen increased attention with reimbursement predicated by quality measures. See *Health Data Analytics* for further discussion.

Medication Use

Safe medication practices, including medication use evaluation, pharmacy and therapeutics, adverse drug reactions, and adverse drug events, are reviewed in healthcare organizations. The types of medications and the setting in which they are used indicate which medications are high risk, high alert, frequently used, and most vulnerable to underuse, overuse, and misuse. Thousands of drugs are currently on the market. Many are hazardous to use but show beneficial effects for patients. The misuse of opioids is a good example of this; nearly half of all opioid deaths involve a prescription opioid.[59] Organizations can identify the drugs they provide in a standard formulary and identify methods to obtain non-formulary items. Then the use of non-formulary medications is monitored, usually by pharmacy staff, to determine cost-effective, safe medications for administration and ways to integrate new medications into use. High-risk medications include antibiotics, opioids, insulin, anticoagulants, and chemotherapy. High-risk populations may include infants and children, frail older adults, immunocompromised patients, critically ill patients, and transplant recipients.

The purpose of medication use monitoring is to improve the efficiency and effectiveness of medication use and the appropriate use of medication. Because of the frequent use of medications in healthcare, ongoing monitoring is needed. Priorities for monitoring are based on the numbers of patients affected (volume), the degree of risk associated with the drug's use (risk), the degree to which the medication is known to be problem prone, and other criteria developed by the medical and professional staff. The usual steps in measuring improvement in the phases of the medication process include

1. prescribing appropriate medication;
2. preparing and dispensing medications;
3. administering medications; and
4. monitoring the effects of medications on patients.

Perhaps a more recent focus in measuring improvement is on the reconciliation of medications prescribed and taken by the patient. "Medication reconciliation is the process of creating the most accurate list possible of all medications a patient is taking—including drug name, dosage, frequency, and route—and comparing that list against the physician's admission, transfer, and/or discharge orders, with the goal of providing correct medications to the patient at all transition points within the hospital."[60(p2)]

Trends and patterns of usage can be presented in several different ways, which may include a description of use in the four steps just listed. Trends can be described in terms of specific medication types, such as antibiotic usage, and compared with antibiograms for specific organisms. Patterns also can be presented relative to overuse, underuse, and misuse. **TABLE 3-6** uses the basic monitoring criteria to illustrate medication monitoring of a specific case that can be used to aggregate the data into trends.

It has been acknowledged in recent years that antibiotics have been overused and overprescribed. Various professional and government organizations have developed strategies to reduce the inappropriate use of antibiotics. Most recently, a partnership of the NQF, National Quality Partners, and the Antibiotic Stewardship Action Team published a *National Quality Partners Playbook: Antibiotic Stewardship in Acute Care.*[61(p5)] It was written to support the call by the Centers for Disease Control and Prevention (CDC) in 2014 to meet the urgent need of improving antibiotic use in hospitals. The core elements of an Antibiotic Stewardship Program include the following:

1. Leadership commitment. Dedicate necessary human, financial, and IT resources.

Table 3-6 Medication Use Monitoring

General Criteria	Specific Criteria
Was the intervention used?	What class or type of medication is being monitored (e.g., antibiotic, opioid, insulin, anticoagulant, psychotropic)?
Was it performed properly according to specific criteria?	Was the medication administered in accordance with policy, criteria, or current evidence (e.g., was the proper antibiotic preoperatively administered and within 1 hour)?
Was it performed safely?	Was the medication administered safely (e.g., should the medication be administered by an infusion device to control the rate, should it be administered in a central vs. peripheral site, was it diluted properly)?
Was there any adverse effect or outcome to the patient?	Were there any adverse effects to patients (e.g., medication reactions or complications, allergies, errors, interactions with other medications or foods)?
Was staff competent to perform the intervention?	Was the staff who administered the medication competent in the procedure (e.g., does the route of administration require special knowledge and skill, does the type of medication require a certain setting for observation, is there a specific staff competency)?
Was it effective?	Did the medication achieve the desired result or an untoward result?
Was there a better alternative to the intervention?	Were there clearly documented indications for use of the medication? If the medication is high risk, high alert, or non-formulary, was there documentation on usage?

2. Accountability. Appoint a single leader responsible for program outcomes who is accountable to an executive-level or patient quality-focused hospital committee.
3. Drug expertise. Appoint a single pharmacist leader responsible for working to improve antibiotic use.
4. Action. Implement at least one recommended action.
5. Tracking. Monitor process measures, impact on patients, antibiotic use, and resistance.
6. Reporting. Report information regularly to doctors, nurses and relevant staff.
7. Education. Educate clinicians about disease state management, resistance, and optimal prescribing.

Blood and Blood Product Use

The administration of blood and blood products is a high-risk aspect of care. Healthcare staff must consider the risk and the therapeutic benefit, including the risk of blood-borne pathogens, transfusion reactions, and transfusion errors. It is also a high-cost item. The key elements to be monitored include ordering, distribution (availability and timeliness of administration), handling and dispensing, administration, and monitoring of the effects on patients. Individual cases are reviewed (**TABLE 3-7**), and then an evaluation of blood usage

practices for providers and the organization can be performed. An evaluation might include blood that is administered when not indicated, not administered when indicated, or administered incorrectly. Specific standards from the College of American Pathologists and the American Association of Blood Banks may be useful for evaluating transfusion services.

Restraints

Restraint use is another high-risk procedure that may be used in certain populations. It is no longer allowed in the long-term care setting but may be used in acute hospitals for medical-surgical populations, for inpatient behavioral health populations, and in the emergency department for highly unpredictable patients and situations. Some national and state organizations are calling for the eradication of restraint use in behavioral health settings altogether because of high-profile adverse events related to their use, and the organization's adoption of trauma-informed principles and practices. Recently developed core measures in inpatient behavioral health include metrics for restraint and seclusion use (The Joint Commission's Hospital-Based Inpatient Psychiatric Services [HBIPS]).

The CMS established specific rules related to restraint usage, and these were adopted by The Joint Commission,

Table 3-7 Blood and Blood Product Usage Monitoring

General Criteria	Specific Criteria
Was the intervention used?	Was blood or blood components administered?
Was it performed properly according to specific criteria?	Was the order for the blood products clear and documented in the medical record? Was blood administration performed using defined policy including vital signs before, during, and after administration? Were proper tubing, filters, and administration devices used?
Was it performed safely?	Was the patient monitored during the administration? Was the rate of administration in accordance with policy, orders, and the patient's condition?
Was there any adverse effect or outcome to the patient?	Were there any adverse reactions to the administration (immediate or delayed)? If there was a reaction, was the response in accordance with policy?
Was staff competent to perform the intervention?	Were the staff who administered the blood products competent in the procedure (is there a specific competency)?
Was it effective?	Was the most appropriate blood product administered for the patient's condition?
Was there a better alternative to the intervention?	Was there a review of lab results, vital signs, and other results before the order to determine whether the particular blood product was indicated (e.g., iron, watchful waiting)? Was there a review of any special considerations before administration, such as religious beliefs?
Was there proper consent and education done?	Was informed consent provided prior to administration? If not were there special exceptions such as trauma or other emergency conditions? Was the patient educated on the process including discharge instructions in the event of delayed reaction?

which has deemed status with CMS. Deemed status refers to the following:

> In order for a health care organization to participate in and receive federal payment from Medicare or Medicaid programs, one of the requirements is that a health care organization meet the government requirements for program participation, including a certification of compliance with the health and safety requirements called Conditions of Participation (CoPs) or Conditions for Coverage (CfCs), which are set forth in federal regulations. The certification is achieved based on either a survey conducted by a state agency on behalf of the federal government, such as the CMS, or by a national accrediting organization, such as The Joint Commission, that has been approved by CMS as having standards and a survey process that meets or exceeds Medicare's requirements. Health care organizations that achieve accreditation through a Joint Commission "deemed status" survey are determined to meet or exceed Medicare and Medicaid requirements.[62(p1)]

The monitoring of this process includes each episode of restraint application (**TABLE 3-8**). When restraints are used, a checklist is employed to ensure that all required components are met and each episode can be easily monitored using criteria. An aggregate utilization summary allows the organization to determine any trends. Such trends may reveal patterns associated with

- time of day or day of week in which restraint use may be higher, such as nights or weekends;
- units in which restraint use may be higher, such as geropsychiatric units or units with higher numbers of patients with tubes and other devices; and
- providers whose ordering practices reveal higher restraint use.

Operative and Invasive Procedures

Operative, invasive, and noninvasive procedures are important diagnostic and therapeutic interventions. They often pose risk to patients and must be monitored systematically (**TABLE 3-9**). Aspects to be considered for monitoring include

- selection of the appropriate procedures;
- patient preparation for procedures;
- performance of the procedure and patient monitoring;
- post-procedure care;
- pre-procedure and post-procedure patient education;
- pre-procedure and post-procedure diagnostic discrepancies;
- moderate sedation monitoring; and
- complications or adverse events related to the procedure.

Procedures always carry the risk of complications even when performed properly. Risk is greater with procedures performed when not indicated, not performed when indicated, and performed poorly or incorrectly. Outcomes are influenced by clinical performance of all pre-procedure processes; clinical performance of the procedure; and patient monitoring before, during, and after the procedure.

Table 3-8 Restraint Use Monitoring

General Criteria	Specific Criteria
Was the intervention used?	Were restraints applied to the patient (what type of restraint and what limb or body part was restrained)? What was the reason for the restraint and was it documented?
Was it performed properly according to specific criteria?	Were restraints applied properly in accordance with policy, Centers for Medicare & Medicaid Services (CMS) regulations, and Joint Commission standards? Was there compliance with requirements for orders, timeliness, trial releases, alternatives, initial face-to-face assessment, and ongoing monitoring?
Was it performed safely?	Were restraints applied safely so that the patient was not at risk for injury or harm?
Was there any adverse effect or outcome to the patient?	Were there any adverse effects (e.g., physical, emotional) to the patient related to the application of restraints?
Was staff competent to perform the intervention?	Were the staff who applied the restraints competent in the procedure (is there a specific competency)?
Was it effective?	Did the use of the restraints achieve the desired result?
Was there a better alternative to the intervention?	Were other alternatives tried before restraints applied (and documented)? Was seclusion used with restraints?

Table 3-9 Operative and Invasive Procedure Monitoring

General Criteria	Specific Criteria
Was the intervention used?	What was the surgical or invasive procedure performed?
Was it performed properly according to specific criteria?	Were there documented indications for the procedure? Was the patient properly informed of risks, benefits, and alternatives and provided consent?
Was it performed safely?	Was the procedure performed using policy, guidelines, or other criteria?
Was there any adverse effect or outcome to the patient?	Was there any adverse effect on the patient before, during, or after the procedure? Was any action taken to prevent, mitigate, or respond to an adverse event (e.g., pre-procedure positioning to prevent injury, post-procedure X-ray if a retained object was suspected)?
Was staff competent to perform the intervention?	Were staff performing the procedure competent? Were providers privileged to perform the procedure?
Was it effective?	What was the result or outcome for the patient?
Was there a better alternative to the intervention?	Was the procedure elective, urgent, or emergent? Were all possible options considered and discussed with the patient? Were specialists consulted if needed? Was the procedure performed in the right setting (e.g., inpatient or outpatient, or in a specialty hospital, or a hospital that performs a high volume of procedures vs. a hospital that infrequently performs a procedure, especially one of high risk and complexity)?

Common errors in the operating room (OR) reported as sentinel events to The Joint Commission include

- wrong patient, wrong site, or wrong procedure;
- unintended retention of foreign objects; and
- operative/postoperative complications.[6]

Kim et al.[58] also identified quality issues in surgery as

- breakdown in communication within and among the surgical team, care providers, patients and their families;
- delay in diagnosis or failure to diagnose; and
- delay in treatment or failure to treat.

Several national databases allow comparisons of organizational data with risk-adjusted surgical cases for observed-to-expected ratios of morbidity and mortality. This allows the organization to use an external comparison or benchmark to assess its rate of complications as a trigger or threshold for action (e.g., National Surgical Quality Improvement Program; Chevron Supplier Quality Improvement Process, Society of Thoracic Surgeons National Database).

Cardiopulmonary Resuscitation

Cardiopulmonary resuscitation (CPR) monitoring and the outcomes are important to include in any QI program (**TABLE 3-10**). Cardiopulmonary resuscitation is defined as the application of chest compressions, defibrillation, and artificial respirations or rescue breathing. One consideration in CPR monitoring is whether the patient exhibited any signs or symptoms that could have been identified for early intervention before a full arrest occurred. If CPR must be performed, there are specific guidelines on chest compressions, airway maintenance and breathing, defibrillation, and medications (i.e., American Heart Association). Advanced care and treatment depend on the setting and patient's underlying condition. A national registry (Get With the Guidelines® Patient Management Tool) for data on CPR events collects detailed information on exact interventions, times, and results (including electrocardiograms). The use of a registry allows comparison of data on process and outcome measures.

Morbidity and Mortality

Review of morbidity and mortality is often based on specific criteria. For mortality, a review of expected or unexpected mortality (observed vs. expected) is performed by condition, within specific time frames (e.g., immediately in the OR, in the hospital setting, or within 30 days after discharge), and based on inclusion and exclusion criteria. For example, patients are usually excluded from review who are expected to die based on a terminal condition with a Do Not Resuscitate/Do Not Intubate/Allow Natural Death orders, who are in hospice, or who have an end-stage condition. Other mortalities are

Table 3-10 Cardiopulmonary Resuscitation (CPR) Monitoring

General Criteria	Specific Criteria
Was the intervention used?	Was CPR performed (defined by defibrillation and chest compressions or similar definition)?
Was it performed properly according to specific criteria?	Was CPR performed correctly and promptly in accordance with basic life support or advanced cardiac life support guidelines including timeliness?
Was it performed safely?	Was CPR performed safely (e.g., consider the location of the victim, defibrillation, and other safety factors)?
Was there any adverse effect or outcome to the patient?	What was the outcome (immediate, defined intervals, at discharge)?
Was staff competent to perform the intervention?	Were staff trained and certified in the proper level of response? Was certification current?
Was it effective?	Were compressions and rescue breathing effective in sustaining perfusion?
Was there a better alternative to the intervention?	Were there early warning signs for rapid response team (RRT) to intervene before full arrest? RRT may be monitored separately for outcomes.

then reviewed as outcomes that can provide information about the quality of care provided. Similarly, complications are also reviewed, and the criteria for cases and conditions to be reviewed are established by the medical and professional staff. Individual cases are then identified and reviewed, and aggregated reports are trended to identify opportunities for improvement. Comparisons of trends can be made internally over time or externally compared with national databases.

Morbidity and mortality data are often risk adjusted to compare similar patients (usually with similar conditions, procedures, or diagnosis-related group [DRGs]). National databases allow comparison of morbidity and mortality using a risk-adjusted model (e.g., all Patient Refined DRGs). Typical occurrence screening examples for mortality include

- death within 24 hours of admission to a hospital;
- death within 72 hours of transfer out of special care unit;
- lack of documentation of deterioration during 48 hours preceding death;
- failure of physician to respond to notification of change in patient's condition during 48 hours preceding death;
- lack of documentation indicating death was expected;
- lack of concordance between premortem and postmortem diagnosis;
- clinically significant incident or occurrence within 72 hours of death;
- clinically significant complication of surgical procedure within 72 hours of death;
- clinically significant complication of invasive procedure within 72 hours of death;
- death during surgery;

- unplanned organ removal during operative procedure within 2 months preceding death;
- surgical procedure to repair a perforation, laceration, or other injury of an organ during an invasive procedure within 2 months preceding death;
- repeat of any surgical procedure within 2 months preceding death;
- myocardial infarction within 24 hours of a surgical or invasive procedure;
- death within 48 hours of elective surgical procedure;
- lack of concordance between preoperative and postoperative diagnosis; and
- was the death preventable?

Infection Prevention, Surveillance, and Control

The goal of the infection prevention and control (IPC) program is to identify and reduce the risks of acquiring and transmitting endemic and epidemic infections among patients, employees, physicians, other IPC professionals, contractors, volunteers, students, and visitors. This includes both direct patient care and support staff. The three major aspects of the IPC program are surveillance, prevention, and control. The usual responsibilities of the IPC program include

- definitions of healthcare-associated infections (HAIs);
- definitions of data elements;
- rationale for surveillance method selected;
- description of patient population studied;
- data collection methods;

- quality control procedures for data validation;
- responsibility;
- systems for reporting and follow-up;
- reporting to public health authorities; and
- documentation of employee infections of epidemiologic significance.

The prevention and control methods used in IPC include

- policies and procedures to protect and prevent infections;
- defined barrier precautions;
- orientation and ongoing education of staff;
- reporting to public health officials;
- methods for screening and documentation of epidemiologically significant infections;
- systems for required waste identification;
- use of personal protective equipment and supplies:
  - patient care supplies and equipment (e.g., sterile and nonsterile supplies, hand hygiene facilities),
  - protective apparel, and
  - engineering controls;
- precautions used to reduce the risk of infection:
  - surveillance, and
  - assessment and analysis of infection rates;
- decontamination, high-level disinfection, and sterilization:
  - reusable medical equipment,
  - policies and procedures, and
  - processes identified:
    - principles of asepsis;
    - disinfection, sterilization;
    - sanitation of rooms, equipment;
    - selection, use, and cleaning of personal protective equipment; and
    - traffic control.

The IPC program is based on a risk assessment of the organization. This assessment includes factors such as

- geographic location of the organization;
- populations within the region or organization and level of risk (e.g., neonates, infants, and children, and patients in various intensive care units [ICUs]);
- volume of patients served and volume of conditions (e.g., number of patients with positive human immunodeficiency virus, tuberculosis, and colonized with methicillin-resistant *Staphylococcus aureus* [MRSA]);
- clinical focus of programs (e.g., types of surgeries and invasive procedures, immunocompromised patients such as patients on chemotherapy, transplant patients);
- number of employees (often encompasses employee occupational health services); and
- scope of services provided (e.g., acute, ambulatory, long-term, and home care).

After the risk assessment is completed, priorities are identified and strategies to prevent or mitigate problems are determined. In many healthcare settings, the prevention of HAIs in high-risk units (ICU, neonatal and pediatric ICU, transplant units, dialysis units, and surgical units) is a key responsibility. These HAIs must be monitored and analyzed to determine trends and ways to reduce their occurrence. The types of surveillance for IPC programs include total house, priority directed, targeted, problem oriented, and outbreak response.

The most important factor in monitoring prevention of HAIs is proper hand hygiene. The monitoring of hand hygiene using either CDC or World Health Organization criteria is a requirement of The Joint Commission and a National Patient Safety Goal. Specific monitoring is performed for surgical-site infections and for device-related infections including ventilator-associated pneumonia, CLABSI, and catheter-associated urinary tract infection.

Another key role is to identify communicable diseases, control outbreaks when identified in patients, and report specific results to the public health department. One preventive measure for controlling certain outbreaks is immunization programs conducted in collaboration with occupational health staff. These might include vaccination for hepatitis B, influenza, pneumonia, and other viral diseases. The infection preventionist is also responsible for monitoring epidemiologically important and multidrug-resistant organisms such as MRSA, *Clostridium difficile,* and vancomycin-resistant *Enterococcus.*

Tools are being developed for collecting data to monitor these high-risk areas for causing adverse events or harm to patients. As conditions or areas of concern for quality and patient safety are identified, healthcare quality professionals need to stay informed of new knowledge, trends, and tools to address infection risk to patients. The models described for specific conditions can be utilized to address key questions about interventions and measures specific to the condition.

Medical Records/Electronic Health Records

The monitoring of the medical record/electronic health record usually includes elements in several categories:

- Required documentation content: The requirements vary by setting, procedure, and even profession. For example, the requirements for a treatment plan/individualized plan of care is different for an acute care hospital and a long-term care facility. The requirements for surgery with general anesthesia are different from those for an outpatient procedure with moderate sedation. Each facility must first identify the required content for the record and then develop a process to monitor important elements. Checklists, databases, or other tools make this process more efficient. This step often reflects the presence or absence of the required content.
- Timeliness of documentation: The next requirement is the time requirement of specific documentation. Most common elements monitored for timeliness include history and physical, preoperative and postoperative notes,

and discharge summaries. This step reflects whether the documentation met or did not meet the required timeline.

- Appropriateness of documentation (clinical pertinence): The monitoring of clinical pertinence requires an assessment of the documentation in terms of the patient's condition, diagnostic results, intervention procedures, vital signs, and other information. This review may determine that documentation was appropriate or not appropriate to the standard of care, key elements of the assessment, treatment plan, interventions, and medication management.

Medical Peer Review

Peer review is an evaluation of an episode of care conducted to improve the quality of patient care or the use of healthcare resources. It is a process protected by statute in most states, although this varies, and by federal statute for federal healthcare facilities. While the protection by statute may vary, the confidentiality of the reviewer and those under review is critical to ensuring the integrity of the process. Healthcare quality professionals often coordinate and facilitate the medical review process on behalf of the medical and professional staff and are responsible for maintaining confidentiality throughout the process.

The first step is to identify an appropriate peer for the specific review. A peer is generally defined as a healthcare professional with comparable education, training, experience, licensure, or similar clinical privileges or scope of practice. The peer review process includes a criteria-based case review. The medical and professional staff establish the criteria. These reviews may include an assessment of the degree to which a standard was met or if providers in the same situation would act in the same manner. These ratings may be noted as a score or level number for tracking purposes or as a trigger for Focused Professional Practice Evaluation when continued quality concerns are identified. Results may be trended by individual provider performance or by organization system. Usually, a peer review committee manages the review and reporting function as a subcommittee of the medical executive committee. Participation in peer review is one way medical staff members are involved in measuring, assessing, and improving performance of licensed practitioners.

Medical staff identify criteria or circumstances that initiate a peer review, set time frames for the review to occur, identify reviewers, and provide mechanisms for participation by the person whose performance is being reviewed. Both outcomes and processes are measured. An effective peer review process includes these elements:

- Consistency: Peer review is conducted using defined procedures.
- Defensibility: Conclusions reached through the process are supported by a rationale.
- Balance: Minority opinions and views of the person being reviewed are considered and recorded.

- Peer review activities are considered in the reappointment process.
- Conclusions from peer review are tracked over time.
- Actions based on conclusions are monitored for effectiveness.
- Findings, conclusions, recommendations, and actions are communicated to appropriate entities.
- Recommendations to improve performance are implemented.

Physician leaders have a role in improving clinical processes used for clinical privileging. Practitioner profiles are extremely important to maintain and are used to evaluate performance and maintain privileges. Some key aspects of these files include the following:

- Profiles are based on performance.
- Profiles are provided to each physician or provider on a regular basis.
- Organizations may use risk-adjusted software.
- EBP determines metrics used.
- Data are timely and accurate.
- Profiles are process focused.
- Physician data are grouped by specialty type or specific diagnoses.
- Data are reported regularly.
- Physician champions talk directly with medical staff about their data.

The physician data must be meaningful to physicians. Data represent major service lines and patient safety issues and include inpatient as well as outpatient data. When available, national targets and benchmarks are used to compare performance. For example, national rates of complications of certain procedures when compared with a specific physician or service can help the organization identify performance concerns about what is expected for the same procedure. Data are easily accessed and shared with the physician to improve performance; the profiles vary by the physician's specialty or area of practice. Some examples of elements that might be found in a physician profile or the Ongoing Professional Practice Evaluation (OPPE). These might include patient volume, length of stay, conformity with system wide initiatives (e.g., use of deep vein thrombosis or pulmonary embolism prophylaxis), legibility of records and use of unapproved abbreviations, and severity-adjusted morbidity or mortality rates. The profile or OPPE is structured according to the current core competencies of the Accreditation Council for Graduate Medical Education Patient Care, Medical Knowledge, Practice-Based Learning and Improvement, Interpersonal and Communication Skills, Professionalism, and Systems-Based Practice.[65]

Finally, profiles are confidential and there must be a mechanism to track activity when they are viewed. Policies and procedures are needed to establish the system for document management. This might include a log or sign-out sheet (e.g., date of request, reason for request, name of person reviewing, and pertinent notes). See *Health Data Analytics* for discussion of privacy and security of protected health information.

Performance Improvement Tools

Described next are methods and tools for decision-making and process improvement. Detailed descriptions and examples of these tools follow. More information on data analysis and SPC are described in *Health Data Analytics.*

Affinity Diagram

The *affinity diagram* (FIG. 3-12) organizes numerous ideas or issues into groupings based on their natural relationships within the groupings. These diagrams typically are used to analyze or chart a process and to structure and organize issues to provide a new perspective.

Brainstorming

Brainstorming (FIG. 3-13) is a free-flowing generation of ideas. This approach can generate excitement, equalize involvement, and result in original solutions to the problem. There is no censoring or discussion of ideas as they are generated, but the team can build upon the ideas of others. It is very important that no judgments are made concerning the idea's worth to the process, or whether the idea is even feasible (money is no object in a brainstorming exercise). Discussion of ideas comes at a later point in the process. This technique works well to generate ideas related to cause and effect or identifying paths toward a goal.

Cause-and-Effect, Ishikawa, or Fishbone Diagram

The *Cause-and-Effect, Ishikawa, or Fishbone Diagram* (FIG. 3-14) is used to display, explore and analyze all the potential causes related to a problem or condition and to discover the root causes of variation.

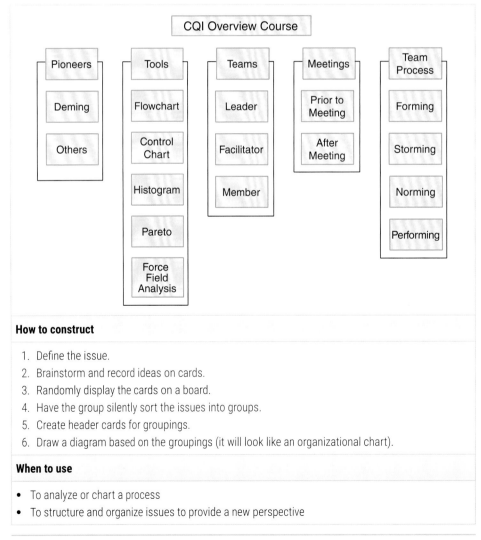

How to construct

1. Define the issue.
2. Brainstorm and record ideas on cards.
3. Randomly display the cards on a board.
4. Have the group silently sort the issues into groups.
5. Create header cards for groupings.
6. Draw a diagram based on the groupings (it will look like an organizational chart).

When to use

- To analyze or chart a process
- To structure and organize issues to provide a new perspective

Figure 3-12 **Affinity diagram.**

How to construct

1. Define the brainstorming topic.
2. Inform participants of the ground rules that (a) "all ideas are good ideas" and (b) "all comments/evaluation should be held in abeyance until the brainstorming is complete."
3. Give everyone a few minutes to think about the topic and write down their ideas.
4. Have the team members call out their ideas. This can be free-flowing, or a structure can be used, such as going around the table with each person verbalizing one idea each time around.
5. As the ideas are generated, one person should write the ideas on a flip chart.

When to use

- Use when a list of possible ideas is needed
- This technique works well to generate ideas for such tools as the cause-and-effect diagram and the tree diagram

Figure 3-13 **Brainstorming.**

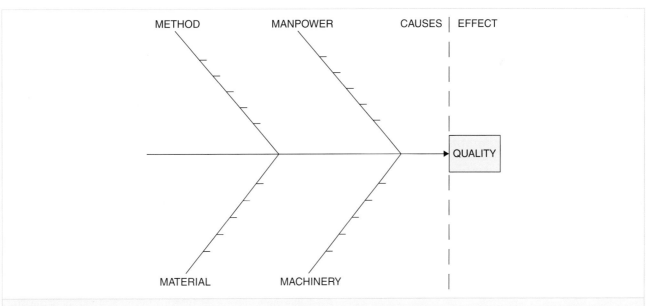

How to construct

1. Determine the effect or the label for the diagram and put it on the far-right side of the diagram.
2. Draw a horizontal line to the left of the effect.
3. Determine the categories (most common categories include the four Ms [Method, Manpower, Material, Machinery] or the five Ps [Process/Procedure, People, Policy, Plant, Price] but these are not the only categories that can be used).
4. Draw a diagonal line for half of the categories above the line and half below the line.
5. Brainstorm the list for each of the categories.
6. Organize each of the causes on each bone (subcategories).
7. Draw branch bones to show the relationships.

When to use

- To identify and organize possible causes of problems
- To identify factors that will lead to success
- As part of a root cause analysis

Figure 3-14 **Cause-and-effect, Ishikawa, or fishbone diagram.**

Checklist

A *checklist* (FIG. 3-15) is a standard way to ensure completion of critical tasks for a process or activity. The checklist ensures accuracy, accountability, completeness, and efficiency. Some ways to organize a checklist include the following:

- Ordered List: a list of tasks needed to be accomplished in a particular order. The checklist is numbered, starting at the first task or step, and proceeding to the last task or step, in increasing numerical order. The ordered list ensures correct and complete processing.
- Itemized List: a list of items to be addressed, with meaningful information alongside; used as a guide or reference. An itemized list provides a complete accounting or reporting of the information present.
- Sub-List: a sub-list is a branch or subset of an ordered list. Sub-lists can exist for almost any of the above types of lists.
- Prioritized List: any of the above lists placed into an order based on a priority scheme. It helps use time effectively, focus energy where it's most needed, and address the important items or tasks first.
- General List: any of the above lists with a space for a check mark, initials, or additional information. As tasks or items are completed, the line is checked or initialed.[66]

Deployment Chart or Planning Grid

A *deployment chart* (FIG. 3-16) is used to project schedules for complex tasks and their associated subtasks. It usually is used with a task for which the time for completion is known. The

Completion	Task

How to construct

1. Identify critical elements or tasks to be completed for a process.
2. Make a list of all elements with a space to indicate completion of the task before moving to the next item.

When to use

- When reliance on memory is not sufficient
- When tasks for a process or activity are critical and omission may cause harm

Figure 3-15   **Checklist.**

tool also is used to determine who has responsibility for the parts of a plan or project. This tool also is called a *planning grid*. The grid helps the group organize key steps in the project to reach milestones and the desired goal. Shaded boxes may be used to indicate the people who primarily are responsible, with ovals indicating an assistant or advisor.

Delphi Method

The *Delphi method* is a combination of the brainstorming, multivoting, and nominal group techniques. This technique is used when group members are not in one location and often is conducted by e-mail when a meeting is not feasible. After each step in the process, the data are sent to one person, who compiles the data and sends out the next round for participants to complete.

Failure Mode and Effects Analysis

Failure mode and effects analysis (FMEA) is a preventive approach to identify failures and opportunities for error and can be used for processes as well as equipment. The traditional techniques for FMEA originated in manufacturing and other industries and were adapted to healthcare. The Veterans Affairs National Center for Patient Safety created the Healthcare FMEA™ (HFMEA). There are six main steps to HFMEA, as displayed in FIGURE 3-17.

Flow Chart or Process Flow Chart

The *flow chart* or *process flow chart* (FIG. 3-18) is a graphical display of a process as it is known to its authors, owners, or team. The flow chart outlines the sequence and relationship of the pieces of the process. Through management of data and information, the team comes to a common understanding and knowledge concerning the process. Information is discussed about the structure (who carries out the specific step in the identified process), the activity that is occurring, and the outcome or the results.

Interrelationship Diagram

This tool organizes numerous complex problems, issues, or ideas by sorting and displaying their interrelations. The *interrelationship diagram* (FIG. 3-19) requires multidirectional thinking when there is not a straight-line cause-and-effect relationship. It is useful to address both operational and organizational issues.

Matrix Diagram

This tool displays the connection between each idea or issue in one group to one or more groups. A *matrix diagram* (FIG. 3-20)

	Bob	Linda	Roy	Sally	Dom
Chart Review at Hospital	X				
Chart Review at MD Office				X	
Interview Drs #123 and #456					X
Interview Office Nurses of Drs #123 and #456		X			
Compile Data			X		
Create Graphics			X		

How to construct

1. Specify the desired outcome.
2. Identify the final step necessary (e.g., a report to a committee with the team's recommendations).
3. Identify the starting point.
4. Brainstorm a list of the necessary steps between the starting and final steps.
5. Refine the list by combining like steps and defining the sequence steps.
6. Design a grid with important items (e.g., who is responsible, due date, budget/cost) listed across the top.
7. Arrange the list of tasks or steps in sequence down the left column.
8. Fill in the appropriate columns, including tentative dates.
9. Revise the planning grid as necessary.

When to use

- Use as a planning tool to identify steps to be taken, timelines, and responsibility for those steps
- Use for project and management teams to determine what needs to be done, in what sequence, who is responsible for what, and how that relates to others

Figure 3-16 **Deployment chart or planning grid.**

How to construct

There are six main steps to HFMEA^{SM}

1. Define a topic and process to be studied.

2. Convene an interdisciplinary team with content and process experts.

3. Develop a flow diagram of the process with consecutive numbering of each step and lettering of all subprocesses.

4. List all possible failure modes of each subprocess, including the severity and probability of the failure mode, and then number these failure modes (brainstorming may be helpful to identify failure modes).

5. After analyzing the failure modes, determine the action for each failure mode to eliminate, control, or accept.

6. Identify the corresponding outcome measure to test the redesigned process.

Figure 3-17 **Healthcare failure mode and effects analysis.**

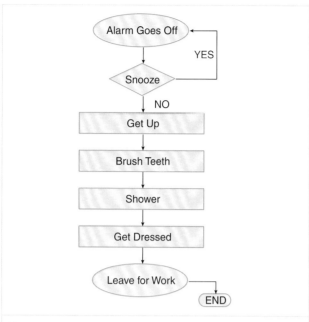

How to construct

1. Define the process that will be represented in the flowchart.

2. Determine all individuals, departments and groups involved in the process.

3. Brainstorm the steps in the process.

4. Construct the flowchart graphically using rows or columns corresponding to the associated work units.

5. Arrange the steps sequentially.

6. Draw arrows between the steps to show the process flow.

7. Review the flowchart and validate its accuracy with other individuals who are involved in the process.

When to use

- To show steps in a process

- To find one or multiple sources of a problem or identify potential areas for improvement

- To examine the handoffs that occur in a process

- To identify personnel, groups, or entire departments that are responsible for processes or tasks

- To demonstrate current processes (current state)

Figure 3-18 Flowchart or process flowchart. (From AHRQ. *Workflow Assessment for Health IT: flowchart.* https://healthit.ahrq.gov/health-it-tools-and-resources/workflow-assessment-health-it-toolkit/all-workflow-tools/flowchart.)

can show the relationship between two items as well as the strength of the relationship. Many matrix diagram formats are available, but the L-shaped matrix is the most common. Other common formats include the T-shaped, Y-shaped, X-shaped, and C-shaped matrices.

Multivoting

Multivoting (FIG. 3-21) is an easy, quick method for determining the most popular or important items from a list. The method uses a series of votes to cut the list in half each time, thus reducing the number of items to be considered.

Nominal Group Technique

This is a group decision-making process for generating many ideas in which each member works by himself or herself. The *nominal group technique* (FIG. 3-22) is used when group members are new to each other or when they have different opinions and goals. This approach is more structured than brainstorming and multivoting.

Plan–Do–Study–Act

The basic *PDSA* model is depicted in FIGURE 3-23. Specific strategies that can be used to test and link tests of change using PDSA cycles and the IHI model[52,67] include the following:

- Plan for multiple cycles of improvement in advance to support rapid-cycle movement;
- Scale the scope and size of tests so that small tests can be done rapidly (e.g., with a few patients, with one provider, in a single day);
- Choose people who want to work on the improvement change process;
- Capitalize on existing resources, best practice, and research. Don't reinvent the wheel;
- Select opportunities for change that are readily achievable ("low-hanging fruit" or easy, visible wins) first. Make the test feasible and practical;
- Don't delay a project because technology is not available; for small projects, paper and pen or other simple methods may be sufficient;
- Collect useful, meaningful measures and review results of every change cycle to determine any modifications that are needed;
- Test the change under a variety of conditions (e.g., different shifts and weekends); and
- Be prepared to stop or abandon the process if no improvement is observed.

Prioritization Matrix

This tool organizes tasks, issues, or actions and prioritizes them based on agreed-upon criteria. The tool combines the tree diagram and the L-shaped matrix diagram, displaying the best possible effect. The *prioritization matrix* (FIG. 3-24) often is used before more complex matrices are needed. This matrix applies options under discussion to the priority considerations of the organization.

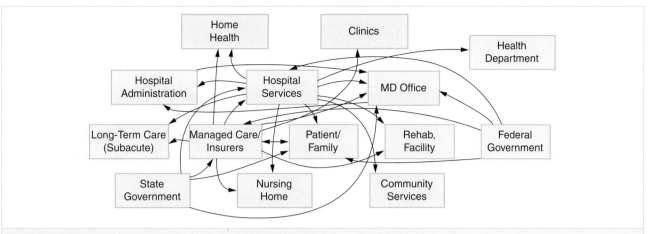

How to construct

1. Determine the issue/problem.
2. Generate ideas through brainstorming and other methods regarding the steps in the processes or issues.
3. Write the steps on cards and arrange them in similar groups (as with the affinity diagram) in cause-and-effect sequence. This technique is most effective when dealing with 15–50 items that may be interrelated. Discussion is appropriate throughout this process to ensure that no steps are missed.
4. Allow at least ½-inch of space between the cards so that relationship arrows can be drawn.
5. Fill in the relationship arrows that indicate what leads to what. This is done one card at a time until all cards have been discussed and relationship arrows drawn. Each card should be examined in terms of what happens when this card (process step) occurs; two-way arrows should be avoided.
6. Review and revise the diagram, transfer the information to a sheet of paper, and distribute it to team members for their review and revision before the next meeting.
7. Identify cards with the most arrows leading to them and cards with the most arrows leading away from them. Cards with incoming arrows represent a secondary issue or bottleneck in a process. Cards with outgoing arrows indicate a basic cause/issue that, if solved or overcome, will affect many other items. Cards with the most arrows are key factors in the process and should be addressed first.

When to use

- When the correct sequencing of events is critical
- When the issue/problem is complex and contains interrelationships among and between ideas/steps

Figure 3-19 **Interrelationship diagram.**

Process Decision Program Chart

This tool maps the identified events and contingencies that can occur between the time a problem is stated and solved. It attempts to identify potential deviations from the desired process, allowing the team to anticipate and prevent the deviation. Use the process decision program chart (FIG. 3-25) when the team is uncertain about a proposed implementation plan. This tool can be displayed in a graphic format combining a tree diagram and a flow chart or as an outline format (the outline format may be more difficult to use when communicating to a group and identifying patterns and simultaneous paths).

Root Cause Analysis

When variation is inherent in the process and a reduction of the variation is desired, the root cause of the variation must be identified to eliminate tampering with the effective

components of the process. The Joint Commission requires a root cause analysis (RCA) in response to sentinel events (unexpected serious adverse events).

1. To start with, identify potential causes of the variation. An interdisciplinary team very familiar with the process can use brainstorming, flowcharting, cause-and-effect diagrams, or some other process to determine these potential causes.
2. The second step is to verify the potential causes by collecting data about the process. After the data are collected and analyzed using the tools discussed in this module, the actual causes of the variation (or at least the most probable causes) can be identified. The following areas are addressed in the analysis:
   ◦ human factors: communications and information management systems;

	Governing Body	Administrative Team	Medical Staff Leaders	Middle Management	Staff Members
Overview Course	▲	▲	▲	▲	▲
Team Training		■	■	■	●
Facilitator Training		■	■	■	●
Just-in-Time Training		●	▲	▲	▲
Systems Thinking	▲	▲	▲	●	
Principle Centered Leadership	▲	▲	▲	●	

How to construct

1. Select the appropriate matrix format (e.g., L-shaped: two sets of items; T-shaped: three sets of items showing both indirect and direct relationships). Place the appropriate items on each axis of the matrix.
2. Determine the relationship symbols to be used (e.g., the following symbols may be selected: ▲ = very important; ■ = moderately important, as appropriate; ● = as needed).
3. Create the matrix and indicate the relationships.

When to use

- When defined tasks are to be assigned to employees
- When comparing tasks to a set of criteria
- When evaluating products or services against certain criteria
- When determining the relationship between patient satisfaction and certain factors

Figure 3-20 **Matrix diagram.**

How to construct

1. Generate a list of items and number them.
2. If the group agrees, combine items that seem to be similar.
3. If necessary, renumber all items.
4. Each member lists on a sheet of paper the items he or she considers the most important (the number of items chosen should be at least one-third of the total number of items on the list).
5. Tally the votes beside each item on the list.
6. Eliminate items with the lowest scores.
7. Repeat the above process until the list is narrowed down to an appropriate number for the group to focus on or the item with the top priority is identified.

When to use

Use after a brainstorming session to identify the key items on which the group will focus

Figure 3-21 **Multivoting.**

- human factors: training;
- human factors: fatigue and scheduling;
- environmental factors;
- equipment factors;
- rules, policies, and procedures; and
- leadership systems and culture.[37]

3. At this point, the team can develop and implement an action plan designed to eliminate or minimize the root causes of the variation.

See *Patient Safety* for more information on RCAs.

6S

6S (FIG. 3-26) is a lean tool. 6S is modeled after the 5S process improvement system designed to reduce waste and optimize productivity with the added pillar of safety. It is used in the workplace to (1) Create and maintain organization and orderliness; (2) Use visual cues to achieve more consistent operational results and (3) Reduce defects and making accidents less likely.[68]

How to construct

1. Define the task as you would for brainstorming.
2. Describe the purpose of this technique and the process to the group.
3. Write the question to be answered for all to see. Be sure to clarify the question as needed for the group.
4. Generate ideas to address the identified question by having the group write down their ideas in silence.
5. List all the items as you would in brainstorming. Only be sure to use a structured approach so that all ideas are listed (again, there is to be no discussion of the items at this time).
6. Clarify and discuss the ideas one at a time.
7. Give each member 4–8 cards or pieces of paper.
8. Members write one selection from the list on each card and assign a point value to each item. The highest value should be assigned to the most important item (i.e., if there are four cards, the most important card is numbered 4, next important 3, etc.)
9. The cards are collected, and the votes are tallied; mark each item on the list with the value on the cards for that item.
10. The item with the largest number becomes the group's selection/priority.

When to use

- Use when team members are new to each other
- Use when dealing with a controversial topic

Figure 3-22 **Nominal group technique.**

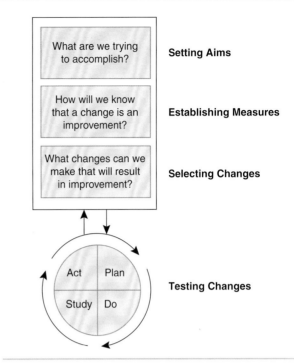

Figure 3-23 **Process improvement model (Plan–Do–Study–Act).** (Reprinted from Langley GL, Moen R, Nolan KM, et al. *The Improvement Guide: A Practical Approach to Enhancing Organizational Performance.* 2nd ed. San Francisco, CA: Jossey-Bass Publishers; 2009, with permission from John Wiley & Sons, Inc.)

	Low Cost	High Strategic Priority	Meets Accreditation Standards	MD Concern	Staff Concern	Totals
Repair roof	3	4	2	3	4	16
Purchase new X-ray machine	5	2	0	1	5	13
Develop skilled nursing	4	1	0	2	2	9
Develop better communications with home health	2	3	1	4	3	13
Develop a staff newsletter	1	5	3	5	1	15

How to construct

1. Create an L-shaped matrix as previously described in the matrix section.
2. Prioritize and assign weights to the list of criteria that will be used in the prioritization.
3. Prioritize the list of options based on each criterion.
4. Prioritize and select the item(s) across all the criteria.

When to use

- When issues are identified and options must be narrowed down
- When options have strong interrelationships
- When options all need to be done, but prioritization or sequencing is needed

Figure 3-24 **Prioritization matrix.**

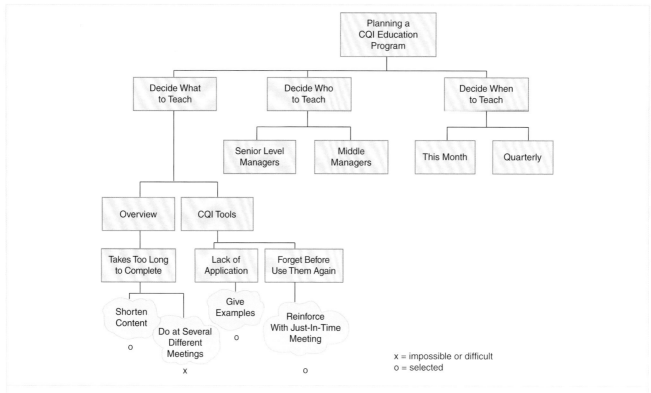

How to construct

1. Determine the proposed flow of a process.
2. Choose the graphic or outline format.
3. Identify the desired goal or improvement.
4. List the first steps in sequence along the first level of the tree diagram, then add a second level of steps to reach the first-level step (refer to how to construct a tree diagram for construction directions).
5. Identify the things that could go wrong at each step and list them as another level below the appropriate step.
6. Brainstorm ideas that could be implemented to prevent the undesired events and display them as clouds branched below the last level.

When to use

- As part of a root cause analysis
- To anticipate any problems before implementing an action plan
- To develop a contingency plan
- To test theories as they are implemented if unable to test a theory before implementation

Figure 3-25 **Process decision program chart.**

Spaghetti Diagram

A *spaghetti diagram* (FIG. 3-27), also called a layout diagram, is a graphic representation of the flow of traffic or movement. It helps an organization visualize flow and figure out how to improve it by looking at how people or materials move from one location to another.[69(p1)]

Supplier Input Process Output Customer

A supplier-input-process-output-customer (SIPOC, FIG. 3-28) is a tool in process management to identify key drivers of a

process. When the healthcare quality professional has a clear understanding of data, types of data, and tools, the process steps may be described with a variety of acronyms (e.g., PDSA; PDCA; assess, plan, implement, evaluate) but include similar components. No specific improvement model is endorsed in this section so that the healthcare quality professional can use tools depending on the improvement question and the organizational context. Regardless of the improvement model, the improvement process seeks to accomplish the following:

- Ensure the project is a priority for the organization and is aligned with the strategic plan.

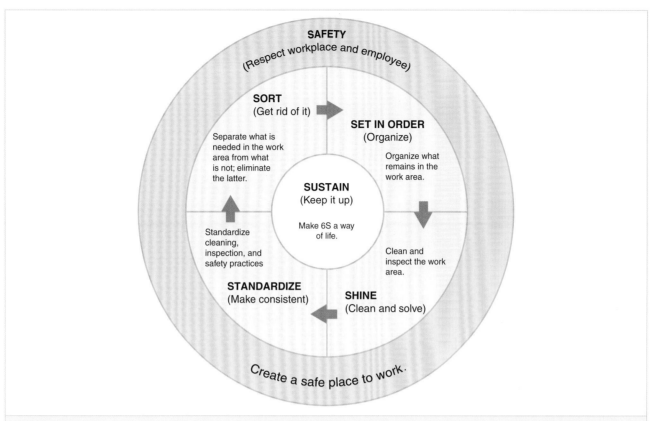

How to construct

1. **Sort (Get rid of it)**: Separate what is needed in the work area from what is not; eliminate the latter.
2. **Set in order (Organize)**: Organize what remains in the work area.
3. **Shine (Clean and solve)**: Clean and inspect the work area.
4. **Safety (Respect workplace and employee)**: Create a safe place to work.
5. **Standardize (Make consistent)**: Standardize cleaning, inspection, and safety practices.
6. **Sustain (Keep it up)**: Make 6S a way of life.

When to use

- To establish orderly flow, eliminate waste, and organize the workplace
- To standardize the work setting

Figure 3-26 **The six pillars of 6S.**

- Ensure leadership support and commitment.
- Assess the priority and feasibility of initiatives based on risks, resources, leadership support, and organizational strategies.
- Clarify the aim, stated in specific measurable terms.
- Present baseline data analysis that illustrates the problem. Use tools and techniques to analyze.
- Demonstrate that the aim is based on the organization's own data and identifies the specific problem to be solved, the program to be enhanced, or the process or system to be redesigned.
- Select an inter-professional team with content and process experts and all key disciplines as members.
- Map the "as-is" or current state process and collect data on key aspects of the process. Continue to use data and tools to identify bottlenecks, constraints, delays, and other barriers.
- Define measures and collect data. Indicate how a change results in improvement.
- Describe the change to be made.
- Implement the change (small tests of change or pilot tests).
- Study the effects of the change and decide: adopt, adapt, or abandon the specific change.
- Map the new "to-be" or future state process.
- Spread the change throughout the organization in a defined implementation plan (include communication plan and education plan).
- Sustain the improvement by monitoring.

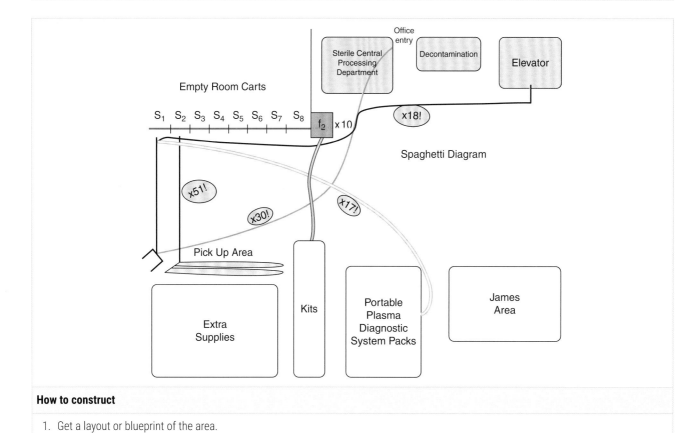

How to construct

1. Get a layout or blueprint of the area.
2. Pick the subject to follow for the flow.
3. Record every movement until completed.

When to use

- To demonstrate flow or movement in a process
- To identify excess or wasted travel or movement

Figure 3-27 **Spaghetti diagram (or layout diagram).**

S	I	P	O	C
Supplier name	Process input	Process step 1	Process output	Customer name
Supplier name	Process input	Process step 2	Process output	Customer name
Supplier name	Process input	Process step 3	Process output	Customer name

How to construct

1. Identify each element of the SIPOC and list across the top of a page.

2. Under each heading of SIPOC list the suppliers, their inputs, the process, the customers, and the outputs.

When to use

To identify internal and external customer needs in a process and to use with other lean tools for process improvement

Figure 3-28 **Supplier input process output customer.**

COPIS (customer-output-process-input-supplier) is also used, which is outward in approach to begin with the customer's viewpoint. Both SIPOC and COPIS are approaches used in Six Sigma and complement DMAIC.

Tree Diagram

This tool maps out the full range of paths and tasks in the process that must be accomplished to achieve a goal. A *tree diagram* (FIG. 3-29) resembles an organizational chart. The tree diagram can be presented as an organizational chart or placed on its side.

Value Stream Mapping

Value stream mapping (FIG. 3-30) is a map of the process in which only value-added steps for the customer are retained and waste removed. This Lean tool analyzes a process from a systems perspective and creates a visual depiction of the sequential steps in a process from beginning to end.

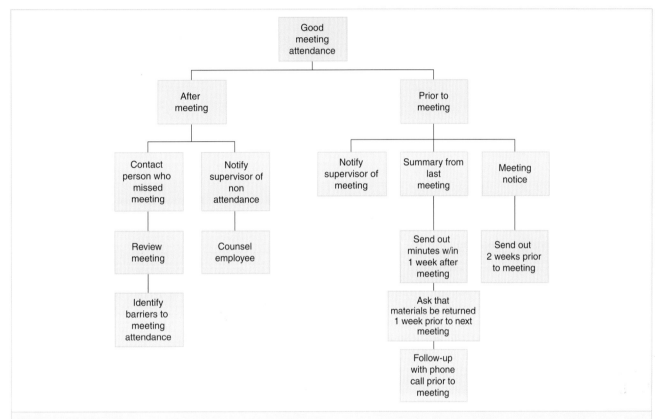

How to construct

1. Identify the overall goal that can be broken down into the steps necessary to achieve it.
2. Position the paper you are working on vertically because the diagram usually is long rather than wide; work from left to right.
3. Select the appropriate tree branches (categories/groups) to investigate (an affinity diagram often is helpful to identify the first level of detail, which always is the broadest level); create headers for each of these branches.
4. For each header, ask: What needs to happen to achieve the header and goal statement? Write ideas on cards and place them to the right of the appropriate first-level idea. This level should have a direct cause-and-effect relationship with the previous level.
5. When complete, ask the following questions to each level of detail: Will these lead to the results? Do we really need to do this task to reach the results?

When to use

- When it is crucial that a step/task not be overlooked
- When a specific task has become the focus, but it is a complicated task to complete
- When there have been numerous roadblocks to implementation

Figure 3-29 **Tree diagram.**

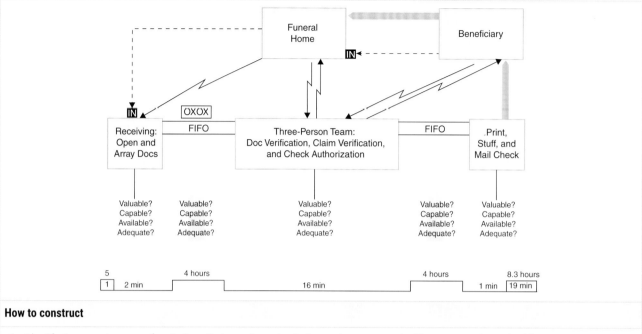

How to construct

1. Identify the current process (mark steps that are of no value to the customer or required by some regulatory body).
2. Identify the ideal process state.

When to use

To improve flow of the process, reduce waste, and implement lean functioning

Figure 3-30 **Value stream mapping.**

Voice of the Customer

Voice of the Customer (VOC) (FIG. 3-31) is a tool conducted at the start (or "Fuzzy Front End") of any new product, process, or service design initiative to understand better the customer's wants and needs. The VOC can serve as key input for new product definition, Quality Function

- What do you like about the current process?
- What do you think needs improvement?
- What would you recommend to improve the current process?
- What could threaten the success of the project?

How to construct

1. Identify customers of a process output.
2. Develop a list of questions to ask customers about the process and their needs.
3. Refine the list to use with the process review and improvement.

When to use

To improve a process

Figure 3-31 **Voice of the customer.**

Deployment, or the setting of detailed design specifications. Four aspects of the VOC are customer needs, a hierarchical structure, priorities, and customer perceptions of performance.[70] The product is a list of needs, wants, and desires of the customer of a process output (e.g., specifications, requirements).

Leading Change and Teamwork

Organizations use teams to work on one or more targeted improvement opportunities. Teams may report up to an established quality operational structure or to a group of individuals with responsibility for the area where the improvement opportunity exists. The composition and size of each team depend on the specific aim of the team. Including the right people on the team is critical to success. IHI[71] identified three categories of team membership with impact on team success:

1. Clinical leadership representation to bring the authority necessary to test and implement the recommended change and to help overcome issues;
2. Technical expertise to ensure relevant understanding of related technical content areas; and

3. Day-to-day leadership to include frontline leadership and physician representation to serve as a driving force during the project and the champion for change during implementation of improvements.

In addition, each team selects a project sponsor or champion with executive authority who serves as liaison to other areas of the organization as well as to other members of senior management. The project sponsor checks in periodically on the team's progress.

What is a team? A *team* is "a group of people who are interdependent with respect to information, resources, and skills and who seek to combine their efforts to achieve a common goal."[72(p2)] An important structural element for healthcare quality is creating a team-based organization. Because patient care involves multiple professional disciplines, the linchpin for improvement is an employee base with regular communication and contact that allows them to coordinate and problem solve to continuously improve quality of care. The organization must develop an infrastructure within which the cycle of improvement can operate. One feature of this infrastructure is teams.

Teamwork in healthcare is "a dynamic process involving two or more health professionals with complimentary backgrounds and skills, sharing common health goals and exercising concerted physical and mental effort in assessing, planning, or evaluating patient care. This is accomplished through interdependent collaboration, open communication and shared decision-making. This in turn generates value-added patient, organizational and staff outcomes."[73(p238)] Nancarrow et al.[74] identified 10 competencies of effective inter-professional teams:

1. Identifies a leader who establishes a clear direction and vision for the team, while listening and providing support and supervision to the team members.
2. Incorporates a set of values that clearly provide direction for the team's service provision; these values should be visible and consistently portrayed.
3. Demonstrates a team culture and interdisciplinary atmosphere of trust where contributions are valued and consensus is fostered.
4. Ensures appropriate processes and infrastructures are in place to uphold the vision of the service (e.g., referral criteria, communications infrastructure).
5. Provides quality patient-focused services with documented outcomes; utilizes feedback to improve the quality of care.
6. Utilizes communication strategies that promote intra-team communication, collaborative decision-making and effective team processes.
7. Provides sufficient team staffing to integrate an appropriate mix of skills, competencies, and personalities to meet the needs of patients and enhance smooth functioning.
8. Facilitates recruitment of staff who demonstrate inter-disciplinary competencies including team functioning, collaborative leadership, communication, and sufficient professional knowledge and experience.
9. Promotes role interdependence while respecting individual roles and autonomy.
10. Facilitates personal development through appropriate training, rewards, recognition, and opportunities for career development.[74(pp5–11)]

Types of Teams

High-functioning teams improve clinical and financial outcomes. The roles that team members assume in the provision of patient care vary depending on philosophical, political, social, communication, and clinical differences about patient care.[75] Inarguably, teams are of great importance. And there are many types of formal and informal teams.

- Temporary project: Teams with a special focus on improvement, problem solving, or product development. There are often both core and resource members. Core members participate throughout the project and have complementary skills needed for the desired work output. Resource members may be critical only for specific phases of the project and may move in and out of the team. Other ongoing or functional work teams are usually permanent or may be longstanding.
- Natural work: These teams involve the people in each work setting who share responsibility for a process, workflow, or type of work. Members are those who work together each day to complete the task. These teams can be cross-functional, as with an OR team, or intact, such as a team of nurses in a unit. Autonomy varies, but there typically is a leader. These teams can be temporary (e.g., brought together to solve a single problem) or permanent (e.g., continuous improvement teams).
- Self-directed: This work team is a type of natural work team that shares many management responsibilities, such as scheduling work, managing budgets, evaluating performance, and hiring new team members.
- Process management: Team focuses on sharing responsibility for monitoring and controlling a work process, such as new product development. Members may rotate on and off the team based on their contributions (expertise).
- Virtual teams: Team typically uses technology-supported communications rather than face-to-face interactions to accomplish their tasks. They may cross boundaries, such as time zones, geography, and organizational units. Virtual teams can be either project teams or ongoing teams.

Steering Committees

Steering committees (often known as quality councils) are permanent QI teams consisting of cross-functional members, and in patient-centered care environments, include patients and family members. These committees are self-managed teams that provide direction and focus by identifying and prioritizing improvement opportunities in the organization. The role of the steering committee or quality council is to sustain, facilitate, and expand the performance and process improvement initiatives based on the strategic plan. It is comprised of top leaders in the organization, including medical staff. The main responsibilities of the quality council include

- lending legitimacy to the quality efforts;
- maintaining organization focus on the identified goals and priorities;
- fostering teamwork for improvement;
- providing necessary resources (e.g., human, financial); and
- formulating organizational policies regarding quality and safety priorities, participation, annual self-assessments, and reward and recognition systems.

When to Use Teams

Three aspects of the required task are examined before deciding whether to use a team: task complexity, task interdependence, and task objectives.[76] Tasks are complex when they involve large amounts of information, they are performed under conditions of high uncertainty, they contain many subtasks that require people with specialized skills and knowledge, and there are no standardized procedures for completing the tasks. Teams are important because they bring larger numbers of specialized individuals (i.e., subject matter experts) to carry the burden and offer greater diverse inputs that are more likely to result in more alternatives generated and more creative solutions. Creativity is particularly important when there are no standardized procedures and the environment is uncertain.

Task interdependence means that the work of one person is highly dependent on the work of others. Patient care typically involves a multitude of disciplines that must coordinate their work, and this requires intense communication. Teams therefore are appropriate, because this type of structure can foster communication between the various disciplines. Finally, teams are appropriate to use when the task objectives are clear and time-bound. One approach for making task objectives clear is to develop a team charter. The charter contains the following information[77]:

- Description of the process, why it needs improvement, and who is affected;
- Development of criteria to demonstrate that the process improved;

- Timeline for meetings;
- Resources available;
- Structure of leadership (e.g., self-managed, leader-directed); and
- Expected communication of progress and results.

How Teams Develop and Grow

Teams develop, mature, and change over time. Tuckman[78] described four stages of development in one popular model with somewhat predictable stages. This classic framework continues to be used to this day.

Stage 1. Forming. During the first stage, the members try to get to know each other, agree on the goal or vision, and delegate tasks. They cautiously explore boundaries to determine acceptable group behavior. Discussions focus on how to accomplish the tasks and the information and resources needed, and the team accomplishes little at this stage. This is a period of testing to find out what kind of behavior is appropriate. Members tend to defer to the leader or dominant member for guidance. In this stage, team leaders need to be directive and provide role clarification. Members get to know each other, agree on goals, and delegate tasks; members may feel anxiety, excitement, and uncertainty, and they may test boundaries of behavior. The team leader needs to be directive, with high-task relationships, and provide role clarification. The team depends on the leader during this learning stage. This stage is short if the tasks are clearly defined and easily achievable.

Stage 2. Storming. This second stage is where conflict typically arises. Members try to express their individuality and resist group pressures and influence. There often are emotional responses to group demands, especially if the group is under pressure to achieve results. To prevent the group from becoming stuck at this stage, leaders need to manage the conflict, not by suppressing it but by using it to energize the team. Conflict and tension often arise, and members assert their individual roles and compete for control. The leader moves to a coaching style of leadership. At this stage, reality sets in. There is the realization that the task may be difficult, they notice their lack of progress, and there is resistance to the task. Resources are applied to the task rather than education about the problem. People are willing to suggest tasks, and the leader then delegates the tasks. People do not take responsibility for problems, yet the team is building cohesion. This is probably the most difficult stage. Arguing, defensiveness, disunity, and tension are often evident.

Stage 3. Norming. In this stage, members develop close ties and a strong identity with the team. There is a shift from "I" to "we" and a willingness to accept the views of others. Team members develop feelings of mutual respect, harmony, and trust. Group standards and members' roles emerge. Leaders need to challenge the team members to continue to grow and guard against too much conformity to group norms. The team develops close ties and a strong identity; members develop harmony by avoiding conflict. Tentative constructive criticism is allowed. A supporting leadership style evolves. Concern moves from silos to the inter-professional group. Members volunteer evidence-based solutions instead of just providing vague suggestions. There is an emerging leadership or ownership of functional roles by the members. There is acceptance of team rules, norms, and roles and finally optimism that things work out. More harmony, cohesion, and discussion of team dynamics occur.

Stage 4. Performing. In the fourth stage, the team works harmoniously toward a common goal and is very productive. The team develops a functional but flexible structure, and roles are interrelated. Interpersonal conflicts are resolved, and the group is highly task oriented. In this stage, the leader needs to develop mechanisms for sharing leadership responsibilities. The team works harmoniously and gains insight into the team's process. Improvement of the team's process and team identification begins to predominate. The team is task oriented and accomplishes its work. Goal orientation is now optimized, and task competency is high. High morale, support, and appreciation come from team members. Roles diminish, and participation by all is encouraged. The team may begin to take on additional responsibilities and is functioning at an optimal level.

Not all teams progress through these four stages, and if they do, they probably move back and forth through the stages as new issues are identified or new members join the team. Nevertheless, the stages point to important developmental issues having implications for team leaders, facilitators, and coaches. Lack of effectiveness often results from leadership and facilitation problems and a lack of clear goals and expectations. Teamwork components of cohesiveness, communication, role clarity, and goal clarity from *The Team Handbook*[79] are integrated into these specific roles found in stages in **TABLE 3-11**.

Table 3-11 Team Roles

Sponsor	Sponsors are the formal leaders and prime movers of the project. They align resources and monitor progress. Sponsors hold others accountable to get on with change. The sponsor inspires the team members to say, "I believe in this project." Some project tasks require sponsors at multiple levels to obtain adequate resources and buy-in from the entire project team.
Champion	Champions are the respected opinion leaders who provide credibility to the project and are integral to the social structure. The champions are respected clinicians or staff with influence through clinical reputation or leadership qualities. Their experience provides credibility for the project team and task. They support the change and work for its implementation by speaking favorably about it and sharing their first-hand knowledge or experience.
Leader	Leaders guide the team to achieve successful outcomes and attain the established goals. They are responsible for guiding the team through the process to achieve the aim or goals. They provide direction and support. The team leader knows meeting procedures and has strong communication and interpersonal skills.
Timekeeper	The timekeeper monitors meeting agendas, ensures the team is aware of the time allotted for each agenda item, and reminds the team when they go over the allotted time.
Process Owner	The process owner is the leader among frontline staff directly involved in the process. This is the team member who is responsible and accountable for sustaining improvements during and after implementation. Ideally, the process owner should be someone with authority over frontline staff directly involved in the process evaluation.
Facilitator	Although facilitators (change agents or coaches) have no formal authority over other team members, they are instrumental in implementing the change through planning, helping, and facilitating. The facilitator is not vested in the project but is skilled in problem solving and adult learning and has good communication and interpersonal skills. As change agents, they are the technical experts on the team; they influence progress by gathering measurable data and information. They listen to the concerns of other team members and help remove barriers. They support the sponsors by advancing the team's work to goal achievement.
	They promote effective group dynamics and are concerned with how decisions are made. They may also serve as coaches or consultants. They keep the team on track. They provide expertise on using tools. Coaches focus on helping the team to learn rather than teaching them. The facilitator needs to have a clear perception of the facts and information and the ability to determine what is relevant. That ability includes an understanding of systems, dynamics, relationships between system components, and psychology. The facilitator, change agent, or coach needs to understand when and how emotions or desires distort one's perception.

(continued)

Table 3-11 Team Roles (*continued*)

Member	A member is an actual representative on the team. Although project team composition varies, in most cases the project team includes the frontline staff (e.g., nurses, physicians, clerks, ancillary services staff) and area supervisors directly affected by the project task. To identify these personnel, consider all relevant stakeholders to the process. The ideal team size is 8–12 people. Unless necessary, team size should not exceed 15 people. They can collect data and information related to the process of focus. For the stakeholders not represented, develop a communication mechanism (team minutes, session report) and designate one or more people to disseminate this information regularly. Chosen team members must be able to commit to attend team meetings and meet their responsibilities.
Scribe	The scribe role may be assigned to one person or rotated between members. The role includes documenting minutes of meetings and other recordkeeping activities.

Characteristics of Effective Teams

It is widely known that teams often fail to produce the results for which they were brought together. What makes a team successful? Abundant research and practice demonstrate the important predictors of team success[80–82]:

- Competent members with technical, problem-solving, interpersonal, and organizational skills;
- Commitment to clear, common goals;
- Standards of excellence;
- Contributions from every member;
- Collaborative environment (culture to support teamwork);
- Leadership support;
- Nonhierarchical structure; and
- External support and recognition.

Characteristics of effective and ineffective teams are further described in **TABLE 3-12**. Four key traits can predict a team's success: (1) Cohesiveness; (2) Communication; (3) Clear roles; and (4) Clear goals.[79]

Cohesiveness is the social glue that binds the team members together as a unit. Cohesiveness can be increased by the establishment of ground rules, or norms, addressing how meetings are run, how team members interact, and what kind of behavior is acceptable. Each member is expected to respect these rules, which usually prevents misunderstandings and disagreements. Balanced participation is encouraged to strengthen the team's cohesion. Because every team member has a stake in the achievements, everyone participates in discussions and decisions, shares the commitment to the project's success, and contributes their talents. The use of brainstorming or a nominal group technique to obtain input from all team members during discussions is one method to encourage members to bond. When a team is cohesive, members are attracted to the team; find membership in the team to be a personally meaningful experience; enjoy the company of the other team members; support, nurture, and care for each other; feel free to share ideas and suggest ways to improve team function; feel they are using their unique skills for the benefit of the team; have a strong "we" feeling; and routinely develop creative solutions to problems.

Communication is the next key component to successful teams. Communication involves a full range of topics, including decision-making and problem solving. Effective communication becomes easier once the team develops a certain level of cohesiveness. Communication is key because further team development and effective functioning cannot occur without team communication. When a team is communicating effectively, team members

- freely say what they feel and think;
- are always direct, truthful, respectful, and positive;
- openly discuss all decisions before they are made;
- handle conflict in a calm, caring, and healing manner;
- openly explore options to solve problems when they arise; and
- do not gossip about each other, have unknown alliances, or hidden agendas.

Effective, clear communication depends on how information is exchanged between team members. Ideally, team members speak clearly, directly, and succinctly. They ask questions in an inviting way. Members listen actively and avoid interrupting when others are speaking. The team encourages all members to use the skills and practices that make discussions and meetings more effective. Team members initiate discussions, seek information and opinions, suggest procedures, elaborate on ideas, complete assignments on time, and summarize.

Team leaders and facilitators act as gatekeepers during communication by managing member participation, keeping discussion focused, and resolving differences creatively. Considering the stage of team development, such as storming, leaders and facilitators may need to ease tension and work through difficulties. Communication also includes well-defined decision-making procedures.

Table 3-12 Team Characteristics

Effective Teams	Ineffective Teams
Mutual agreement and identification with respect to the team goal	Does not distinguish between facts, opinions, and feelings
Open communication between members	Does not separate idea generation from idea evaluation
Mutual trust and support	Prematurely closes discussion before all alternatives are identified
Management of human differences	Dominated by aggressive members
Selective use of the team	Fails to assign specific responsibilities
Appropriate member skills	Does not review minutes, tasks, or due dates
Leadership	Works on problems that are outside the scope of the team
Values and goals of the members interpreted as needs and values of the team	Exhibits uncertainty about the team's direction
Team believes it can accomplish the impossible	Launches many improvement projects without clear objectives
Understands the value of constructive team cohesiveness and how to use it	Fails to apply discussion skills
	Hides a secret agenda
Mutual influence between members and the leader	Relies on one person to manage discussion without sharing responsibility
Exhibits clear goals, purposes, discussions, and decisions	Discusses the project outside the meeting rather than bringing issues to the team
Agrees on the goal	
Has formally defined roles	Repeats points of discussion
Revises plan as needed	Concedes to opinions rather than fact-based data
Uses tool to map the process and project steps	Uses majority rule rather than consensus in disagreements
Effectively uses talents of members	Uses decision by default, with silence assumed as consent
Balances participation of all members	Avoids certain topics
Discusses issues openly	Does not acknowledge ground rules
Clarifies ideas or issues	Has recurring differences on acceptable behavior
Uses consensus-based decision-making	Has conflicting expectations
Uses data for problem solving	Does not attend to clues or shifts in the team mood
Applies resources and training throughout the project	Makes remarks that discount someone's behavior or contribution

The role of champion can greatly benefit engagement in a quality or safety effort. The ideal champion is perceived as credible and able to influence others to adopt or implement a new process as part of the patient safety or quality effort. Physician champions are especially effective in improving physician engagement in quality and safety efforts. Champions are also critical for successful teams in healthcare settings. They can contribute to the success of projects, innovations and other organizational change initiatives.

A team is always aware of the different ways it reaches consensus. The team discusses how decisions are made, explore important issues by polling, test for agreement, and use data as the basis for decisions. Occasionally, the team may want to designate a member to observe team interactions and give feedback on how decisions are made so the group can talk about any changes it needs to make. Team members are also sensitive to nonverbal communication. This includes seeing, hearing, and feeling the team dynamics.

Role clarity is the next area to facilitate team success. The roles are common among teams but they may differ slightly depending on the type of team that is convened. The role of team member supersedes individual professional roles. Although professional roles brought to the team give the team its potential strength, it is also important for team development that individuals feel equally valued. In addition, team members know who is doing what and what other team members expect of them. When a team achieves role clarity, members feel that accomplishments of the team are placed above those of individuals, understand the roles and responsibilities of all other team members, and there is a clear understanding of what other team members expect of them. A team facilitator is clearly identified. Facilitation requires skills that are both art and science. A skilled facilitator guides group process in an unbiased manner ensuring that the meeting agenda is carried out and decisions are responsibly reached with independent contributions from all team members.

The final component of team development to become a fully functioning and high-performing team is clearly defining team goals and the means used to reach these goals. When a team achieves goal clarity, team members agree on what the real work of the team is, clearly understand the goals, agree on how to reach the goals, and agree on clear criteria for evaluating the outcomes of the team. Teams operate most efficiently when they tap everyone's talents and when all members understand their duties and know who is responsible for what issues and tasks. Goal clarity begins with a charter.

Successful teams are one of the most important aspects of effective organizational functioning and quality, safety and PI efforts. Two special team types have patient safety as their focus but include essential elements of teams that increase their ability to address patient safety and error reduction. The first is Team Strategies and Tools to Enhance Performance and Patient Safety (TeamSTEPPS®), a teamwork system designed for healthcare professionals. This is an evidence-based teamwork system designed to improve communication and teamwork skills. Team members learn four primary teamwork skills: leadership, communication, situation monitoring, and mutual support. Three types of team outcomes are desired: performance, knowledge, and attitudes.

The TeamSTEPPS model is based on lessons learned, change models, the literature of quality and patient safety, and culture change. Phase 1 assesses an organization's readiness for undertaking the initiative. Phase 2 includes planning, training, and implementation; options in this phase include tools and strategies. Phase 3 sustains and spreads improvements in teamwork performance, clinical processes, and outcomes.[83] See the section *Patient Safety* for more information on TeamSTEPPS.

The second special type of team is Crew Resource Management (CRM). A specific CRM training program based on airline safety was developed for healthcare. Although the team is focused on patient safety, the effectiveness of team functioning is a first critical component.[84] Additional elements include a focus on the patient safety mindset and high-reliability functioning. The team learns skills in decision-making under stressful situations through continued practice, simulation, and use of checklists to embed teamwork behaviors into daily work and provide numerous opportunities to practice the desired behaviors.

For those organizations employing Six Sigma or Lean methods, a *Workout* is a fast track change acceleration process developed originally at General Electric. The *Workout* is conducted by a group of team members in a short time (hours or days).[85] With well-defined team roles and clear direction defined in a challenge statement and goal the *Workout* is a good example of the effective use of teams for rapid PI. This process has also been called Rapid Process Improvement Workshop in some organizations.

Evaluating Team Performance

Evaluating team performance is important to the overall effectiveness of an organization's operations and improvement efforts. Three key actions determine the success of any team and are used for evaluation:

1. Developing shared goals and methods to accomplish outcomes;
2. Developing methods and skills to communicate and make decisions across systems and organizations; and
3. Engaging leadership that balances getting input and making decisions, so work moves ahead.

Team performance also requires formal evaluation. In general, evaluation of a team includes three criteria:

1. Productivity or results: The extent to which the goals were met. Did the team accomplish what it set out to do and within the defined time frame?
2. Satisfaction of team members: It is important that team members can work together in the future. To the extent that members are satisfied with the team, they are more likely to work well together in the future.
3. Individual growth: The extent to which individual members developed professionally by serving as team members.

A more formalized manner of evaluating team performance includes the following process criteria:

- Organizational alignment:
  - Does the team have statements of mission, vision, values, structures, roles, and goals?
  - Does the team have a charter? Are the purpose and goals important to the organization's strategic priorities?
- Goal clarity: Are there clearly stated goals, and do actions exist to achieve the goals?
- Leadership: Is there clear leadership support of the team?
- Roles: Are team roles been defined?
- Norms: Does the team define ground rules and abide by them?
- Team participation: Do all members of the team participate and share tasks?
- Team meetings: Are team meetings organized with agendas, time frames, action plans, and decisions?
- Competency to perform tasks: Are members trained to work on tasks?
- Communication: Is communication open, honest, and constructive?
- Atmosphere: Is the atmosphere warm, accepting, and supportive for all team members?
- Decision-making: Does the team achieve consensus on decisions and look at multiple alternatives before reaching a decision?
- Problem solving: Is the team able to validate problem identification before moving to a solution by using sound data and tools?
- Conflicts: Does the team have a process for constructively managing interpersonal conflict?

- Performance management: Does the team manage its performance, or must management intervene?
- Work tools and training: Has the team been trained on tools and data management to function effectively?
- Boundary management: Has the team developed relationships with other teams, stakeholders, and customers?

Healthcare quality professionals play an important role in leading or facilitating PI projects. Many different types of improvement projects may be chartered. They vary in breadth, scope, and duration. There are also different names that may be assigned to projects, but they all can be categorized under the umbrella of quality and safety. For example, there may be rapid process improvement teams, green belt project teams, black belt project teams, Lean projects, Six Sigma projects, and redesign projects. They are similar in their basic approach. The types of tools and level of statistical analysis may vary by type of team. Depending on the complexity of the project, a simple action plan may be sufficient, or the use of a Gantt or Program Evaluation Review Technique chart for project management might be more helpful.

A basic approach and actual steps in a PI project include the following:

1. Alignment with priorities and strategic goals and objectives.
   a. This first step ensures the leaders support this project because it aligns with the strategic goals and PI priorities and are willing to devote resources to it.
2. A team charter is usually written at this point and describes the scope, boundaries, expected results, and resources used by a process improvement team.
   a. The individual or group who formed the team usually provides the charter.
   b. Sometimes the process owner or the team members develop a charter.
   c. A charter is always needed for a team working on a process that crosses departmental lines.
   d. A charter may not be necessary for a team that is improving a process found solely within a work center or office space.
3. Basic team functions are identified
   a. members of the team.
   b. roles within the team.
   c. meeting schedule.
   d. project timeline.
   e. resources available and needed to complete the improvement project.
   f. expected communication of progress and results.
4. Clear, defined aim for the team to work toward a common goal.
5. Analysis of baseline performance and problem identification is needed to determine the level of improvement.
6. A map of the process (current and ideal) is developed.

7. Description of the process: why it needs improvement and who is affected.
8. Development of criteria to demonstrate that the process is improved.
9. Measurement of success; this includes the numerator and denominator for a percentage, rate, or other weighted measure.
10. Changes to be tested and implemented.
    a. Tests of change supported by data collection, analysis, and reporting.
    b. Control or methods to sustain the change.
11. Results or outcomes of the project.
12. Reporting of the project and results to leaders, the organization, or others.
13. Evaluation tools for the team process.

Aligning Incentives to Advance Quality

Reward systems are critical to the success of quality, safety and PI initiatives. In fact, "The most damaging alignment problem to which many total quality failures have been attributed is the lack of alignment between expectations that arise from total quality change processes and reward systems."[86(p362)] Rewards are important because they can motivate people. Motivating people to provide excellent customer service is a top priority for most organizations. Therefore, before discussing rewards, it is important to understand motivation.

Basics of Motivation

Work motivation is "the psychological forces that determine the *direction* of a person's behavior in an organization, a person's level of *effort,* and a person's level of *persistence*."[87(p181)] There are many theories of motivation and each has somewhat different but complementary implications for actions that motivate employees. Therefore, a basic understanding of major theories is important.

Need Theories. Need theories center on what employees are motivated to obtain from work (outcomes). These theories include Maslow's hierarchy of needs, McClelland's need theory, and Hertzberg's two-factor theory.

Maslow's[88] need theory was first published in 1943. Maslow, a psychologist, believed that human needs could be arranged in a hierarchy from the most basic to higher order needs, as follows:

- Physiologic or survival needs (basic survival needs such as food and water);
- Safety or security needs (protection from harm or physical deprivation);
- Belongingness or social needs (the need for interaction with others, companionship, belonging, and friendship);

- Esteem or status needs (needs for recognition and appreciation); and
- self-actualization needs (the need for self-fulfillment or to reach one's highest potential).

Maslow believed that basic needs had to be met before higher order needs. For example, basic survival needs are met (e.g., working in a safe environment) before employees focus on esteem needs. In addition, Maslow maintained that only unsatisfied needs served to motivate people; people want what they do not have.

McClelland proposed a concept like Maslow's, narrowing the number of needs to three types: achievement, power, and affiliation.[89]

Finally, Herzberg's two-factor theory classified the elements of motivation into two categories: motivators and hygiene factors.[90] Motivators are the elements of a job that increase job satisfaction, including challenging work, achievement, recognition, growth, and advancement. Hygiene factors, on the other hand, do not contribute to motivation, but their absence leads to dissatisfaction. Hygiene factors include company policy and administrative issues such as supervision, working conditions, interpersonal relations, safety, salaries, morale, and productivity. Herzberg expanded on Maslow's theory, making a distinction between factors that motivate and factors that maintain motivation.

At least two managerial implications for motivation are clear from need theories:

- There are many different needs, and these differ between employees.
- If employees are not motivated, managers seek to determine the needs of employees and which are satisfied or dissatisfied.

The relationship between Maslow's Hierarchy of Needs and employee engagement is shown as FIGURE 3-32.

Expectancy Theory. Expectancy theory is concerned with how people decide which behaviors to engage in and how much effort they give to that behavior. This theory focuses on the person's perception of effort-to-performance and performance-to-outcome links. Essentially, a person asks, "If I work hard (effort), will I be able to perform?" Motivation is improved by strengthening that link. Managers want to be certain that employees believe that if they work hard, they will achieve high performance. Thus, providing training and education so that they have the appropriate skills to perform the work would improve motivation. In accordance with this theory, managers do the following:

- Be certain employees possess the necessary skills to perform well.
- Coach employees to believe that if they work hard they will be successful.
- Know what outcomes employees perceive as important (as detailed by needs theory).
- Establish clear policies about what levels of performance are rewarded (result in outcomes) and which levels are not.

Individuals also ask themselves, "If I perform at a high level, will there be an outcome, and is it something I care about?" To strengthen this performance-outcome link, managers want employees to believe that if they perform at a high level, there is an outcome that they desire. Managers can strengthen this link by having valid performance appraisal systems to capture quality and safety performance. Systems should also be in place to reward such performance. For example, when an employee reports an adverse event, there should be an immediate outcome that is positive in the eyes of that employee.

Equity Theory. Equity theory centers on the input and outcomes part of the motivation equation. The overall idea is that employees are motivated when there is fairness in the workplace. This theory contends that employees determine

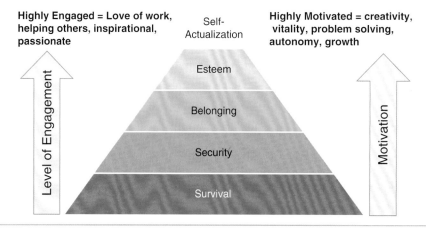

Figure 3-32 **Maslow's hierarchy of needs applied to employee engagement.**

fairness by looking at the ratio of their inputs (work effort) to their outcomes (e.g., rewards, benefits). For example, Employee A may be motivated if he or she receives a financial bonus that he or she perceives to be equitable given his/her effort on the PI project. However, employees also compare the ratio of their inputs to outcomes with others' inputs and outcomes. Therefore, if Employee B in the same department is awarded a larger financial bonus for the same amount of effort, Employee A's motivation would probably drop. Some ways for managers to motivate employees include the following:

- Acknowledge different performance levels with different levels of rewards.
- Employ just culture principles and practices (see the section *Patient Safety*).
- Periodically check employees' perceptions about their own input and outcomes as well as those of others (through annual employee engagement surveys).
- Know what outcomes are desirable and tie those to performance in a timely manner.

Procedural Justice. *Procedural justice* is a theory of motivation that focuses on fairness with respect to processes or procedures used to allocate outcomes. Research demonstrates that people are more likely to see outcome allocations as fair when the following conditions exist:

- Input from employees is sought and considered when decisions are made.
- There is an opportunity for performance errors to be corrected.
- Rules and policies for allocation of outcomes are applied consistently.
- Decisions are made in an unbiased manner.

What Employees Say

There is research support for these various motivation theories. In the past 25 years, the Gallup Organization undertook two extremely large studies. The first asked, "What do the most talented employees need from their workplace?" For this part of the research, Gallup interviewed more than 1 million people who were employed across a broad range of companies, industries, and countries. This study's "most powerful" conclusion is that the retention and performance of an employee is determined "by his relationship with his immediate supervisor."[91] So, what makes a good supervisor? Gallup's data indicate that there are 12 factors critical to the retention and performance of employees:

- Do I know what is expected of me at work?
- Do I have the materials and equipment I need to do my work correctly?

- Do I have the opportunity at work to do what I do best every day?
- In the last 7 days, did I receive recognition or praise for doing good work?
- Does my supervisor, or someone at work, seem to care about me as a person?
- Is there someone at work who encourages my development?
- Do my opinions seem to count at work?
- Does the mission or purpose of my work organization make me feel my job is important?
- Are my coworkers committed to doing high-quality work?
- Do I have a best friend at work?
- In the last 6 months, has someone at work talked to me about my progress?
- This past year, have I had opportunities at work to learn and grow?

More recently, Harter and Adkins[92] discussed the fact that employees want more from their managers. They found that

1. managers account for up to 70% of variance in engagement;
2. consistent communication is connected to higher engagement; and
3. managers must help employees develop their strengths.

These factors clearly are consistent with the theories of motivation discussed previously.

Setting Up an Incentives and Reward System

Given the role rewards play in employee motivation, setting up an effective reward system is important. Seven steps are fundamental to a reward system[93]:

- Determine priorities and values; rewarded behaviors are prioritized.
- Identify the criteria or milestones.
- Establish a budget for recognition.
- Determine who is accountable for managing the recognition.
- Develop specific procedures and features of the rewards and recognition.
- Obtain feedback from employees on desired rewards and recognition.
- Modify program based on feedback.

The most important step is to reward the desired behavior.[94]

Sharing Successes of Teams, Projects, and Initiatives

Sharing organization success stories internally and externally is important for several reasons. As described earlier, it motivates employees and serves as both reward and recognition to them. The value is demonstrated to the employees in increasing knowledge transfer, learning from experience, sharing best practices, and stimulating innovation within the organization. Value is next demonstrated to the customer in showcasing successful processes and outcomes to the people served. Communicating successes also demonstrates accountability and transparency to the community and public served. There may be other stakeholders for whom communicating success is also important.

Externally, sharing of lessons learned with other organizations, professional groups, online communities, and the public might be performed in different ways. Some of the more common groups for sharing are professional conferences, committees, and professional organizations. The report format often includes

- abstract,
- title,
- objectives,
- outline,
- content,
- results, and
- references.

In addition, sometimes the A3 format is used (FIG. 3-33) to address an improvement process. This format is usually standardized from Lean/Six Sigma projects. This usually includes the background; current condition; goal; analysis; proposal/recommendation/countermeasure; plan; follow-up.[95]

The form in which communication takes place can also include face-to-face presentations, webinars, posters and storyboards, publications, and social networking tools. Publications may be local newsletters, peer-reviewed journals, or online forums including blogs. It is necessary to follow specific submission guidelines for a poster, abstract, or article. The publishing organization defines poster measurements, labeling design, and key elements for text and graphics. Abstract criteria focus on topics of interest, maximum and minimum word limits, and categories to include. Journal articles must conform to author guidelines and use a specific writing style. In preparing for any of these external communication methods, it is essential to have samples of the work product reviewed to increase the chances of acceptance.

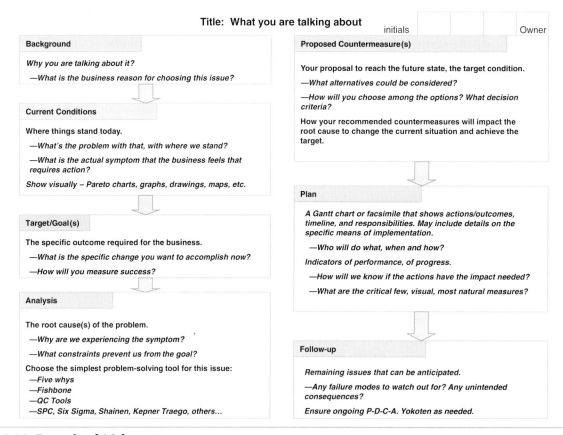

Figure 3-33 Example of A3 format. (From Shook, John Y. *Managing to Learn: Using the A3 Management Process*. Cambridge, MA: Lean Enterprise Institute. Copyright © 2010, Lean Enterprise Institute, Inc., Cambridge, MA, lean.org. Lean Enterprise Institute, is a registered trademark of Lean Enterprise Institute, Inc., All rights reserved. Used with permission.)

Recognition and Quality Awards

Quality professionals are often instrumental in completing applications for external quality awards as well as addressing internal quality awards. One framework used to understand PI in complex systems is the Baldrige National Health Care Criteria for Performance Excellence Framework (https://www.nist.gov/baldrige). The Baldrige Award was created in 1987, named for former U.S. Secretary of Commerce Malcolm Baldrige in tribute to his managerial ability. The award is given to organizations demonstrating a commitment to quality excellence. This model displays the principles of PI and shows the relationships between the structural, process, and outcome factors. Other common quality awards or designations are shown in **TABLE 3-13**.

Table 3-13 Common Quality Awards or Designations

Award	Sponsoring Organization	Eligibility	Recognition
Baldrige Performance Excellence Program	National Institute of Standards and Technology	National organizations (different sectors eligible, e.g., healthcare, education, business, government)	Performance excellence in 7 Baldrige categories
Beacon Award for Excellence	American Association of Critical-Care Nurses	Critical care hospital units (high acuity and critically ill patients)	Hospital nursing units
Deming Prize	Union of Japanese Scientists and Engineers	Japan	Business total quality management performance Individuals, business units, organizations
Healthcare Quality Recognition Awards	National Association for Healthcare Quality	Individual professional recognition, state recognition	Healthcare quality and safety
Hospital Rankings and Reports	U.S. News & World Report	Hospitals	Rankings by scores based on data that include survival, patient safety, nurse staffing and other factors
John M. Eisenberg Patient Safety and Quality Awards	National Quality Forum and The Joint Commission	Organizations whose accomplishments are clearly linked to the principles Dr. Eisenberg promoted throughout his career	Healthcare quality and safety
Long-term care national quality awards	American Health Care Association (AHCA)/National Center for Assisted Living (NCAL)	Long-term care and assisted living facilities	Commitment, achievement excellence
Magnet Recognition Program (includes Pathway to Excellence)	American Nurses Credentialing Center	Healthcare organizations and systems	Nursing services and empirical outcomes for patients and nursing
Nicholas E. Davies Award of Excellence	Health Information and Management Systems Society	Healthcare organizations	Utilization of health information technology to substantially improve patient outcomes and value
Robert W. Carey Performance Excellence Award	Department of Veterans Affairs	Veterans Affairs organizations	Based on Baldrige criteria Performance excellence in 7 categories

(continued)

Table 3-13 Common Quality Awards or Designations (*continued*)

Award	Sponsoring Organization	Eligibility	Recognition
Medtronic Safety Culture & Technology Innovator Award	NPSF Lucian Leape Institute	Individuals and teams	Recognizes extraordinary and innovative initiatives to drive successful implementation of technology through culture change in healthcare
Safety Grade	The Leapfrog Group	Hospitals	Better systems in place to prevent medication errors, higher quality on maternity care and high-risk procedures, and lower readmission rates
Shingo Prize for Operational Excellence	Utah State University	Any industry Any part of world	Customer focus and business results
State quality awards	States (public–private partnerships)	Individual states	Baldrige-like criteria or criteria set by states

There are other external awards not necessarily called quality awards but acknowledge high-performing organizations that demonstrate evidence of that performance per defined criteria. Usually through a rigorous evaluation process, the organization is selected for the award, prize, or designation.

Steps in evaluating readiness to apply for external quality awards include the following:

1. Demonstrate ownership and commitment to the cultural transformation for performance excellence.
2. Make the pursuit of quality an organizational commitment for the sake of intrinsic improvement, not just to win an award.
3. Create the organization cultural transformation by upholding the standards in daily practice.
4. Identify the specific quality reward or recognition program and requirements.
5. Review the standards and criteria.
6. Determine eligibility.
7. Develop a team approach to self-assessment (facilitator or coordinator and subject matter experts).
8. Perform a self-assessment or gap analysis of current performance compared with the standards or criteria (**TABLE 3-14**).
9. Identify strengths or evidence of compliance for each criterion.
10. Identify opportunities for improvement based on the criteria.
11. Prioritize findings from the self-assessment or gap analysis.
12. Plan a course of action to meet the standards; perform benchmarking (see *Health Data Analytics* for more information on benchmarking).
13. Develop an action plan based on the priority for each criterion.
14. Perform ongoing feedback and update evidence of compliance.
15. Determine who coordinates the application submission process.
16. Complete an application.
17. Submit the application.
18. Plan for a site visit and documentation of evidence.
19. Maintain an infrastructure to sustain the process.
20. Integrate/hardwire into daily operations.
21. Celebrate successes.
22. Plan for redesignation (Baldrige, Magnet).

Recognition of Internal Customers

An important structural element in the quality, safety and PI program is recognizing internal customers. Every process has both internal and external customers. Most people readily understand the concept of being a supplier of goods to an external customer. However, the idea of internal customers is equally important.

An employee can be a customer when they receive material, information, or services from others in the organization. Conversely, an employee also can be a supplier when they provide material, information, or services to others in the organization or to external customers. For example, when a nurse sends a specimen to the laboratory, the nurse is the supplier and the laboratory is the customer. When the laboratory sends a report back to the nurse, the laboratory is the supplier and the nurse is the customer. Just as there are suppliers to

Table 3-14 Sample Framework for Performing a Gap Analysis

Standard	Importance (High, Medium, Low)	For High-Importance Areas			
		Stretch (Strength) or Improvement Goal	What Action Is Planned?	By When?	Who Is Responsible?
Standard					
Strength or Evidence					
1.					
2.					
Opportunity for Improvement					
1.					
2.					
Standard					
Strength or Evidence					
1.					
2.					
Opportunity for Improvement					
1.					
2.					

From Healthcare Criteria for Performance Excellence: Optional self-analysis worksheet. NAHQ thanks the Baldrige Performance Excellence Program at the National Institute of Standards and Technology for use of text/graphics from the Criteria for Performance Excellence. Gaithersburg, MD: Baldrige Performance Excellence Program; 2011. www.nist.gov/baldrige/publications/hc_criteria.cfm.

internal customers, those internal customers can, in turn, be suppliers to external customers. This approach can help to

- remind departments without direct contact with external customers that they are still a critical link to customer satisfaction;
- improve relationships;
- acknowledge the complexity of the work;
- make the work process flow smoothly; and
- avert potential bottlenecks.

TABLE 3-15 provides an example of an approach one organization followed to ensure the recognition of internal customers. Notice that the customer service standard pledge reflects the values necessary to make quality a reality (e.g., teamwork, information sharing).

In most healthcare organizations and as above, service excellence is as important as clinical excellence. For example, Sharp HealthCare, a Malcolm Baldrige award recipient,

implemented several initiatives that formed the foundation of service excellence—what they refer to as The Sharp Experience.[96] These include the following:

1. AIDET: Acknowledge, Introduce, Duration, Explanation, Thank you.
2. Behavior Standards:
   - attitude is everything,
   - reward and recognition,
   - courteous communication,
   - teamwork,
   - service recovery,
   - zero harm,
   - performance matters,
   - service excellence,
   - privacy and confidentiality,
   - electronic communication manners,
   - mutual respect, and
   - diversity.

Table 3-15	Customer Service Standards and Pledge		
Respect Me and My Job	**We Are All Professionals**	**Work and Communicate with Me**	**Smile—It's Contagious**
Our need: Respect. *Our response:* I understand the need to be respectful, and I will • acknowledge you, • be sensitive to your point of view, • thank-you for a job well done, • value your time and priorities, • discuss my concerns with you in private, • value your job and its contribution to the organization, • treat you as I would like to be treated, and • speak to you in a pleasant tone in person or on the phone.	*Our need:* Professionalism. *Our response:* I understand the need to represent the hospital in a professional manner, and I will • take responsibility for my actions, • protect confidential information about patients and fellow employees, • look professional in dress, grooming, and manner, • coach others when necessary, and • follow through on my promise to you.	*Our need:* Teamwork. *Our response:* I understand the need for teamwork, and I will • pitch in and offer to help you whenever possible, • ask for your input before making a decision that may affect you, • talk to you directly instead of talking to others secretly if I have a concern, • listen to you, offer positive advice, and not interrupt until you are finished, • recognize that everyone has a valid opinion, and • seek out information and share what I have learned.	*Our need:* Positive attitude. *Our response:* I understand the need for a positive work environment, and I will • be sensitive to the effects my actions have on others, • replace criticism with positive ideas, • try to see things through the other person's eyes, • attempt to leave any personal problems at home, • coach my coworkers in portraying a positive attitude, and • project a caring and concerned attitude.

Reprinted from Baird K. *Customer Service in Health Care: A Grassroots Approach to Creating a Culture of Service Excellence.* New York, NY: Wiley; 2000. Copyright 2000 by Jossey-Bass, with permission of John Wiley & Sons, Inc.

3. Must Haves
   - Greet people with a smile and "Hello," using their name when possible.
   - Take people where they are going, rather than pointing or giving directions.
   - Use key words at key times: "Is there anything else I can do for you? I have the time."
   - Foster an attitude of gratitude. Send thank-you notes to deserving employees.
   - Round with reason to better connect with staff, patients, family, and other customers.

Storytelling is also part of the Sharp culture. The development and sharing of stories can be a potent means or promoting values and beliefs in an organization. StoryCorps, a nonprofit organization, helps organizations

> remind one another of our shared humanity, to strengthen and build the connections between people, to teach the value of listening, and to weave into the fabric of our culture the understanding that everyone's story matters. At the same time, we are creating an invaluable archive for future generations.[97(p2)]

The measurement of customer perception, satisfaction, engagement and loyalty is important for healthcare organizations to determine how their customers like the services provided. There are many vendors who survey these customers and provide data back to the organization for tracking, trending, and benchmarking performance.

The CMS identified customer perception as a key component of measuring hospital performance and developed the Hospital Consumer Assessment of Healthcare Providers and Systems[98] (CAHPS) survey as a standardized method to compare performance and link payment to performance. The Hospital Consumer Assessment of Healthcare Providers and Systems (HCAHPS) is the first national, standardized, publicly reported survey of patients' perspectives of hospital care. Before the advent of HCAHPS, there was no national standard for collecting and publicly reporting information about patient experience of care that allowed comparisons across hospitals locally, regionally, and nationally.

The survey is designed to produce data about patients' perceptions of care that allow objective comparisons of hospitals on topics that are important to consumers. Public reporting of the survey results increases accountability by increasing transparency in the quality of care. The CMS and the HCAHPS Project Team take steps to ensure the survey is credible, useful, and practical.

In 2002, CMS partnered with the AHRQ to develop and test the HCAHPS survey. In May 2005, the HCAHPS survey was endorsed by the NQF, and approval for the national implementation for public reporting occurred in March 2008. The survey, methods, and results are in the public domain.

The Deficit Reduction Act of 2005 created an additional incentive for acute care hospitals to participate in HCAHPS. As of July 2007, hospitals must collect and submit HCAHPS data to receive their full Inpatient Prospective Payment System annual payment update. Inpatient Prospective Payment System hospitals that fail to publicly report the HCAHPS survey may receive an annual payment update that is reduced by 2 percentage points. The Patient Protection and Affordable Care Act of 2010 (P.L. 111-148) includes HCAHPS among the measures to be used to calculate value-based incentive payments in the Hospital Value-Based Purchasing program, with discharges since October 2012. HCAHPS results are published on the Hospital Compare website four times a year.[99] The survey consists of both inpatient and outpatient items depending on the population assessed.

Instruments are available for other settings such as for long-term care, but there are no comparative data collected or published for this setting and NCQA uses CAHPS version 5.0H survey as part of their HEDIS measures in evaluating health plan performance and accrediting plans.

Organizational Learning and Training

Everyone in the organization is responsible for quality and safety. Therefore, educating staff at all levels of the organization is critical to the success of quality and PI. Because the most common cause of failure in any performance or process improvement effort is uninvolved or indifferent top and middle management, it is essential that all leaders be educated from the start. Training begins at the top and cascades down through the organization. Ultimately, senior and middle management are part of the teaching team; this demonstrates to employees that they are committed to quality and safety.

The method of education or training must be tailored to the audience and use tools and methods to match the audience needs and learning styles. Governing body or board members must also be included in understanding and their accountability for quality of care in the organization. Some form of board training is often included for new members. A comprehensive program for all levels of employees, management, board, and physicians is designed to meet the needs of these different groups. For example, board member training includes

- a review of oversight responsibility for the organization's quality and safety performance;
- some form of quality, safety and PI committee or review function;
- use of quality performance as a criterion in rating executive performance; and
- trends and public reporting of the organization's data and its image in the community.

Determining Education and Training Needs

There are many ways to determine the educational needs of the healthcare workforce. Methods to obtain information include

- evaluating knowledge and skills contained in the job description;
- asking participants;
- asking participants' supervisors;
- asking others who are knowledgeable about the job (e.g., customer, peers, experts in quality, safety and PI);
- testing participants on their skills and knowledge; and
- analyzing the participant's past performance appraisals.[93,100,101]

Fundamentals of Performance Improvement Curriculum

The PI curriculum includes the following elements:

- Explanation of the need for organizational improvement, including individual and collective benefits of performance and process improvement;
- Development and use of common quality language or taxonomy;
- Discussion of the organization's quality and safety goals;
- Definition of the program structure;
- Articulation of the organization's philosophy and a model for improvement;
- Description of the improvement process;
- Description and clarification of responsibilities;
- Tools and techniques to participate in teams and to manage work processes;
- Description of how change may affect the individual's job and work relationships;
- Metrics and successful past projects in the organization; and
- Reporting structure for leaders and staff.

Tailor training to the specific needs of each group (i.e., top management, middle management, frontline staff). **TABLE 3-16** offers a comparison of topics addressed across major groups in a quality, safety, and PI curriculum. There are some common reasons why managers are often reluctant to support training in quality, safety and PI. These barriers must be overcome for the organization to develop the infrastructure necessary to support healthcare quality and safety. Barriers include no results from the training, too costly, no involvement in the process, no time for staff to participate, and lack of preparation of programs.[102(pp2–4)]

Another approach to considering training is the IHI Improvement Advisor Professional Development Program,[71] which includes the following agenda for training:

- science of improvement (includes high-reliability organizations),

Table 3-16 Education and Training Topics

Top Management Topics	Middle Management Topics	Staff Topics "What Everyone Should Know"
• Quality as a strategic advantage • Role of leadership in creating and sustaining quality vision • Integrating quality values into day-to-day leadership • Indicators for measuring, evaluating and improving quality and organizational performance • Components of performance excellence and implementation process • Basic quality and performance improvement tools • Role as team leaders • Awareness of accreditation standards • Role as team champion	• Key concepts of quality and performance management (e.g., customer satisfaction, process management, teamwork, continuous improvement methods) • Management practices for building teamwork, employee involvement and recognition for customer service • Team building and contributions for quality, team leadership skills, conflict resolution • Communication skills, listening and giving feedback • Principles of customer service • Managing process performance (measurement, quality and performance improvement tools, variation, problem solving, data collection and analysis) • Measurement of quality outcomes • Accreditation/regulatory standards	• Organization's mission, vision, and performance improvement plan • Quality awareness, definition of quality • Fundamental training in quality and performance improvement, including process improvement tools and techniques • Concepts of quality management: customer satisfaction, process improvement, teamwork, continuous improvement • Promoting cooperation between coworkers within and between departments • Communication skills • Customer service • Relevant accreditation standards and regulatory requirements

- model for improvement,
- scoping improvement efforts,
- understanding systems and processes,
- using data for improvement,
- understanding relationships,
- gathering information,
- organizing information,
- developing powerful ideas for change,
- testing changes,
- implementing changes,
- decision-making,
- working with people, and
- planned experimentation.

The IHI's Open School is a free resource to National Association for Healthcare Quality (NAHQ) members, students and faculty. It offers exceptional training resources for quality, safety and PI. Also, see the section *Patient Safety* for more information on learning systems and learning organizations.

Requisite Skills to Lead Performance and Process Improvement Efforts

The key operating assumption of capacity building is that different groups of people have different levels of need for knowledge and skills. A teaching plan ensures each group receives the knowledge and skill sets they need, when they need them, and in the appropriate amounts. FIGURE 3-34 shows a pyramid model in which experts need a high level of specific knowledge on PI, quality management, and tools, whereas most staff need a much lower level of knowledge in this area. For skill development, *HQ Essentials* from NAHQ offers a roadmap for achieving mastery in performance and process improvement. FIGURE 3-35 shows the dimension for cultural and process change management. Finally, being able to demonstrate financial and clinical outcomes requires planning and program development skills. Wiseman et al.[103] offer a simple model for what is needed to get to outcomes by linking processes to improvement—planning, implementing, and evaluating (FIG. 3-36).

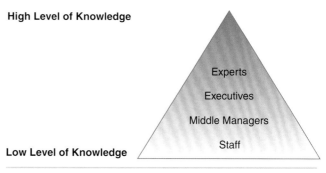

High Level of Knowledge

Experts
Executives
Middle Managers
Staff

Low Level of Knowledge

Figure 3-34 **Levels of knowledge.**

	Proficiency Levels and Descriptors	
Competency	**Proficiency 1: Advanced**	**Proficiency 2: Master**
3.3. Use meaningful metrics to articulate return on investment of PPI project.	3.3.1a. Identify meaningful process and outcome measures. 3.3.1b. Explain the origin, reliability, validity, and accuracy of data and the sources used for benchmarking and comparison. 3.3.lc. Optimize decisions through the analysis of information and development of alternative hypotheses and action plans. 3.3.1d. Aid interpretation and communication of data and information by using visual display techniques.	3.3.2a. Advise the organization on the adoption of metrics to achieve value-based results.
3.4 Mitigate barriers that impede sustainable change.	3.4.1a. Assess the status of workflow changes in identifying barriers to optimum adoptions. 3.4.1b. Develop plans to overcome barriers utilizing change management techniques.	3.4.2a. Apply organizational development principles and practices involving adaptive innovation. 3.4.2b. Implement strategies to address barriers within units and across the organization.
3.5. Monitor accountability structures and controls required to achieve improved performance.	3.5.la. Monitor adherence to workflows and policies and report compliance to the governance authority. 3.5.1b. Analyze the improved workflow and policy changes, recommending changes to continually advance performance improvement.	3.5.2a. Establish governance structures and processes to ensure accountability for adherence to workflows and policies. 3.5.2b. Investigate industry best practices to recommend innovations to continually advance performance improvement.
3.6. Provide the education, training, and tools necessary for effective implementation of process and workflow changes.	3.6.1a. Prepare training curricula and materials to train process owners on revised work processes and policies. 3.6.1b. Assist with training, process owners, team members, and sponsors on implementation and control plans.	3.6.2a. Implement a work process optimization training program. 3.6.2b. Provide an infrastructure for peer learning. 3.6.2c. Share the organization's lessons learned and improvement results with external audiences.

Figure 3-35 **Performance and process improvement competency (culture and change management).**

National Association for Healthcare Quality. Performance and Process Improvement. HQ Essentials: Competencies for the Healthcare Profession (2017).

Through skill acquisition, healthcare quality professionals can lead performance and process improvement efforts and ensure appropriate methods and measures are used to achieve organizational goals and improve the health of individuals and populations.

Section Summary

A formal quality, safety, and PI program and infrastructure are required to ensure quality and safety. Models of PI, acquired from industry, have been adopted and applied to the healthcare setting. The tenets of quality and safety must first be developed through strategic planning. Strategic planning is supported by the establishment of priorities for performance and process improvement activities, translating strategic goals into quality outcomes, and aligning culture and structure. Various PI tools can be used within a team to make significant changes to core processes, and ultimately ensure good clinical outcomes by using evidence-based principles and practices.

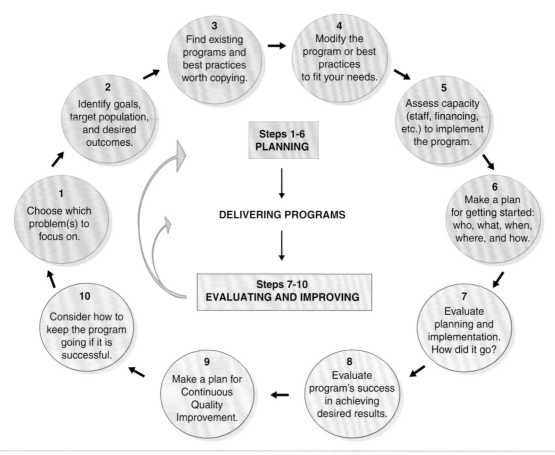

Figure 3-36 Getting to outcomes: 10 steps to achieving accountability. (Reprinted from Wiseman S, Chinman M, Ebener PA, et al. *Getting to Outcomes™: 10 Steps for Achieving Results-Based Accountability.* Santa Monica, CA: RAND Corporation; 2007, with permission. https://www.rand.org/pubs/technical_reports/TR101z2 .html.)

References

1. Gaucher EM, Coffey RJ. *Transforming Healthcare Organizations: How to Achieve and Sustain Organizational Excellence.* San Francisco, CA: Jossey-Bass Publishers; 1991.

2. The W. Edwards Deming Institute. Deming the man: Dr. W. Edwards Deming; 2016. https://deming.org/deming-the-man/. Accessed April 30, 2017.

3. Deming WE. *Out of the Crisis.* Cambridge, MA: MIT Press; 2000.

4. Deming WE. *The New Economics for Industry, Government, Education.* Cambridge, MA: MIT Press; 2000.

5. The Juran Institute. About us: 2017. https://www.juran.com/about-us. Accessed April 30, 2017.

6. Juran JM. *Juran on Leadership for Quality: An Executive Handbook.* New York, NY: The Free Press; 1989.

7. Crosby PB. *Quality Is Free: The Art of Making Quality Certain.* New York: McGraw-Hill; 1979.

8. Hunt VD. *Quality in America: How to Implement a Competitive Quality Program.* Homewood, IL: Business One Irwin; 1992.

9. Westcott RT. *The Certified Manager of Quality/Organizational Excellence Handbook,* 4th ed. Milwaukee, WI: American Society for Quality; 2013.

10. Codman EA. *A Study of Hospital Efficiency.* Ann Arbor, MI: University Microfilms; 1916 & 1972.

11. Roberts JS, Redman RR, Coate JG. A history of the Joint Commission on Accreditation of Hospitals. *J Am Med Assoc.* 1987;258:936–940. doi:10.1001/jama.1987.03400070074038

12. Donabedian A. *The Definition of Quality and Approaches to Its Assessment.* Ann Arbor, MI: Health Administration Press; 1980.

13. Berwick DM. Continuous improvement as an ideal in health care. *N Engl J Med.* 1989;320(21):53–56. doi:10.1056/NEJM198901053200110

14. Batalden PB, Buchanan. Industrial models of quality improvement. In: N Goldfield, DB Nash, eds. *Providing quality care.* Philadelphia: American College of Physicians; 1998.

15. Berwick DM, Godfrey AB, Roessner J. *Curing Health Care.* San Francisco, CA: Jossey-Bass Publishers; 1990.

16. James BC. *Quality Management for Health Care Delivery.* Chicago: The Hospital Research and Education Trust; 1990.

17. White SV. Interview with a quality leader: Brent James on reducing harm to patients and improving quality. *J Healthcare Qual.* 2007;29(5):35–44. doi:10.1111/j.1945-1474.2007.tb00211.x

18. Institute of Medicine, Committee on Quality of Health Care in America. *To Err is Human: Building a Safer Health System,* (L. T. Kohn, J. M. Corrigan, & M. S. Donaldson, Eds.). Washington, DC: National Academies Press; 2000.

19. Berwick DM, Nolan TW, Whittington J. The triple aim: care, health and cost. *Health Affairs.* 2008;27(3):759–769. doi:10.1377/hlthaff.27.3.759.

20. Epstein RM, Street RL. *Patient-Centered Communication in Cancer Care: Promoting Healing and Reducing Suffering.* Bethesda, MD: National Cancer Institute; 2007.

21. Pelletier LR, Stichler JE. Patient-centered care and engagement: nurse leaders' imperative for health reform. *J Nurs Admin.* 2014;44(9):473–480. doi:10.1097/NNA.0000000000000102

22. American Hospital Association. The patient care partnership: understanding expectations, rights and responsibilities; 2003. http://www.aha.org/content/00-10/pcp_english_030730.pdf. Accessed April 30, 2017.

23. Center for Advancing Health. *A New Definition of Patient Engagement: What Is Engagement and Why Is It Important?* Washington, DC: Author; 2010.

24. Glascow R. *Technology and Chronic Care.* Paper presented at the Congress on Improving Chronic Care: Innovations in Research and Practice. September 8–10, Seattle, WA; 2002.

25. Kaplan S, Greenfield S, Ware JE. Assessing the effects of physician-patient interactions on the outcomes of chronic disease. *Med Care.* 1989;27(3, supplement):S110–S127. doi:10.1097/00005650-198903001-00010

26. Von Korff M, Gruman J, SchaefferJ, Curry SJ, Wagner EH. Collaborative management of chronic illness. *Ann Intern Med.* 1997;127(12):1097–1102.

27. Robbins SP. *Organizational Behavior.* 8th ed. Upper Saddle River, NJ: Prentice Hall; 2001.

28. Kotter JP. What leaders really do. *Harvard Bu Rev.* 1990;68:103–111.

29. Kouzes JM, Posner BZ. *Leadership: The Challenge.* San Francisco, CA: Jossey-Bass; 2002.

30. American Hospital Association. Accountability: the pathway to restoring public trust and confidence for hospitals and other healthcare organizations; 1999. http://www.aha.org/content/00-10/AHAPrinciplesAccountability.pdf. Accessed May 1, 2017.

31. American Hospital Association and American Medical Association. Integrated leadership for hospitals and health systems: principles for success; 2015. https://www.ama-assn.org/sites/default/files/media-browser/public/about-ama/ama-aha-integrated-leadership-principles_0.pdf. Accessed May 1, 2017.

32. U.S. Department of Health & Human Services, Health Resources & Services Administration. Performance measurement and management; 2011. https://www.hrsa.gov/quality/toolbox/508pdfs/performancemanagementandmeasurement.pdf. Accessed May 1, 2017.

33. Kaplan R, Bower M. The balanced scorecard and quality programs. *Balanced Scorecard Report* [Newsletter], 3–6. Cambridge, MA: Harvard Business School Publishing; March 15, 2001.

34. Kaplan R, Norton D. Using the balanced scorecard as a strategic management system. *Harvard Bus Rev.* 1996;74:75–85.

35. Studer Group. https://az414866.vo.msecnd.net/cmsroot/studergroup/media/studergroup/pages/who-we-are/about-studer-group/studergroup_infographic.pdf. Accessed May 2, 2017.

36. Provost L, Miller D, Reinertsen J. *A Framework for Leadership for Improvement.* Cambridge, MA: Institute for Healthcare Improvement; 2006.

37. White SV. Interview with a quality leader: David Brailer on information technology and advancing healthcare quality. *J Healthcare Qual.* 2004;26(6):20–25. doi:10.1111/j.1945-1474.2004.tb00531.x

38. Rosati RJ. Creating quality improvement projects. In: EL Siegler, S Mirafzali, JB Foust, eds. *A Guide to Hospitals and Inpatient Care* (pp. 326–338). New York, NY: Springer; 2003.

39. Reinertsen JL, Bisognano M, Pugh MD. *Seven Leadership Leverage Points for Organization-Level Improvement in Health Care.* 2nd ed. Cambridge, MA: Institute for Healthcare Improvement; 2011.

40. Sackett D, Rosenberg WMC, Muir-Gray JA, Haynes RB, Richardson WS. Evidence-based medicine: what it is and what it isn't. *Br Med J.* 1996;312(13):71–72. doi:10.1136/bmj.312.7023.71

41. Tonelli M. The limits of evidence-based medicine. *Respir Care.* 2001;46(12):1435–1440. doi:10.1097/00001888-199812000-00011

42. Greenhalgh T. Narrative-based medicine in an evidence-based world. *Br Med J.* 1999;318:323–325. doi:10.1136/bmj.318.7179.323

43. Institute of Medicine, Committee on Quality of Health Care in America. *Crossing the Quality Chasm: A New Health System for the 21st Century.* Washington, DC: National Academies Press; 2001.

44. Deaton C. Outcomes measurement and evidence-based nursing practice. *J Cardiovas Nurs.* 2001;15(2):83–86.

45. Zander K, Bower K. *Nursing Case Management, Blueprint for Transformation.* Boston, MA: New England Medical Center Hospitals; 1987.

46. Every NR, Hochman J, Becker R, Kopecky S, Cannon CP, for the Committee on Acute Cardiac Care, Council on Clinical Cardiology, American Heart Association. Critical pathways: a review. *Circulation.* 2000;101:461–465. doi: 10.1161/01.CIR.101.4.461. http://circ.ahajournals.org/content/101/4/461.full.

47. Rotter T, Kinsman L, James EL, et al. Clinical pathways: effects on professional practice, patient outcomes, length of stay and hospital costs. *Cochrane Database Syst Rev.* 2010;17(3), CD006632. doi:10.1002/14651858.CD006632

48. Institute of Medicine. *Clinical Practice Guidelines We Can Trust.* Washington, DC: The National Academies Press; 2011. http://www.iom.edu/Reports/2011/Clinical-Practice-Guidelines-We-Can-Trust.aspx. Accessed May 2, 2017.

49. Agency for Healthcare Research and Quality. National Guideline Clearinghouse. https://www.guideline.gov. Accessed May 1, 2017.

50. Resar R, Griffin FA, Haraden C, Nolan TW. *Using Care Bundles to Improve Health Care Quality.* IHI Innovation Series white paper. Cambridge, MA: Institute for Healthcare Improvement; 2012. http://www.ihi.org/resources/Pages/IHIWhitePapers/UsingCareBundles.aspx. Accessed May 2, 2017.

51. U.S. Department of Health & Human Services and Department of Justice. Health Care Fraud and Abuse Control Program Annual Report for Fiscal Year 2016; 2017. https://oig.hhs.gov/publications/docs/hcfac/FY2016-hcfac.pdf. Accessed May 2, 2017.

52. Institute for Healthcare Improvement. How to improve: Science of improvement: testing multiple changes; 2017. http://www.ihi.org/resources/Pages/HowtoImprove/ScienceofImprovementTestingMultipleChanges.aspx. Accessed May 2, 2017.

53. Chassin MR. Is health care ready for six sigma quality? *Milbank Quart.* 1998;76(4):565–591. doi:10.1111/1468-0009.00106

54. Ahmed S, Manaf NH, Islam R. Effects of lean six sigma application in healthcare services: a literature review. *Rev Environ Health.* 2013;28(4):189–194. doi: 10.1515/reveh-2013-0015.

55. Lean Enterprise Institute. Principles of lean. www.lean.org/Whats Lean/Principles.cfm. Accessed May 2, 2017.

56. MoreSteam. Lean six sigma online training; 2012. www.moresteam.com/lean-six-sigma/green-belt.cfm. Accessed May 2, 2017.

57. Naik T, Duroseau Y, Zehtabchi S, et al. A structured approach to transforming a large public hospital emergency department via lean methodologies. *J Healthcare Qual.* 2012;34(2):86–97. doi:10.1111/j.1945-1474.2011.00181.x

58. Chassin MR, Loeb JM. High-reliability healthcare: getting there from here. *The Milbank Quart.* 2013;91(3):459–490.

59. Centers for Disease Control and Prevention. 2017. Opioid overdose. https://www.cdc.gov/drugoverdose/. Accessed May 1, 2017.

60. Institute for Healthcare Improvement. Medication reconciliation to prevent adverse drug events; 2017. http://www.ihi.org/Topics/ADEsMedicationReconciliation/Pages/default.aspx. Accessed May 1, 2017.

61. National Quality Forum. *National Quality Partners Playbook: Antibiotic Stewardship in Acute Care.* Washington, DC: Author; 2016. http://www.qualityforum.org/Publications/2016/05/National_Quality_Partners_Playbook__Antibiotic_Stewardship_in_Acute_Care.aspx. Accessed May 2, 2017.

62. The Joint Commission. Facts about federal deemed status and state recognition; 2016. https://www.jointcommission.org/facts_about_federal_deemed_status_and_state_recognition/. Accessed May 1, 2017.

63. Stempniak M. Patient safety in the OR. *Hospitals and Health Networks;* 2012. http://www.hhnmag.com/articles/6184-patient-safety-in-the-or. Accessed May 2, 2017.

64. Kim FJ, da Silva RD, Gustafson D, Nogueira L, Harlin T, Paul DL. Current issues in patient safety in surgery: a review. *Patient Saf Surg.* 2015;9:1–26. doi:10.1186/s13037-015-0067-4

65. Swing SR. The ACGME outcome project: retrospective and prospective. *Med Teach.* 2007;29:648–654. doi:10.1080/01421590701392903

66. Safer Healthcare. Checklists: a critical patient safety tool & guide. http://www.saferhealthcare.com/high-reliability-topics/checklists/. Accessed February 16, 2017.

67. Langley GL, Moen R, Nolan KM, et al. *The Improvement Guide: A Practical Approach to Enhancing Organizational Performance.* 2nd ed. San Francisco, CA: Jossey-Bass Publishers; 2009.

68. U.S. Environmental Protection Agency. *Lean & Environment Toolkit: Chapter 5.* https://www.epa.gov/lean/lean-environment-toolkit-chapter-5#definition. Accessed May 3, 2017.

69. Daley AT. *Using Spaghetti Diagrams to Improve Process Flow.* Chi Solutions, Inc.; 2009. https://www.chisolutionsinc.com/wp-content/uploads/2015/01/2009_10_Spaghetti-Diagrams-E-Postcard-Article.pdf. Accessed May 2, 2017.

70. Gaskin SP, Griffin A, Hauser HR, Katz GM, Klein RL. Voice of the Customer. Massachusetts Institute of Technology. http://www.mit.edu/~hauser/Papers/Gaskin_Griffin_Hauser_et_al%20VOC%20Encyclopedia%202011.pdf. Accessed February 16, 2017.

71. Institute for Healthcare Improvement. Improvement advisor professional development program. www.ihi.org/offerings/Training/ImprovementAdvisor/Pages/default.aspx

72. Thompson L. *Making the Team: A Guide for Managers.* Upper Saddle River, NJ: Prentice Hall; 2000.

73. Xyrichis A, Ream E. Teamwork: a concept analysis. *J Adv Nurs.* 2008;61:232–241. doi:10.1111/j.1365-2648.2007.

74. Nancarrow SA, Booth A, Ariss S, et al. Ten principles of good interdisciplinary work. *Hum Resour Health.* 2013;11:1–19.

75. Andreatta PB. A typology for health care teams. *Health Care Manage Rev.* Oct–Dec 2010;35(4):345–354. doi:10.1097/HMR.0b013e3181e9fceb

76. Luecke R. *Creating Teams with an Edge: The Complete Skill Set to Build Powerful and Influential Teams.* Harvard Business Essentials Series. Boston, MA: Harvard Business School Press; 2004.

77. Schwarz M, Landis S, Rowe J. A team approach to quality improvement. *Fam Pract Manage.* April 1999;6:25–31.

78. Tuckman W. Developmental sequence in small groups. *Psychol Bull.* 1965;63:384–399. doi:10.1037/h0022100

79. Scholtes PR, Joiner BL, Streibel B. *The Team Handbook.* 3rd ed. Madison, WI: Joiner/Oriel; 2003.

80. Borrill C, West M, Shapiro D, Rees A. Team working and effectiveness in health care. *Br J Healthcare Manage.* 2000;6(8):364–371.

81. Lemieux-Charles L, McGuire ML. What do we know about health care team effectiveness? A review of the literature. *Med Care Res Rev.* June 2006;63(3);263–300. doi:10.1177/1077558706287003

82. Mitchell P, Wynia M, Golden R, et al. *Core Principles & Values of Effective Team-Based Health Care.* Washington, DC; IOM; October 2012.

83. Agency for Healthcare Research and Quality. About Team-STEPPS. http://teamstepps.ahrq.gov/about-2cl_3.htm. Accessed May 1, 2017.

84. American Combatives, Inc. Airline crew safety training program; 2009. www.americancombatives.com/index.php?option=com_content&view=article&id=66&Itemid=79. Accessed May 1, 2017.

85. Zuzelo PR. *The Clinical Nurse Specialist Handbook.* 2nd ed. Sudbury, MA: Jones & Bartlett; 2010.

86. Evans JR, Dean JW. *Total Quality: Management, Organization and Strategy.* 3rd ed. Mason, OH: Thomson South-Western; 2003.

87. George JM, Jones GR. *Organizational Behavior.* 3rd ed. Upper Saddle River, NJ: Prentice Hall; 2002.

88. Maslow A. *Motivation and Personality.* New York, NY: Harper and Row; 1954.

89. McClelland DC, Atkinson JW, Clark RA, Lowell EL. *The Achievement Motive.* New York, NY: Irvington; 1976.

90. Herzberg F, Maysner B, Snyderman B. *Works and the Nature of Man.* New York, NY: John Wiley & Sons; 1966.

91. Buckingham M, Coffman C. *First, Break all the Rules: What the World's Greatest Managers Do Differently.* New York, NY: Simon & Schuster; 1999.

92. Harter J, Adkins A. Employees want a lot more from their managers. *Gallup Business J.* 2015. http://www.gallup.com/businessjournal/182321/employees-lot-managers.aspx. Accessed May 2, 2017.

93. Gaucher EJ, Coffey RJ. *Total Quality in Healthcare: From Theory to Practice.* San Francisco, CA: Jossey-Bass; 1993.

94. Gunawardena I. Reward management in healthcare. *Br J Healthcare Manage.* 2011;17(11):527–530.

95. Shook J. *A3 templates from Lean Enterprise Institute.* Ambridge, MA: Lean Enterprise Institute; 2010. http://www.lean.org/common/display/?o=1314. Accessed May 2, 2017.

96. Sharp HealthCare. The Sharp experience; 2017. http://www.sharp.com/about/the-sharp-experience/. Accessed May 1, 2017.

97. StoryCorps. About us. http://storycorps.org/about. Accessed May 2, 2017.

98. Centers for Medicare & Medicaid Services. HCAHPS: Patients' perspective of care survey; 2012. www.cms.gov/HospitalQualityInits/30_HospitalHCAHPS.asp. Accessed May 1, 2017.

99. Centers for Medicare & Medicaid Services. HCAHPS: Hospital care quality information from the consumer perspective; www.hcahpsonline.org. Accessed May 2, 2017.

100. Kirkpatrick DL. *Evaluating Training Programs.* 2nd ed. San Francisco, CA: Berrett-Koehler; 1998.

101. Phillips J, Stone R. *How to Measure Training Results: A Practical Guide to Tracking the Six Key Indicators.* New York, NY: McGraw-Hill; 2002.

102. Phillips JJ, Phillips PP. Manager's role in learning and performance; 2003. http://www.roiinstitute.net/wp-content/uploads/2014/03/2014-ManagersRoleinLeaningandPerformance.pdf. Accessed May 2, 2017.

103. Wiseman S, Chinman M, Ebener PA, et al. *Getting to Outcomes™: 10 Steps for Achieving Results-Based Accountability.* Santa Monica: RAND Health; 2010:p. 2.

Suggested Reading & Other Resources

Almoosa KF, Luther K, Resar R, Patel B. Applying the new Institute for Healthcare Improvement inpatient waste tool to identify "waste" in the intensive care unit. *J Healthcare Qual.* 2016;38(5):e29–e38. doi:10.1097/JHQ.0000000000000040

American Association of Critical Care Nurses. Beacon Award for Excellence.™ https://www.aacn.org/nursing-excellence/beacon-awards. Accessed May 2, 2017.

American Nurses Credentialing Center. Magnet Recognition Program®; 2017. www.nursecredentialing.org/Magnet.aspx. Accessed May 2, 2017.

Bailit M, Dyer M. *Beyond Bankable Dollars: Establishing a Business Case for Improving Healthcare.* New York, NY: The Commonwealth Fund; 2004.

Barry R, Murcko AC, Brubaker CE. *The Six Sigma Book for Healthcare.* Chicago, IL: Health Administration Press; 2002.

Becher EC, Chassin MR. Improving the quality of healthcare: Who will lead? *Health Affairs.* 2001;20:164–179. doi:10.1377/hlthaff.20.5.164

Berwick DM. Continuous improvement as an ideal in health care. *New Engl J Med.* 1989;320:53–56. doi:10.1056/NEJM198901053200110

Berwick DM, Godfrey AB, Roessner J. *Curing Health Care.* San Francisco, CA: Jossey-Bass; 1990.

Berwick DM, Nolan TW, Whittington J. The triple aim: care, health and cost. *Health Affairs.* 2008;27(3):759–769. doi:10.1377/hlthaff.27.3.759

Blackmore CC, Williams BL, Ching JM, Chafetz LA, Kaplan GS. Using lean to advance quality improvement research. *J Healthcare Qual.* 2016;38(5):275–282. doi:10.1097/01.JHQ.0000462684.78253.a1

Brackett T, Comer L, Whichello R. Do lean practices lead to more time at the bedside? *J Healthcare Qual.* 2013;35(2):7-14. doi:10.1111/j.1945-1474.2011.00169.x

Brown MJ, Kor DJ, Curry TB, Marmor Y, Rohleder TR. A coordinated patient transport system for ICU patients requiring surgery: impact on operating room efficiency and ICU workflow. *J Healthcare Qual.* 2015;37(6):354–362. doi:10.1111/jhq.12019

Centers for Medicare & Medicaid Services. Partnership for patients and hospital engagement networks: continuing forward momentum on reducing patient harm; September 25, 2016. https://www.cms.gov/Newsroom/MediaReleaseDatabase/Fact-sheets/2015-Fact-sheets-items/2015-09-25.html. Accessed May 2, 2017.

Crawford B, Skeath M, Whippy A. Multifocal clinical performance improvement across 21 hospitals. *J Healthcare Qual.* 2015;37(2):117–125. doi:10.1111/jhq.12039

Denny DS, Allen DK, Worthington N, Gupta D. The use of failure mode and effect analysis in a radiation oncology setting: The Cancer Treatment Centers of America experience. *J Healthcare Qual.* 2014;36(1):18–28. doi:10.1111/j.1945-1474.2011.00199

Donabedian A. *Exploration in Quality Assessment and Monitoring.* Ann Arbor, MI: Health Administration Press; 1980.

Farrokhi FR, Gunther M, Williams B, Blackmore CCL. Application of lean methodology for improved quality and efficiency in operating room instrument availability. *J Healthcare Qual.* 2015;37(5):277–286. doi:10.1111/jhq.12053

Fottler MD, Ford RC, Heaton CP. *Achieving Service Excellence: Strategies for Healthcare.* Chicago, IL: Health Administration Press; 2002.

Fried BJ, Johnson JA. *Human Resources in Healthcare: Managing for Success.* Chicago, IL: Health Administration Press; 2001.

Gardner W, Morton S, Tinoco A, et al. Is it feasible to use electronic health records for quality measurement of adolescent care? *J Healthcare Qual.* 2016;38(3):164–174. doi:10.1097/01.JHQ.0000462675.17265.db

Gaucher EJ, Coffey RJ. *Breakthrough Performance: Accelerating the Transformation of Health Care Organizations.* San Francisco, CA: Jossey-Bass; 2000.

Griffith JR, White KR. *Thinking Forward: Six Strategies for Highly Successful Organizations.* Chicago, IL: Health Administration Press; 2003.

Hadelman J. *The Impact of Strategic Healthcare Leadership: Top Ten Leadership Trends in Health Care in the 21st Century.* Oak Brook, IL: Witt/Kieffer; 2000.

Helmrich RL, Merritt AC. *Culture at Work in Aviation and Medicine.* Aldershot: Ashgate; 1998.

Horak BJ. *Strategic Planning in Healthcare: Building a Quality-Based Plan Step-by-Step.* Portland, OR: Book News; 1997.

James BC. *Quality Management for Health Care Delivery.* Chicago, IL: The Hospital Research and Education Trust; 1990.

Johnson D, Snedeker K, Swoboda M, et al. Increasing therapist productivity: using lean principles in the rehabilitation department of an academic medical center. *J Healthcare Qual.* 2015;[Epub ahead of print]. Post Author Corrections: December 15, 2015. doi:10.1097/JHQ.0000000000000013

Juran JM. The QC circle phenomenon. *Industrial Control.* 1967 January;23:329–336.

Michael M, Schaffer SD, Egan PL, Little BB, Pritchard PSL. Improving wait times and patient satisfaction in primary care. *J Healthcare Qual.* 2013;35(2):50–60. doi:10.1111/jhq.12004

National Association for Healthcare Quality (NAHQ). *NAHQ Code of Ethics and Standards of Practice for Healthcare Quality Professionals.* Glenview, IL: Author; 2011. www.nahq.org/Quality-Community/content/codeethicspractice.html

Plsek P, Omnias A. *Juran Institute Quality Improvement Tools: Problem Solving/Glossary.* Wilton, CT: Juran Institute; 1989.

Rever H. Applying the DMAIC steps to process improvement projects "Define, Measure, Analyze, Improve, Control" is the roadmap to improving processes; n.d. http://www.iil.com/emailfiles/downloads/ApplyingtheDMAICSteps_Harry%20Rever.pdf. Accessed May 2, 2017.

Singprasong R, Eldabi T. An integrated methodology for process improvement and delivery system visualization at a multidisciplinary cancer center. *J Healthcare Qual.* 2013;35(2):24–32. doi:10.1111/j.1945-1474.2011.00174.x

Tyler JL, Biggs E. *Practical Governance.* Chicago, IL: Health Administration Press; 2001.

Wilkinson C, Champion JD, Sabharwal K. Promoting preventive health screening through the use of a clinical reminder tool: an accountable care organization quality improvement initiative. *J Healthcare Qual.* 2013;35(5):7–19. doi:10.1111/jhq.12024

Young T, Brailsford S, Connell C, et al. Using industrial processes to improve patient care. *Br Med J.* 2004;328:162–164. doi:10.1136/bmj.328.7432.162

Online Resources

Agency for Healthcare Research and Quality (AHRQ)

- **Patients & Consumers**
  www.ahrq.gov/consumer/index.html
- **Performance Improvement (PI) Plan & Template**
  https://innovations.ahrq.gov/qualitytools/performance-improvement-pi-plan-and-template
- **Quality and Patient Safety**
  www.ahrq.gov/qual/pips/issues.htm

- **CLABSI**
  https://www.ahrq.gov/professionals/education/curriculum-tools/clabsitools/index.html
- **Talking Quality**
  www.talkingquality.ahrq.gov/content/about/default.aspx

American Heart Association

- **Get With the Guidelines Patient Management Tool**
  http://www.heart.org/HEARTORG/Professional/GetWithTheGuidelines-Resuscitation/Get-With-The-Guidelines-Resuscitation_UCM_314496_SubHomePage.jsp
- **Americans for Quality Health Care Quality Tool Box: Consumer Engagement**
  www.nationalpartnership.org/site/PageServer?pagename=qcn_ToolBox_ConsumerEngagement

ANCC Magnet Recognition Program
  www.nursecredentialing.org/Magnet.aspx

Association for Professionals in Infection Prevention and Epidemiology
  http://www.apic.org/

Baldrige Performance Excellence Program

- **Baldrige-Based State, Local and Regional Award Programs**
  www.nist.gov/baldrige/community/state_local.cfm
- **Baldrige Excellence Builder**
  https://www.nist.gov/sites/default/files/documents/baldrige/publications/Baldrige_Excellence_Builder.pdf
- **National Institute of Standards and Technology**
  www.nist.gov/baldrige/

Centers for Disease Control and Prevention

- **Surgical-Site Infection**
  https://www.cdc.gov/HAI/pdfs/toolkits/SSI_toolkit021710SIBT_revised.pdf
- **Sepsis**
  https://www.cdc.gov/sepsis/clinicaltools/

Institute for Healthcare Improvement (CLABSI, Ventilator, Obstetrics, Sepsis)
  http://www.ihi.org/topics/bundles/Pages/default.aspx

The Commonwealth Fund
  http://www.commonwealthfund.org/

The Leapfrog Group Hospital Ratings and Reports
  http://www.leapfroggroup.org/ratings-reports

National Association for Healthcare Quality

- **Performance and Process Improvement Essential Competencies**
  http://nahq.org/education/hq-essentials
- **Quality Review and Accountability Essential Competencies**
  http://nahq.org/education/hq-essentials

Office of Inspector General—U.S. Department of Health & Human Services
  https://oig.hhs.gov/

Quality Prizes and Awards

- **AHCA/NCAL National Quality Award Program**
  www.ahcancal.org/quality_improvement/quality_award/pages/default.aspx
- **American Association of Critical-Care Nurses Beacon Award for Excellence**
  www.aacn.org/wd/beaconapps/content/mainpage.pcms?menu=beaconapps
- **National Association for Healthcare Quality—Professional Recognition Awards**
  www.nahq.org/membership/leadership/prorecognition.html (Members only)
- **National Quality Forum and Joint Commission John M. Eisenberg Patient Safety and Quality Awards**
  www.jointcommission.org/topics/eisenberg_award.aspx
- **U.S. Department of Veterans Affairs Robert W. Carey Performance Excellence Award**
  www.va.gov/OP3/docs/Carey/Robert_W_Carey_Performance_Excellence_Award.asp
- **Union of Japanese Scientists and Engineers Deming Prize**
  http://www.juse.or.jp/english/
- **University of Utah Shingo Prize for Operational Excellence**
  www.shingoprize.org/model-guidelines.html

Partnership for Patients
  https://partnershipforpatients.cms.gov/

Society for Healthcare Epidemiology of America (SHEA; CAUTI)
  http://www.jstor.org/stable/10.1086/675718

United Kingdom National Health Service

- **Falls Prevention**
  http://www.knowledge.scot.nhs.uk/fallsandbonehealth/the-national-falls-programme/the-prevention-and-management-of-falls-in-the-community-a-framework-for-action-for-scotland-2014-2016/falls-care-bundles-for-the-community-setting.aspx

U.S. Department of Health & Human Services, Health Resources & Services Administration
  https://www.hrsa.gov/quality/toolbox/methodology/quality improvement/

U.S. Environmental Protection Agency

- **Lean Practices @ EPA**
  https://www.epa.gov/lean

U.S. News & World Report

- **Best Hospitals Rankings & Ratings**
  http://health.usnews.com/best-hospitals

Section 4

Health Data Analytics

Robert J. Rosati

SECTION CONTENTS

Abstract

Data analytics is a major component of quality improvement across the continuum of healthcare delivery. Organizations are investing heavily in building the infrastructure to enhance capabilities to analyze and report valid and reliable quality, safety, and performance data. The impetus for change came from external and internal pressures (e.g., demonstrating value and delivering optimal care). This section describes the foundational steps to plan and deploy a data management system to support the quality improvement (QI) program, measure identification, measurement selection, sampling, balanced scorecards, dashboards, incorporating external data sources, identifying appropriate benchmarks, data collection, and data validation. Information is provided on the characteristics of data management systems, tools to display data, the application of statistical analysis, and how to interpret and compare data. How to interpret data is fundamental to the success of the organization. Finally, the principles presented throughout the section are applicable to reporting and setting goals to improve performance.

Learning Objectives

1. Acquire knowledge about the historical progression of science and data analytics used for quality and performance improvement in healthcare.
2. Develop an understanding of activities required for the data collection design and data management (e.g., activities, records, reports, and committee meetings).
3. Recognize tools and approaches useful in designing and constructing quality and performance improvement activities (e.g., principles of qualitative and quantitative data collection).
4. Apply process analysis tools, basic statistical techniques and methods for statistical process control (e.g., sampling, measures, dashboard).
5. Interpret data to support decision-making and promote change to advance quality and performance excellence in healthcare.

Historical Perspectives on Quality

The need for quality has always existed. However, the means for meeting that need—the processes of managing and improving for quality—have undergone extensive and continuing change.[1] Before the 20th century, managing quality was based on ancient principles that included product inspection by consumers, which is still widely used in today's villages, and marketplaces concept, with which buyers rely on the skill and reputation of trained, experienced craftsmanship.

As commerce expanded beyond village boundaries and with the growth of technology, additional methods and tools were invented to assist in managing for quality such as specifications by sample and quality warranties in sales contracts. In large towns, the craftsmen organized into monopolistic guilds, which generally were strict in their enforcement of product quality. Their strategies included mandated specifications for input materials, processes, and finished goods; audits of the performance of guild members; and export controls on finished goods.

The early approach to managing for quality in the United States followed the prevailing practice in European countries that had colonized the North American continent. Apprentices learned a trade, qualified to become craftsmen, and in due course might become masters of their own shops. The Industrial Revolution, which originated in Europe, created the factory system. The factory out-produced the small independent shops and made them largely obsolete. The craftsmen became factory workers, and the masters became factory foremen. Quality was managed as before, through the skills of the craftsmen, and supplemented by departmental inspection or supervisory audits.

When the Industrial Revolution spread to the United States, Americans again followed European practice. The Industrial Revolution also accelerated the growth of additional strategies, including written specifications for materials, processes, finished goods, and tests; measurement and the associated measuring instruments and testing laboratories; and standardization in many forms.

During World War II, U.S. industry was faced with the added burden of producing enormous quantities of military products. A part of the war strategy was to shut down production of many civilian products such as automobiles, household appliances, and entertainment products. A massive shortage of goods developed amid a huge buildup of purchasing power. It took the rest of that decade (the 1940s) for supply to catch up with demand. In the interim, manufacturing companies gave top priority to meeting delivery dates, so quality of products suffered. The practice of giving top priority to delivery dates persisted long after the shortages ended.

A new strategy emerged during World War II—statistical quality control (SQC). To improve the quality of military goods, the War Production Board sponsored numerous training courses on the statistical techniques developed by the Bell System during the 1920s. W. E. Deming,[2] who became widely known in quality improvement during the 1980s, was one of the lecturers at some of the War Production Board courses. Many training course attendees became enthusiastic and organized the American Society for Quality Control (now known as American Society for Quality [ASQ]). In its early years ASQ was strongly oriented toward SQC, thereby stimulating further enthusiasm for the method.

After World War II, the Japanese embarked on a course of reaching national goals through trade rather than military means. The major manufacturers, which had been extensively involved in military production, were faced with converting to civilian products. A major obstacle to selling these products in international markets was a reputation for shoddy merchandise, created by the export of poor-quality goods before World War II.

To solve their quality problems, the Japanese learned how other countries managed for quality, sending teams abroad to visit foreign companies and study their approaches. They also invited foreign lecturers to Japan to conduct training courses for managers. As the result of this educational process, the Japanese devised unprecedented strategies to create a revolution in quality. Several of those strategies proved crucial:

- Upper managers personally took charge of leading the revolution.
- All levels and functions underwent training in managing for quality.
- QI was undertaken at a continuing, revolutionary pace.
- Quality circle (QC) involved employee participation in decision-making and problem solving to improve the quality of work.

During the early postwar period, American companies logically considered competition from the Japanese to be based on price rather than quality. Their response was to shift the manufacturing of labor-intensive products to low-labor-cost areas, often offshore. As time went on, price competition declined while quality competition increased.[3] During the 1960s and 1970s, numerous Japanese manufacturers greatly increased their share of the American market; a major reason was the superior quality of their products. Numerous industries were affected (e.g., consumer electronics, automobiles, steel, and machine tools).

U.S. companies generally failed to notice the trend, continuing to believe that competition from the Japanese primarily was price-based rather than quality-based. Some observers sounded warning signals: "The Japanese are headed for world quality leadership and will attain it in the next two decades because no one else is moving there at the same pace."[4] The alarm was sounded at the conference of the European Organization for Quality Control in Stockholm in June 1966.

The most obvious effect of the Japanese quality revolution was the massive export of goods. The impact on the United States was considerable, especially in sensitive areas such as manufacturing, steel, and electronics. The affected manufacturing companies were damaged by the resulting loss of sales. The workforce and their unions were damaged by the resulting "export of jobs." The national economy was damaged by the resulting unfavorable trade balance.

In healthcare, the major drivers for data analytics and information systems were Medicare and Medicaid in the 1960s. Communication between departments and the need for discrete departmental systems were drivers in the 1970s. The 1980s drivers were diagnosis-related groups (DRGs) and reimbursement. Integration due to mergers and consolidation was the major driver of analytics in the 1990s; and in the 2000s, a focus on value and outcomes-based reimbursement are major drivers for health data analytics and information systems.[5]

New Era of Data Analytics

The use of data in healthcare delivery, monitoring, and improvement is rapidly evolving. Davenport[6] championed the concept that if organizations were going to succeed, they needed to compete on analytics. This meant exploring Big Data with a recent emphasis on population health and value-based care. The strategy would use all the data captured by the organization's disparate systems (e.g., medical records, human resources, finance, imaging) to support improvements in staffing, customer relationships, financial performance, services provided, product development and managing the supply chain. Further, Davenport proposed that being successful would require an executive commitment to recognizing the importance of analytics capabilities, sophisticated information systems, and employing people with analytical skills. Big Data has three main characteristics and some added a fourth (veracity):

1. Volume: The physical size of the data and number of records are dramatically higher than what is typically managed on a traditional data system.

2. Velocity: Data are received in near or real time or as a continuous stream and should be made available to inform decisions as quickly as possible (predictive, prescriptive analytics).

3. Variety: Data include structured records, unstructured text, images (medical imaging), audio, video, and biomedical sensor traces.

4. Veracity: The vast amounts of structured and unstructured data come from sources that may be uncertain or imprecise.[7(p1),8]

By 2013, McKinsey & Company reported that the Big Data revolution was substantially under way in healthcare.[9] Several major health systems were using data to deliver better care, provide increased value, and innovate. Today almost every segment of the healthcare industry invests in Big Data. The scale of the investment varies depending on how much the organizations can afford to allocate to expand their analytic capabilities but they recognize that "competing on analytics" is necessary to survive in the current healthcare environment. This becomes particularly evident with the shift to population health and value-based care.

With the proliferation of electronic health records (EHRs) and health information exchanges (HIEs), large data sets are now available to healthcare professionals and health services researchers. The National Institutes of Health define biomedical Big Data as the "complexity, challenges and new opportunities presented by the combined analysis of data. In biomedical research, these data sources include the diverse, complex, disorganized, massive, and multimodal data being generated by researchers, hospitals, and mobile devices around the world."[10(p1)] Their Big Data to Knowledge or "BD2K" initiative acknowledges that there is a lack of appropriate tools, poor data accessibility, and insufficient training about Big Data in healthcare, which impedes rapid translation of data into useful information at the service level.[11] The BD2K initiative has four aims to assist healthcare professionals in using Big Data:

1. Facilitate broad use of biomedical digital assets by making them Findable, Accessible, Interoperable, and Reusable (FAIR).

2. Conduct research and develop the methods, software, and tools needed to analyze biomedical Big Data.

3. Enhance training in the development and use of methods and tools necessary for biomedical Big Data science.

4. Support a data ecosystem that accelerates discovery as part of a digital enterprise.[11(p3)]

By utilizing Big Data, infrastructure organizations can monitor populations (e.g., people with diabetes and asthma) to determine if the right care is being provided and assess health outcomes. Further, it is possible to drill down to specific providers and benchmark their performance. Hospitals that manage clinical bundles can use the data to evaluate the care delivered prior to discharge and to assess which post-acute providers deliver the best outcomes at the lowest cost. For example, a hospital could look at 30-, 60-, 90-day readmission rates for heart failure patients with care transitions to skilled nursing facilities (SNFs), home healthcare, or home with no services. Choosing the organizations to partner with in the future might rely on performance.

With a focus on data comes the need to accelerate the adoption of health IT. Technology is widely recognized and was singled out as a key goal by the Health Care Delivery and Information Technology (HCDIT) Subcommittee of the President's Information Technology Advisory Committee.[12] Studies suggest that the quality of healthcare can improve with the appropriate use of technology.[13,14] These studies specifically highlight the need to facilitate the transmission of clinical information contained in the medical record between healthcare providers. A second goal identified by the HCDIT subcommittee is use of health IT to achieve substantial economic and social benefits (such as reducing medical errors, eliminating unproductive healthcare expenditures, and improving quality of care). As cited above, most hospitals adopted EHRs. In ambulatory care, only 54% had adopted a basic EHR and 78% of office-based physicians reported using an EHR.[15]

A lack of standards hindered the adoption of IT tools in the healthcare industry.[13] The National Committee on Vital and Health Statistics (NCVHS) began to standardize formats and data for the electronic exchange of patient health record information in 2002,[16] which progressed to the Healthcare Information and Management Systems Society (HIMSS) developing a set of principles to support IT interoperability in the United States.[17] In addition, other organizations and task forces continue to work on international protocols and frameworks for data exchanges between heterogeneous systems in the healthcare industry. The industry Health Level 7 (HL7), the Systemized Nomenclature of Medicine (SNOMED), and Extensible Markup Language (XML) special interest groups were leaders in defining EHR standards. As these standards evolved, more comprehensive EHRs were developed and shared among all the providers in the healthcare system. EHRs sometimes are referred to as personal health records (PHRs). There is a distinction between the two types of records: PHRs are geared more toward consumers and EHRs pertain to records used and held by healthcare providers.

Federal support increased since the 2004 announcement of the U.S. Department of Health & Human Services 10-year plan to create a new national health information infrastructure that will include an EHR for every American and a new network to link health records nationwide. Health IT and interoperable systems are requisites for healthcare delivery in the 21st century. Health IT potentially includes products such as EHRs, patient engagement tools such as PHRs and secure, private Internet portals, and HIEs. An IOM report[18] that examined the state of the art in system safety and opportunities to build safer systems concluded as follows:

- Safety is an emergent property of a larger system that considers not just the software but also how it is used by clinicians.
- The "sociotechnical system" includes technology (software, hardware), people (clinicians, patients), processes (workflow), organization (capacity, decisions about how health IT is applied, incentives), and the external environment (regulations, public opinion).
- Safer implementation and use of health IT is a complex, dynamic process that requires a shared responsibility between vendors and healthcare organizations.
- Poor user-interface design, poor workflow, and complex data interfaces threaten patient safety.
- Lack of system interoperability is a barrier to improving clinical decisions and patient safety.
- Constant, ongoing commitment to safety—from acquisition to implementation and maintenance—is needed to achieve safer, more effective care.[18(ppS2–S4)]

The Health Information Technology for Economic and Clinical Health Act (HITECH Act) was enacted under Title XIII of the American Recovery and Reinvestment Act of 2009 (Pub.L. 111–5). Under the HITECH Act, the U.S. Department of Health & Human Services authorized spending $25.9 billion to promote and expand the adoption of health IT. The HITECH Act also established meaningful use of interoperable EHR adoption in the healthcare system as a critical national goal and incentivized EHR adoption.

Title IV of the Act included incentive payments ($63,750) for Medicaid providers who would adopt and use "certified EHRs" over 6 years beginning in 2011 Eligible professionals had to begin receiving payments by 2016 to qualify for the program. For Medicare, the maximum payments were set at $44,000 over 5 years. To receive the EHR stimulus money, the HITECH Act required providers to show "meaningful use" of an EHR system. Meaningful use is defined as using certified EHR technology to

- improve quality, safety, and efficiency; reduce health disparities;
- engage patients and family;
- improve care coordination, and population and public health; and
- maintain privacy and security of patient health information.[19]

Meaningful use compliance results include better clinical outcomes, improved population health outcomes, increased transparency and efficiency, empowered consumers, and more robust research data on health systems. Meaningful use sets specific objectives that eligible professionals and hospitals must achieve to qualify for the financial incentive programs. These objectives are defined as the "Stages of Meaningful Use."

- Stage 1 (2011 to 2012)—Data capture and sharing;
- Stage 2 (2014)—Advance clinical processes;
- Stage 3 (2016)—Improved outcomes.

The impact of the federal initiatives that supplied the stimulus funding and the requirements for meaningful use benefit the use of data for quality, safety, and performance improvement efforts. Certified EHRs can potentially be a rich source of standardized and structure information that can be used by quality, safety, and performance improvement teams to measure the impact of improvement activities and assess patient clinical outcomes.

Data and Information

Healthcare professionals are constantly challenged to sift and interpret the vast amount of data available and then distinguish what is relevant, meaningful, and important to plan a course of action. Nutley and Reynolds[20] described eight activities to encourage and improve the use of health data to strengthen health systems. These include the following:

1. Assess and improve the data use context. Organizational and behavioral factors influence whether an organization uses data to inform decision-making; whether it promotes a culture of information.
2. Engage data users and data producers. Lack of communication is a barrier in those who produce data and those who need data to make decisions.
3. Improve data quality. For managers to make sound decisions for improving processes, they need to be confident that the data they are relying on is sound—accurate, complete, and timely.
4. Improve data availability. This includes data synthesis, data communication, and access to data. Management information systems (MISs) can facilitate data being available to decision-makers.
5. Identify information needs. Various stakeholders have various data and information needs, and their audiences may be different. Healthcare quality professionals can help managers prioritize those data that will be useful in monitoring and evaluating a program or service.
6. Build capacity in the data use core competencies. Frontline staff and managers need to be competent in data analysis, interpretation, synthesis, and presentation, and how to develop data-informed recommendations.
7. Strengthen the organization's data demand and use infrastructure. Data-informed decision-making requires that the culture supports the use of data, that an infrastructure exists to ensure data quality, and processes are in place to obtain and report data-rich outcomes.

8. Monitor, evaluate, and communicate results of data use interventions. Data must be top of mind in an organization, and value placed on using data to make important decisions. Successes in using data to improve performance must be explicitly shared in management meetings.

The key to all performance improvement activities is the collection of meaningful data and the communication of useful information. The art of quality, safety, and performance improvement is to communicate the right information the right way at the right time to the right people. There is a distinction between data and information.

- *Data* are the representation of things, facts, concepts, and instructions that are stored in a defined format and structure on a passive medium (e.g., paper, computer, microfilm). For leadership to be confident that the data they are using to make decisions are sound, there must be an emphasis on data quality. The American Health Information Management Association (AHIMA) defined 10 characteristics of data quality (see **TABLE 4-1**). The top four characteristics are accuracy, accessibility, comprehensiveness, and consistency.
- *Information* is created when meaning is attached to data, for which is translated into results and useful statements decision-making. For information to be meaningful, data must be considered within the context of how they have been obtained and intent for their use.[21,22]

The information contained in data helps leaders to focus on goals and proof points as well as demonstrating value.[7] See **TABLE 4-2** for more information on the value of data for leaders.

The Quality Measurement and Management Project developed the following seven basic concepts related to quality-management information:

1. Healthcare data must be carefully defined and systematically collected and analyzed in their full context before they can be useful in quality-management.
2. Tremendous amounts of healthcare data and information are available, but not all of it is useful for quality management.
3. Mature information revolves around clearly established patterns of care, not individual cases. Patterns identify a consistent process that can be studied and improved.
4. Most quality indicators currently available are useful only as indicators of potential problems and not as definitive measures of quality.
5. Multiple measures of quality need to be integrated to provide a clear picture of quality of care in an institution or managed care organization.

Table 4-1 Data Quality Characteristics

Characteristic	Meaning
Accuracy	Data represent correct values, valid, and attached to the correct patient record.
Accessibility	Data items are easily obtained and legal to access with strong protections and controls built into the process.
Comprehensiveness	All required data items are included; entire scope of the data is collected and documents intentional limitations.
Consistency	Value of the data is reliable and the same across applications.
Currency	Data are up-to-date.
Definition	Clear definitions provided so that current and future data users will know what the data mean. Each data element has clear meaning and acceptable values.
Granularity	Attributes and values of data are defined with the correct level of detail.
Precision	Data values are just large enough to support the application or process.
Relevancy	Data are meaningful to the performance of the process or application for which they are collected.
Timeliness	Timeliness is determined by how the data are being used and their context.

Adapted from The American Health Information Management Association (AHIMA). *Statement on quality healthcare data and information*; 2007. http://bok.ahima.org/doc?oid=101304#.WSXX5WgrKM8

6. Developing outcomes information without monitoring the process of care, when warranted, is inefficient because it cannot lead directly to improvement in quality.
7. Cost and quality are inseparable issues.[23(p28)]

Bader and Bohr[23] translated the seven concepts to a seven-step strategy for the interpretation and use of quality-of-care information, which are still relevant today. These steps are outlined below.

Step 1. Planning and Organizing for Data Collection, Interpretation, and Use. Planning for collection and utilization of internally and externally generated data leads to a higher likelihood of success. Anticipating barriers, identifying responsibilities, and laying the groundwork for multidisciplinary

Table 4-2 How Data Help Leaders

Better Care

Mission and Vision	Assess the extent of how the mission and values are being achieved.
	Develop a vision and evaluate program achievements.
Clinical Quality	Understand the mechanism for physician appointment and recredentialing while knowing their performance review process is effective.
	Decide on individual credentialing recommendations effectively.
Performance Improvement	Determine priorities for continuous improvements.
	Monitor aspects of organizational performance and take corrective action.
	Help the governing body evaluate and improve its performance.

Smarter Spending

Strategic Planning	Prioritize strategic goals, including programs, to support or discontinue.
	Judge progress toward strategic goals and objectives.
	Identify the need for policy implementation effectiveness.
Resources	Understand changes in community needs, financial resources, and technology.
	Weigh long and short-term financial viability.
	Weigh the impact of budgetary decisions on quality of care/service.
	Secure an organization's resources, efficiency, and effectiveness based on accurate information.

Healthier People

Health Improvement	Determine goals for improving the health status of the community.
	Evaluate the effectiveness of programs designed to improve health.

Table constructed using information from O'Rourke LM, Bader BS. An illustrative quality and performance report for the governing board. *Quality Lett Healthcare Leaders.* 1993;5(2):15–28.

and inter-professional collaboration can more smoothly guide the process toward improvement. Consideration needs to be given to whether the data will be quantitative (e.g., clinical values) or qualitative (e.g., a review of clinical notes). Qualitative data require a rigorous process that delineates exactly where to look for the data and what needs to be captured.

In addition, a data dictionary that defines all data elements and calculations of indicators can be an invaluable element to improve the communication of information.

Step 2. Verifying and Correcting Data. The purpose of verifying data is to identify data limitations and opportunities to improve internal systems that lead to better data quality, provide an opportunity to correct data (e.g., find missing data), and to review data to become familiar with it. For qualitative data, it is necessary to establish interrater reliability to ensure staff who reviewed clinical records consistently captured the same information.

Step 3. Identifying and Presenting Potentially Important Findings. The first step in this process is to perform preliminary data analysis, often descriptive analyses. When conducting this type of analysis, it is recommended that several questions be addressed.

- How do these data compare with other organizations' (as with mortality rates) or with previously trended internal data (for example, healthcare-associated infection rates)?
- What is the trend over time? Is it static, improving, or worsening?
- How are data likely to be interpreted (or misinterpreted)?
- Is there an opportunity for improvement?
- Who receives the data? For what purpose?

Data must be translated into meaningful information. Several techniques are used to present information in a clear and concise manner.

Step 4. Continuing to Study and Develop Recommendations for Change. If further study of the data is warranted, a variety of methods are available. These include variation analysis, review of additional data, retrospective medical reviews, and process analysis. Variation analysis seeks an explanation for statistically significant differences in the data. These differences may reflect clinical factors, patient characteristics, data collection (such as sampling characteristics), or organizational characteristics (such as staffing).

Additional data may need to be collected and reviewed to completely understand variations in data. For example, a hospital may show a steady increase in mortality rates. Additional data related to hospital case mix, diagnostic categories, mortality within a specified time from date of hospital admission, and other hospital characteristics may be used to fully interpret the data. Focused/intensive retrospective review refers to an activity for which processes or outcomes use pre-established criteria or indicators. Findings may be presented in peer review or other settings. Process analysis refers to a method of analyzing data using industrial performance improvement techniques. Process analysis occurs when a group diagrams a healthcare process. The group then measures process variations and looks for ways to improve the process and the administrative or clinical outcome.

Step 5. Taking Action. "Taking action" implies that people, teams, departments, and committees are empowered to make decisions and implement changes based on information discovered through data analysis. Actions may occur in several forms: education and training of staff, simulation, education and reporting of findings to outside vendors or the public, changes in organizational or departmental policies and processes, and changes in practice patterns.

Step 6. Monitoring Performance. Monitoring performance entails monitoring the influence and effectiveness of a quality, safety, or performance improvement action and involves the collection of additional data. Questions to be considered include the following:

- Have the proposed changes been implemented? To what extent?
- How could compliance with the changes be enhanced?
- What effect are the changes having on patient outcomes? Are these desirable effects?
- Are changes modified and then tested further, communicated on a wider scale, tested for a longer period before drawing conclusions, or ended because they are ineffective?

Step 7. Communicating Results. There are three basic barriers to the interpretation and use of information: human factors, statistical factors, and organizational factors.

1. Human factors include fear of the data; resentment of external data; unrealistic expectations about data (including the myth that all data must be perfect); and lack of training related to planning, organizing, and analyzing data.
2. Statistical factors include flawed data, missing data, untimely data, poorly displayed data, and data that are difficult to integrate with other organizational data.
3. Organizational factors include data overload; a poor data retrieval system; lack of resources (time, people, money); and poor relationships among administration, physicians, and staff.

Communication is an integral component in each of the previous steps. Striving for healthcare quality is a journey. Performance improvement begins with the communication of where an organization is and where it is going. Effective communication requires providing information to the appropriate staff so they can act. Consider which audiences and methods of communication will be most effective in bringing about change. Depending on the findings, audiences may include frontline clinical staff for patient issues, administration for service delivery failures, or the human resources department for staffing concerns.

Design and Management

Quality, safety, and performance improvement activities and research exist on a continuum of rigor and may be viewed more like a soft science (**TABLE 4-3**). The scientific approach is the most sophisticated method of acquiring knowledge and involves inductive and deductive reasoning, which might

Table 4-3 Continuous Quality Improvement (Soft Science) and Research (Hard Science)

	Applied		Theoretical	
Soft				**Hard**
Social Sciences		Biological Sciences		Physical Sciences
Descriptive		Inferential		Predictive
Problem Solving		Fundamental Functions		Hypothesis Testing
Observational data	**Integrative data**	**Survey data**	**Secondary data**	**Output data**
Qualitative studies	CQI studies	Program evaluations	Efficacy research	Experimental studies
Focus groups	Meta-analysis	Epidemiological investigations	Case-control studies	Randomized clinical trials
Retrospective chart reviews	Methodologic reviews	Practice change evaluations	Quasi-experimental research	Longitudinal experimental studies
CQI Studies	**Evaluation Research**	**Outcomes Research**	**Health Services Research**	**Clinical Research**

Updated in 2017 for HQ Solutions by CL Beaudin from Byers JF, Beaudin CL. The relationship between continuous quality improvement and research. *J Healthcare Qual*. 2002;24(1):8.

be considered superior to those arrived at through reliance on tradition, authority, and experience. The underlying assumptions of design, measurement, and interpretation are similar. Research utilization is a key aspect of the QI process and critical to achieving healthcare quality as defined by the local, state, and federal regulations and standards. Healthcare quality professionals use the level of research rigor that best answers the specific performance improvement question and area of study balancing rigor and practicality. Research studies and systematic reviews can be evaluated for usefulness to a practice setting using critical appraisal tools. These tools guide healthcare quality professionals through the research critique process, allowing effective evaluation and synthesis of research findings for use in performance improvement activities.[24] When the healthcare quality professional begins the design process for activities, the goodness of project fit (QI process versus research process) by examining the question to be answered, data collection, analysis plan, and application of findings. See **TABLE 4-4** for an overview of the processes.

Table 4-4 Quality Improvement and Research Processes

QI Process	Research Process
Identify the process improvement, survey the literature, and flowchart the process.	Identify information need(s) or ask the question to be investigated.
Define the customers and problem.	Define the variable(s) or the elements for which data are required.
Formulate a plan.	Formulate a plan of study or hypotheses.
Choose one or a combination of basic or quality-management and planning tools.	Choose or design the research design and collection tools/instruments.
Collect the data.	Collect the data.
Analyze the data and look for root causes.	Analyze the data.
Display the data.	Display the data.
Report the data and findings.	Report the data and findings.
Draw conclusions.	Draw conclusions.
Act upon recommendations deduced from the conclusions.	Act upon recommendations deduced from the conclusions.
Continue to monitor the process.	Continue to monitor the process.
Evaluate and communicate conclusions.	Evaluate and communicate conclusions.
Hold the improvement.	

Quality Measurement

Performance outcomes measurement or decision support systems can provide a primary focus to determine the quality of healthcare services provided to consumers. By analyzing data and information generated by an effective performance outcomes measurement system, healthcare quality professionals will be able to help identify areas in which to improve quality and resources in their organizations. Other uses for outcomes systems include helping to identify how an organization measures up in relation to its competitors, identifying individual providers and practitioners who meet acceptable levels of quality, allowing providers to respond more rapidly to market changes, paying for exceptional performance, and justifying value-based services.

Chassin et al.[25] suggested that quality, safety, and performance improvement programs can focus explicitly on maximizing health benefits to patients and, to achieve the goal, measures must be included that advance knowledge about whether the goal is being achieved. They note four criteria for accountability measures (i.e., process measures; if met, there will be a higher likelihood of improving patient outcomes). The criteria include the following:

- Strong evidence base shows that the care process leads to improved outcomes.
- Measure accurately captures the provision of evidence-based care.
- Measure addresses a process with few intervening steps that must occur before the improved outcome is realized.
- Implementing the measure has little or no chance of inducing unintended adverse consequences.

Healthcare quality professionals facilitate analysis and interpretation of outcomes data for an organization. The reference point for the outcomes data are always kept in mind whenever the results of such data are analyzed. The overall goals for use of outcomes and decision-support data are to improve quality, reduce costs and resource consumption, increase organizational profitability, and develop an information-based strategic plan. Comparisons of length of stay (LOS), costs, complications, and mortality cannot be made legitimately without adjusting severity at the patient level. Severity adjustment and clinical case mix permit effective analysis and eliminate practitioners' concerns that "their patients are sicker." Evidence to support the focus of measurement is shown as **TABLE 4-5.**

Risk Adjustment

Risk adjustment is a technique used to consider or to control the fact that different patients with the same diagnosis may have additional conditions or characteristics that can affect how well they respond to treatment. Analysis of outcomes data

Table 4-5 Evidence to Support the Focus of Measurement

Measure Type	Evidence	Example of Measure Type and Evidence
Health Outcome An outcome of care is the health status of a patient (or change in health status) resulting from healthcare, desirable or adverse. In some situations, resource use may be considered a proxy for a health state (e.g., hospitalization may represent deterioration in health status).	A rationale supports the relationship of the health outcome to at least one healthcare structure, process, intervention, or service.	#0230: Acute myocardial infarction (AMI). 30-day mortality. Survival is a goal of seeking and providing treatment for AMI. Rationale linking healthcare processes or interventions (aspirin, reperfusion) to mortality or survival. #0171: Acute care hospitalization (risk-adjusted) [of home care patients]. Improvement or stabilization of condition to remain at home is a goal of seeking and providing home care services. Rationale linking healthcare processes (e.g., medication reconciliation, care coordination) to hospitalization of patients receiving home care services. #0140: Ventilator-associated pneumonia for intensive care unit and high-risk nursery patients. Avoiding harm from treatment is a goal when seeking and providing healthcare. Rationale linking healthcare processes (e.g., ventilator bundle) to ventilator-acquired pneumonia.
Intermediate Clinical Outcome An intermediate outcome is a change in physiologic state that leads to a longer-term health outcome.	Quantity, quality, and consistency of a body of evidence that the measured intermediate clinical outcome leads to a desired health outcome.	#0059: Hemoglobin A1c management (A1c > 9). Evidence that hemoglobin A1c level leads to health outcomes (e.g., prevention of renal disease, heart disease, amputation, mortality).
Process A process of care is a healthcare-related activity performed for, on behalf of, or by a patient.	Quantity, quality, and consistency of a body of evidence that the measured healthcare process leads to desired health outcomes in the target population with benefits that outweigh harms to patients. Specific drugs and devices should have Food & Drug Administration approval for the target condition. If the measure focus is on inappropriate use, then quantity, quality, and consistency of a body of evidence that the measured healthcare process does *not* lead to desired health outcomes in the target population.	#0551: Angiotensin-converting enzyme (ACE) inhibitor and angiotensin receptor blocker (ARB) use and persistence among members with coronary artery disease at high risk for coronary events. Evidence that use of ACE inhibitor and ARB results in lower mortality or cardiac events. #0058: Inappropriate antibiotic treatment for adults with acute bronchitis. Evidence that antibiotics are not effective for acute bronchitis.
Structure Structure of care is a feature of a healthcare organization or clinician related to its capacity to provide high-quality healthcare.	Quantity, quality, and consistency of a body of evidence that the measured healthcare structure leads to desired health outcomes with benefits that outweigh harms (including evidence of the link to effective care processes and the link from the care processes to desired health outcomes).	#0190: Nurse staffing hours. Evidence that increasing nursing hours results in lower mortality or morbidity or leads to provision of effective care processes (e.g., lower medication errors) that lead to better outcomes.

(continued)

Table 4-5 **Evidence to Support the Focus of Measurement (*continued*)**		
Special Considerations by Topic		
Patient Experience with Care	Evidence that the measured aspects of care are those valued by patients and for which the patient is the best or only source of information (often acquired through qualitative studies). Or, evidence that patient experience with care is correlated with desired outcomes.	#0166: HCAHPS. Evidence that patients or consumers value the aspects of care being measured (e.g., communication with doctors and nurses, responsiveness of hospital staff, pain control, communication about medicines, cleanliness and quiet of the hospital environment, and discharge information).
Efficiency Measures of efficiency combine the concepts of resource use and quality.	Efficiency measured with combination of quality measures and resource-use measures. Quality measure component: Evidence for the selected quality measures as described in this table. Resource-use measure component: Does not require clinical evidence as described in this table.	Currently, there are no NQF-endorsed efficiency measures that combine quality and resource use. Potential measure: Diabetes quality measures or composite used in conjunction with a measure of resource use per episode. Evidence for diabetes quality measures as described in this table.

Reprinted from National Quality Forum. *Guidance for evaluating the evidence related to the focus of quality measurement and importance to measure and report.* Washington, DC: NQF; 2011:15–16. www.qualityforum.org/WorkArea/linkit.aspx?LinkIdentifier=id&ItemID=70941. Copyright © 2011 National Quality Forum, with permission.

using statistical techniques considers and controls for patient characteristics or conditions that are clinically meaningful and demonstrates a statistical effect on the rates for each condition. This removes the bias effect that can result when practitioners primarily treat patients who are more likely to experience desirable outcomes, such as those with fewer risk factors or co-occurring illnesses (morbidities).

Some outcomes measurement systems define the differences between *risk adjustment* and *severity*, whereas other systems use the terms interchangeably. However, there is a difference. Patients in a study population may respond with either "yes" or "no" when asked if they have had certain outcomes; the outcomes variable in this case is binary. The probability of a "yes" answer is the risk of the outcome.

Statistical methodologies to adjust for risk are applied to the outcomes data to predict patient-specific variables such as certain diagnoses that are risk factors. The validity of each risk adjustment model is assessed based on the choice of risk factors, including both potential risk factors and those included in the model, and through measures of how well the predictions match overall experience. This assessment includes indicators such as measures of patient subpopulations, including patients with more than one risk factor, and the concordance statistic, which shows, in percentages, how accurate the model is at predicting the outcome.

The yes-or-no nature of outcomes data means that outcomes can refer to clinical outcomes, such as inpatient C-section complication rates. Outcomes also can be defined by using LOS and charges or cost, such as when an LOS

exceeds a certain number of days and results in a "yes" or "no" answer. When the categories are in two or more groups, a set of outcomes can be defined and the risk adjustment methodologies can be applied to the full set of outcomes at the same time.

An important distinction must be made between the statistical analysis of binary and continuous data. Risk adjustment methodologies do not apply to dependent variables that are continuous, like cost or LOS. The answer could be any number on a continuum, not "yes" or "no." Severity adjustment methodologies are applied to the cost of LOS data to predict severity by using patient-specific variables, called *severity factors*. Frequently, the presence of additional diagnoses helps to define the severity of a group of patients within a DRG, on an individual patient level, or both. Both risk-adjusted and severity-adjusted data are extremely important outcomes system tools. Using unadjusted or raw data means that all patients in the clinical topic category, regardless of their health status or the existence of varying clinical conditions, are included in the rate calculation. Both raw and risk-adjusted data can be made available on the same outcomes topic because payers frequently use risk-adjusted data in their initial decision-making.

Healthcare quality professionals also must be familiar with the ways in which their decision-support databases handle statistical "outliers." Are all patients included, or are patients more than two standard deviations (SDs) from the mean removed from data analysis? Most decision-support databases have a consistent approach regarding patients who are outliers. It is critical during data comparisons to make sure that all data sources managed patient outliers in a consistent fashion. For example, a hospital physician group was trying to compare its performance on resource utilization and LOS for community-acquired pneumonia. One patient was hospitalized for more than 100 days because the patient was ventilator-dependent and did not have adequate resources to be placed in an extended care facility. This patient's record needed to be removed from the raw data before a fair comparison could be made.

Another factor to consider in the analysis and interpretation of outcomes data is the level of detail. The best system includes clinical and financial information for every payer and practitioner and the patient. This integrated data repository can mine data for

- benchmarking quality performance against established standards;
- comparing physician performance within given outcome topics;
- examining details at the patient level;
- viewing patient diagnoses, procedures, and other information;
- determining the impact of managed care on costs and outcomes; and
- analyzing product lines to evaluate their effectiveness and to increase or downsize service offerings.

Evidence-Based Practice

Evidence-based medicine is the "conscientious, explicit and judicious use of current best evidence in making decisions about the care of individual patients."[26(p71)] Because multiple disciplines are involved in healthcare delivery, however, the term *evidence-based practice* (EBP) is more appropriate than *evidence-based medicine* from a healthcare quality perspective. Clinicians base their care not only on experimental evidence but also consider experiential evidence, physiologic principles, patient and professional values, and system features in their decision-making. This practice allows individualized application and diffusion of aggregate research evidence.[27,28] There are many benefits to using EBP including the following:

- Promotes quality and patient safety through the provision of effective and efficient healthcare resulting in less variation in care and fewer unnecessary or nontherapeutic interventions.[29]
- Iterative with outcomes measurement; one facilitates the other.[30]
- Complements the principles of continuous quality, safety, and performance improvement.

Outcomes evaluation at the individual and aggregate level is an essential step in evaluating the EBP influence.

EBPs and QI are based on clinical research and health services research. Clinical research evaluates the impact of interventions on patient outcomes. Outcome measures may include clinical outcomes, functional outcomes, and patient satisfaction or engagement. This type of research helps healthcare quality professionals determine clinical evidence-based best practices. Health services research evaluates the health system at the micro and macro levels. Results from this type of research guide healthcare quality professionals in improving work processes and systems of care.

Epidemiological Principles

The influence of quality, safety, and performance improvement can be enhanced through the application of clinical epidemiology (e.g., case-control studies, cohort studies, propensity score matching) to data collected on many patients for relatively little cost. This comports to a recent emphasis in the healthcare industry related to "population health." Comprehensive linked databases have enormous potential to provide information on the influence of tests and treatments on health. The potential value of these data can be realized if (1) actual receipt of these interventions, health outcomes, and potentially confounding variables can be ascertained accurately for individual patients; and (2) selection bias can be minimized by identifying an appropriate basis for comparison.[31] For example, it is possible to assess changes in patient outcomes after an "improvement intervention" on a specific nursing unit by comparing those outcomes to a matched group of patients from other units in a hospital or over a prior period for the same unit when adjusting for any confounding variables. Using data available in electronic records and appropriate statistical methods makes it possible to test for statistical differences related to a quality, safety, or process improvement initiative compared to current practice. This level of analysis generally makes the results more robust, leading to wider acceptance across an organization and broad adoption of the improvement effort (also known as "spread").

Population Health

Healthcare is moving beyond the episode of care to determine health outcomes. Population health is defined as "the health outcomes of a group of individuals, including the distribution of such outcomes within the group."[32(p380)] It considers all the determinants of health, including medical care, social and physical environments and related services, genetics, and individual behavior. An inherent byproduct of population health is the identification, reduction, or elimination of inequity and health disparities.[33] With healthcare reform emerged population health management, which requires many different types of data to guide population care delivery and to understand the value of these programs. Population health management (or population medicine) "is the design, delivery, coordination, and payment of high-quality healthcare services to manage the Triple Aim for a population using the best resources available within the healthcare system."[33(¶11)]

Population health is another area where data are large volume and high velocity. When the data are available, organizations can assess how they are managing high-risk and high-volume patients, as well as the general population. For example, it is often helpful to know what percentage of the population are high utilizers in terms of hospitalizations or emergency room visits and to determine the characteristics of these patients so they can be better managed (e.g., more visits to their primary care provider, better diet, behavioral health referrals). In another example, Boult and Wieland found that these four features contributed to better population management of primary care for older adults with chronic illnesses:

1. comprehensive assessment of the patient's health conditions, treatments, behaviors, risks, supports, resources, values, and preferences;
2. evidence-based care planning and monitoring to meet the patient's health-related needs and preferences;
3. promotion of patients' and family caregiver's active engagement in care; and
4. coordination and communication among all the professionals engaged in a patient's care, especially during transitions from the hospital.[34]

These population management activities are amenable to measurement and analytics. As payment shifts toward value versus volume, it is more prevalent for organizations to be evaluated based on how they are managing entire populations. Payers are putting providers at-risk to achieve the best outcomes for these groups of patients. Without good data and analytics, it is almost impossible to achieve the goal of being a high-performing organization in meeting the needs of specific populations.

Information Systems

Information systems can be used to support a variety of activities within healthcare organizations. Effective processes for information gathering and dissemination include considerations such as

- identify who needs to know the information (this may include various stakeholders such as senior management, board members, customers, physicians, etc.);
- determine which information stakeholders need to know to make decisions related to improving the quality of care; and
- develop a system that ensures the right people receive the right information at the right time in the right way.[35]

Areas commonly supported include quality, safety, and performance improvement, cost control, and productivity; patient registration; utilization management; program planning and evaluation; external reporting; research; and education. Information systems can be grouped into the following: clinical, administrative, imaging, human resources, financial, patient experience, and decision support.

An organization needs to select the best health information system and technology that supports quality, safety, and performance improvement practices such as

- measurement,
- tracking,
- sharing healthcare delivery performance measures,
- monitoring refinements to clinical workflow processes (both internal and external),
- effects of change on overall patient experience and care coordination across care settings, and
- reducing costs and improve patient health outcomes.[36(pp4–5)]

An organization can use a checklist to evaluate various system options. Rarely do organizations build their own information management systems. If an organization chooses to buy or build its own, there are considerations when looking at functionality, developing the architecture, and implementing and maintaining the system. See **TABLE 4-6** for a buy or build checklist. Different information systems are described below.

Administrative Support Information Systems

Administrative support information systems aid day-to-day operations in healthcare organizations, including

- financial information systems (payroll, accounts payable, patient accounting cost accounting, forecasting, budgeting and asset management);
- human resources information systems (employee record, time and attendance, position and performance management, labor analysis, turnover, and absenteeism); and
- office automation systems (word processing, e-mail, scheduling, facsimile/scanning, and spreadsheets).

Management Information Systems

A MIS can contain both the manual and the automated methods that provide information for decision-making. Other names for an MIS, which are used interchangeably, include data-processing structure, medical information system, hospital information system, or decision support system. The term, as it commonly is used, refers to an automated or computerized system. Information plays a key role in decision-making in each stage of the management process.

Table 4-6 Information Systems: Buy or Build Checklist

Buy	Build
Does the system provide for capture, storage, and retrieval of clinical and financial information from a variety of sources (e.g., health information management [HIM], medical records/EHRs, admission, discharge, transfer, billing, laboratory, pharmacy, blood bank, operating room schedule, and radiology)?	What expertise does the organization have in-house to develop the system, database software, analytic tools, and hardware? How much money and time must be invested to procure this expertise?
Does the system interface with the organization's existing information systems?	Do either HIM or quality, safety or performance improvement staff have the full industry knowledge required to develop and deploy the information system to support clinical and financial needs of the organization (architecture, nomenclature, and other national standards)?
Does the system allow for the establishment of "triggers" or thresholds for important measures of performance and signal an alert when these thresholds have been exceeded?	Can staff provide necessary documentation, training, support, and maintenance for the system on an ongoing basis? If so, will changing priorities interfere with the sustainability of the program?
Does the system have critical alerts such as abnormal laboratory values, drug interactions, and others to promote patient safety (e.g., identifying serious reportable or "never" events)?	How will the organization be able to sustain the system? Are resources available to keep the program up to date in an ever-changing clinical, regulatory and accreditation environment?
Does the system have "rules-based" processing or an algorithm (i.e., the system automatically provides a complete list of cases that meet or fail criteria)?	Is there a true understanding of the future data demands of accreditation organizations, regulatory agencies, third-party payers, employers, and other external data demands?
Is the system flexible enough to allow for concurrent and retrospective reviews?	Will there be long-term dedicated resources to enhance such an application for quality, safety and performance improvement (including various functions such as credentialing, provider profiling)?
Does the system support accreditation and regulatory reporting requirements?	What would be gained by being part of an established vendor network or user group addressing the needs of credentialing and quality, safety, and performance improvement?
Does the system have the capability for data mining reporting or statistical analysis?	Is it more cost-effective alternative to develop such applications in-house or would the facility be better served by purchasing software dedicated to these needs?
Does the system allow for multiple users to access the same programs at the same time?	
Is it an "open operating system" (a system that enables users to operate on a variety of different hardware platforms)?	
Does the system have networking capabilities?	
Will the system display data in graphic form?	
Is there the capability for drill-down analysis of underlying causes of outcomes?	
Does the system allow access to reports via a secure Intranet website within the organization?	

Whether a staff member or manager is trying to establish goals, estimate resources, allocate resources, evaluate a quality, safety or performance process, or monitor a system, access to accurate and timely information is an ongoing requirement of any MIS. The quality of judgments and decisions directly correlates with availability and reliability of data and its synthesis into meaningful, timely information.

Choices for the design or flow of information are so important that they can be a determining factor in the survival of a patient or organization. Although accurate and timely healthcare information provides the rationale for management decisions, this often is not the case. O'Rourke and Bader[37] explain that information often is incomplete, confusing, and not sufficiently relevant to the organization's mission, strategic goals, or customer and stakeholder needs when it is presented in many governing body reports. Organizations clarify the difference between data and information. And, data must be carefully selected, validated, and formatted to make reports useful. This often is easier to mandate than accomplish. However, the goal remains that governing body reports contain only the critical information needed for effective decision-making. Achieving this goal would eliminate healthcare data being presented as a pile of computer printouts and various fragmented reports.

Clinical Information Systems

Designed to support direct patient care processes, automated clinical information systems have great potential for analyzing and improving the quality of patient care. Barriers to healthcare leaders' and healthcare organizations' implementation of MIS include normal resistance to change, the mindset that patient care is best managed by people, lack of exposure to the application of information science and computers in healthcare educational and training programs, and inadequate resources. In 2008, only 9.4% of non-federal acute care hospitals had a basic EHR system; in 2014, that percentage rose to 75.5%, due in large part to the passage of the HITECH Act of 2009.[38] Nearly all reported hospitals had a certified EHR, one that met the technological capability, functionality, and security requirements adopted by the U.S. Department of Health & Human Services, Office of the National Coordinator for Health Information Technology (ONC).[38(p1)]

From a managed care perspective, Rontal[39] outlined the following criteria as being needed for an MIS: appropriate use, place of service, specific procedures, preventive care, cost-effectiveness, patient satisfaction, chronic illness management, access to care, and patient education. Also needed are outcomes of care for mortality, morbidity, complications, readmissions, quality of life, and disability. Clinical information systems often depend on integration with administrative information systems for some data.

Currently, expanded clinical information systems include EHRs and their retrieval systems, computer-assisted medical decision-making for history and physicals and antibiotic selection, clinical application programs for health-risk programs, health maintenance organization encounter data, clinical algorithms, predictive modeling, and simulation. To analyze and interpret outcomes data, EHR-based systems allow healthcare providers to identify positive and negative outcomes so that appropriate action can be taken. Both types of systems serve to focus users on areas of concern regarding outcomes performance. Cost savings occur because energy can be focused on analyzing and controlling deviations from the baseline.

Decision Support Systems

Decision-support data facilitate cross-functional analyses to improve patient care processes and outcomes. Decision support systems address strategic planning functions. Included in this area are

- strategic planning and marketing,
- resource allocation,
- performance evaluation and monitoring,
- product evaluation and services, and
- medical management (e.g., EBP, clinical guidelines and pathways).

By integrating financial and clinical data, there is an opportunity to perform highly sophisticated data analysis involving predictive outcome management. These data help healthcare quality managers and executive leadership evaluate current operations and the feasibility of the development of new product lines and services. Healthcare quality managers coordinate outcome and decision-support data by posing the following pertinent questions:

- What kinds of comparative analyses will be most important?
- With whom can we compare ourselves?
- How can we be sure the data are comparable?
- What do we do when the data reveal significant differences in our outcomes and the outcomes of the peer or benchmark?

Organizations use decision support systems to develop an outcomes information management plan, which includes evaluating performance outcomes measurement systems. Outcomes are viewed in terms of various clinical topics including mortality, complication rates, infection rates, Cesarean section (C-section) rates, fall rates, and other clinical outcomes measurement categories. Categories may or may not reflect the resources (cost, charges, LOS), associated with a given outcome.

Bright and colleagues[40] assessed healthcare process measures and clinical outcome measures associated with commercially and locally developed clinical decision support systems (CDSSs). This study found that a CDSS is effective in improving healthcare process measures across diverse settings. "Effect of Clinical Decision-Support Systems: A Systematic Review" explained the benefits of CDSS and suggested more research is required to promote the use of CDSS and to increase the clinical effectiveness of the systems. However, evidence is limited about the impact on certain outcome measures (i.e., economic and financial). This research expands on the 2012 Agency for Healthcare Research and Quality (AHRQ) evidence report "Enabling Health Care Decisionmaking Through Clinical Decision Support and Knowledge Management," which discussed key features for successful CDSS implementation.

Registries

Registries are part of the bigger picture of health date integration to generate new ideas and drive innovations in individual and population health management. A disease registry is an information tool for tracking the clinical care and outcomes of a defined population. Most disease registries support care management for groups of patients with one or more chronic diseases, such as diabetes, coronary artery disease, or asthma.

Data registries include information about the health status of patients and the healthcare they receive over varying periods of time. Data registries typically focus on patients who share a common reason for receiving healthcare (e.g., specific procedure performed or primary diagnosis). Registries allow healthcare professionals and others to see how patients with different characteristics respond to various treatments. The information is often used to inform patients and their providers about the best course of treatment for a patient. Information from registries is often utilized to compare the performance of healthcare providers regarding their outcomes. Registries are another tool to evaluate the care being delivered and identify opportunities for improvement. The challenge with registries is that some are designed for submission of the information to a national or state database and may have very limited local reporting capabilities.

Patient Data

Healthcare facilities and clinical staff who treat patients are required to maintain adequate medical/health records to serve as a basis for planning care and for communicating about patients' conditions and treatments with other healthcare providers. The medical or health record serves other purposes as well. For example, medical records are reviewed by administrative staff performing quality, utilization, and risk management (RM) functions and by physicians engaged in peer review. Outside organizations also use the medical record for matters relating to payment and accreditation. In malpractice cases, the medical record serves as the major source of evidence about the care the patient received. Information contained in

medical records also is used in retrospective clinical research. If protected health information (PHI) is collected for research, institutional review board approval is needed.

Healthcare organizations have a clear policy about who can access medical records, whether those records are written, computerized, or otherwise maintained. Policy statements make clear what, other than actual medical records, constitutes a portion of the record. For example, with the advent of and frequent use of photography, videotaping of procedures or fetal heart monitoring strips, it is important to address (based on state law and legal advice) whether such media are part of the medical record. Information is often exchanged for the purposes of health treatment and payment.

Organizations are required by federal and state statutes to maintain the security, integrity, and confidentiality of patients' personal data and other information. An organizational plan for health information management (HIM) addresses the critical balance between data sharing and data confidentiality. Although timely, easy access to data and information is required, organizations also must ensure that data and information are safeguarded. The organization is responsible for protecting records against loss, defacement, tampering, and unauthorized use.

Each organization must determine the level of security, integrity, and confidentiality for different categories of information. Access to each category of information must have a functioning mechanism designed to preserve the confidentiality of data and information identified as sensitive or requiring extraordinary means to protect patient privacy. Organizations must follow the standards developed by their accreditation organization (e.g., CARF International [CARF], The Joint Commission, National Committee for Quality Assurance [NCQA], URAC, Community Health Accreditation Partner [CHAP]). Training programs must be in place to educate staff about these requirements and consequences of not adhering to institutional policies. The organization also must identify sanctions for employees who breach confidentiality.

Healthcare organizations must keep confidential all PHI pertaining to medical peer review, quality, safety, and performance improvement, and the monitoring and evaluation of patient care. PHI is defined in the Health Insurance Portability and Accountability Act (HIPAA) of 1996. All records that can be identified by patient or provider are kept secure and confidential so that the patient's and provider's privacy can be maintained. This includes the medical record (in any format, hard copy or electronic) and may also include reports, data abstracts, and supplies. Effective information management security and confidentiality policies and procedures in a healthcare organization contain the following elements:

- identification of people with access to information;
- delineation of specific information to which people have access;

- requirements for people with access to information to keep that information confidential;
- HIPAA requirements for release of health information;
- requirements for removal of medical records (a patient's medical record is the property of the healthcare facility); medical records are removed from the organization jurisdiction and into safekeeping only in accordance with a court order, subpoena, or statute;
- protection of PHI[41];
- handling the root cause analysis (RCA) reporting requirement if the organization is Joint Commission-accredited; and
- mechanisms for securing information against unauthorized intrusion, corruption, and damage.

The elements of PHI in the HIPAA regulations are listed in FIGURE 4-1. Examples of information management confidentiality and security methods include the following:

- Portions of medical records may be stored separately, for example, if the record contains information regarding certain types of psychiatric and addictions treatment.
- The complete medical record would have to be available as needed for medical care and follow-up, utilization

review, or in quality, safety, and performance improvement activities.

- Organizations can restrict access to computer files or portions of computer files with the use of security codes or by restricting certain computer operations to specific devices or people.
- An organization relying on computerized information has an adequate backup plan for each computer application and extensive security firewalls.

The legal basis for confidentiality derives from the physician–patient privilege, set forth by statute in almost all states. This is one of several relationships recognized as special by law. The preservation of confidentiality is viewed as essential to the maintenance of the relationship. The need for confidentiality in the physician–patient relationship gives rise to a legal privilege. This means that, absent a patient authorization or waiver or an overriding law or public policy, medical information about a patient is protected from the process known as *discovery*, through which parties to a lawsuit normally can compel disclosure of relevant evidence. In certain states, the physician–patient privilege is extended beyond physicians to protect the patient's relationship with other healthcare practitioners (e.g., psychologists, clinical social workers, clinical nurse specialists, nurse midwives, nurse anesthetists, and nurse practitioners). Information that is privileged must satisfy the following conditions:

- It must have been communicated in the context of the physician–patient relationship.
- It must have been given with the expectation that it remains confidential.
- It must be necessary for the diagnosis and treatment of the patient.

In understanding the function of the medical record to provide information about the patient's care, treatment, and services and to serve as the method of sharing this information between caregivers, there are monitoring processes to ensure the integrity, accuracy, and completeness of the record and reflect the pertinent clinical documentation. The medical record may be a hard copy document or electronic (or a combination). With legislation demanding that healthcare organizations implement EHRs, the use of electronic records increased.

A written consent is required for an organization to release patient information to anyone outside the organization. A typical release of information form contains the following elements:

- patient name;
- name of individual/organization requesting information;
- reason for release of information;
- anticipated use of information released;
- exact material to be released, including reference to PHI;
- period during which the release of information is valid;

- All geographic subdivisions smaller than a state, including street address, city, county, precinct, zip code, geocodes (in some instances, the first three numbers of a zip code may be collected)
- Birth dates, admission dates, discharge date, date of death, all ages over 89 unless aggregated to 90 or older; only year data may be collected
- Telephone and fax numbers
- Electronic mail addresses, Web universal resource locators (URLs), and Internet protocol (IP) addresses/numbers
- Medical record, health plan beneficiary, and account numbers
- Certificate/license numbers
- Vehicle identification and license plate numbers
- Device identifiers and serial numbers
- Biometric identifiers, including finger and voice prints
- Full-face photographic images and any comparable image
- Any other unique identifying number, characteristic, or code that could be used alone or in combination to identify a person:
  - Patient name
  - Name of individual/organization requesting information
  - Reason for release of information
  - Anticipated use of information released
  - Exact material to be released, including reference to PHI
  - Period during which the release of information is valid
  - Documentation that information is released only to the individual/organization named above
  - Signature and date of the patient or legal representative (as defined by policy/state law).

Figure 4-1 Health Insurance Portability and Accountability Act of 1996. (From U.S. Code of Federal Regulations. www.gpo.gov/fdsys/pkg/CFR-2002-title45-vol1/xml/CFR-2002-title45-vol1-sec164-514. xml; 2002.)

- documentation that information is released only to the individual/organization named above; and
- signature and date of the patient or legal representative (as defined by policy/state law).

Authorized Release of Information

Information from medical records and studies may be released without written authorization from patients to individuals or groups who have need for information for treatment, payment, or healthcare operations. Release of information is regulated by national and state statutes. These people may include the

- representatives from the governing body;
- organization director (chief executive);
- healthcare personnel involved in the care of a patient;
- people responsible for quality, safety, and performance improvement activities; and
- people in the HIM/medical records department.

HIPAA requires healthcare providers (e.g., doctors and health plans) to obtain written authorization from patients to share medical record information. This may be for purposes unrelated to treatment, payment, or routine healthcare operations. The authorization form can originate from the hospital, physician, or health plan, or it can come from the organization requesting the data, such as a researcher, employer, or insurance company. There is no mandated form but a valid form must include several core elements such as the name, purpose of disclosure, and expiration date.

Mechanisms are established to inform patients of utilization management policies and procedures. A common method to inform and obtain consent is to include a statement on the admission consent form or consent for treatment form. Of concern is provision of the reason for hospitalization, such as treatment of substance use disorders, treatment of mental health disorders, HIV/AIDS, and other PHI as identified by HIPAA or special considerations (e.g., Substance Abuse Confidentiality Regulations, 42 CFR Part 2 Revised). These policies must be communicated to the third-party payer as part of the contract review process.

Medical Peer Review

Policies and procedures ensure confidentiality during the medical peer review process. They are consistent with organizational policies and procedures (usually within the HIM/medical records department) and may include completion of a confidentiality statement signed by staff and practitioners involved in the peer review process. The nature of the data contained in a medical record is highly confidential. Policies and procedures clearly define who may have access to a medical record and under what circumstances in accordance with medical staff

bylaws, hospital policy, and applicable laws and regulations. Because of the complexity of those issues, consultation from general counsel regarding national and state statutes is critical. Practitioner profiles can be maintained as a part of the credentials file or in a separate locked file. Most states have laws governing medical peer review and its activities. When applicable, files and their contents and meeting minutes are marked as "Confidential—peer review according to statute X." A simple "CONFIDENTIAL" stamp also will suffice.

Policies and procedures define the circumstances under which copies of medical peer review information are made, such as individual physician request. In accordance with medical staff bylaws and rules and regulations, a mechanism is developed for release of information with specification of contents to be disclosed. This mechanism is in place in response to the need to evaluate a practitioner's competence for appointment and reappointment to other healthcare institutions.

Committee minutes of quality, safety, and performance improvement activities usually are protected under medical peer review statutes. Consequently, maintaining confidentiality of records extends beyond credentialing to the entire quality, safety, and performance improvement program within an organization. Therefore, maintenance of confidentiality of records extends beyond credentialing to the entire QI program across the organization.

A mechanism is developed to track activity on each individual practitioner profile. A log or sign-out sheet attached to each file contains the date of request, reason for request or review, name of person reviewing, and any pertinent notes such as requests for copies of the contents. Policies and procedures define the circumstances under which copies of practitioner files are made, such as individual physician requests. In accordance with medical staff bylaws and rules and regulations, a mechanism is developed for release of information with specification of contents to be disclosed. This mechanism is in response to evaluation of a practitioner's competence for appointment and reappointment to other healthcare institutions.

Study Design

Healthcare quality professionals and their quality, safety, and performance improvement teams prioritize quality and performance improvement activities based on the quantitative and qualitative data available to them. The initiatives with the most opportunity for improvement are tackled first. The initiatives selected usually focus on core processes, high-risk processes, high-risk patients and populations, high-risk medications, or high-risk actions/interventions. The level of risk is based on the potential consequences of injury or harm to patients. Managing high-risk patients and processes will significantly affect morbidity and mortality. Examples of high-risk processes include

- core processes: admission, transfer, discharge;
- high-risk processes: medication delivery/administration, surgery;
- high-risk patients: patients with reduced renal function, patients who are immunocompromised, neonates, patients in critical care units;
- high-risk medications: heparin, insulin, chemotherapy, opiates; and
- high-risk actions/interventions: blood transfusions, use of restraints, extracorporeal circulation.[42]

Key steps to implementing quality, safety, and performance improvement activities are as follows.[42,43] These steps ensure success of the quality, safety, and performance improvement models described earlier.

1. Ensure leadership support and commitment for the quality, safety, and performance improvement initiative.
2. Assess priority and feasibility of initiatives based on risk, resources, leadership support, and organizational strategies and goals.
3. Identify the aim of the initiative and include the topic, process, or problem to be improved (have a good and justified rationale).
4. Convene an interdisciplinary team of content and process experts with all key disciplines as participants (involve all the right people and have a leadership sponsor and champion for the change).
5. Use tools and techniques to analyze processes, best practices, research, and consensus-based evidence for the desired change.
6. Develop the change to be implemented and add timelines and individual accountability for the project.
7. Identify the measure(s) that will demonstrate that the change resulted in improvement and set performance goals.
8. Educate staff on the desired change.
9. Implement and test the change via the redesigned processes.
10. Collect, analyze, and evaluate data on the redesigned process.
11. Make additional changes based on findings and disseminate to all areas.
12. Report and display results to reward staff on improvements.
13. Continue to monitor performance to ensure that the change is sustained.
14. Compare performance internally and externally.
15. Celebrate successes internally and externally.

Today, quality, safety, and performance improvement projects call for perspectives beyond unit-based or team activities regardless of healthcare setting. The use of epidemiologic principles in healthcare quality grows as healthcare reform focuses on improving the health of the population, advancing quality of care for the individual, and containing costs—the Triple Aim[44] and more recently, workforce engagement and workforce safety.[45] This requires looking at the distribution and determinants of health status and disease states. Various methods can be used to carry out quality, safety, and performance improvement projects and epidemiological studies: surveillance, descriptive studies, analytical studies, and systematic review. Outcomes of interest can include injury, disability, and health-related quality of life.[46] Project results can contribute to changing clinical practices and policies at the point of care, developing/validating EBP, implementing population-based interventions, and preventive medicine targeting health conditions (e.g., cancer, cardiovascular disease, obesity, and diabetes).

There are different types of performance measures. Before selecting a measure, one must understand what purpose each measure serves. It is helpful to scan existing quality measures to identify those that are valid and reliable (e.g., the Centers for Medicare & Medicaid Services [CMS], AHRQ, National Quality Forum [NQF], and NCQA). Look for measures vetted through consensus-driven processes involving various stakeholders, including patient and families. The benefit of using an existing and tested measure is there is evidence to support the fidelity in assessing the structure, process, or outcome of care.

- Structure: measures of infrastructure, capacity, systems, and processes (e.g., nurse staffing ratios).
- Process: measures of process performance. They tell whether the parts or steps in the system are performing as planned. This can be "in process" or "end of process" (e.g., timely administration of prophylactic surgical antibiotics).
- Outcome: measures that show results of overall process or system performance (often risk adjusted, e.g., mortality).

Further guidance on evaluating and selecting quality measures is offered by McGlynn[47(p9)] and summarized below.

- Important—is the measure assessing an aspect of efficiency that is important to providers, payers, and policymakers? Has the measure been applied at the level of interest to those planning to use the measure? Is there an opportunity for improvement? Is the measure under the control of the provider or health system?
- Scientifically sound—is the measure reliable and reproducible? Does the measure appear to capture the concept of interest? Is there evidence of face, construct, or predictive validity?
- Feasible—are the data necessary to construct this measure available? Is the cost and burden of measurement reasonable?
- Actionable—are the results interpretable? Can the intended audience use the information to make decisions or act?

McGlynn further explains that the ideal healthcare quality measure does not exist and that tradeoffs must be made when selecting measures for quality assurance, quality control, quality management, or QI.

There are many quality measures that are vetted and readily available for use by healthcare quality professionals to employ in their improvement efforts. For example, clinical quality measures (CQMs) were designed to be measures of process, access, outcome, structure, and patient experience to assess the quality of care provided by physicians and other healthcare professionals for Medicare and Medicaid populations. Implementation of these measures was a requirement for providers to attain both Stage 1 and Stage 2 Meaningful Use. CMS provides annual updates that document specifications for an evolving set of electronic CQMs that can be gathered from EHRs.[48] These measures can help providers and organizations report on quality, advancing care information and improvement activities. Further, CMS Conditions of Participation require a data-driven performance improvement program in hospitals and within the next few years will include all healthcare providers.

The AHRQ developed a suite of measures: AHRQ Quality Indicator modules.[49] Software is available for users to apply AHRQ QI to their organization's administrative data. AHRQ QI modules include prevention, inpatient, patient safety, and pediatric. AHRQ also maintains a National Quality Measures Clearinghouse, a resource of evidence-based quality measures and measure sets. Other efforts funded by AHRQ have also brought a focus on more rigorous quality and performance-based data, analytics, improvement science, and implementation research.

Another major source of quality measures can be found at the NQF. The NQF endorsed over 300 measures that are used in federal public reporting and pay-for-performance programs as well as in private-sector and state programs. Measures that focus specifically on health plans are published by NCQA. NCQA's Healthcare Effectiveness Data and Information Set (HEDIS) are measures used by more than 90% of America's health plans to assess performance on multiple dimensions of care and service. CMS is working with health plans, purchasers, physicians, provider organizations and consumers on a Core Quality Measures Collaborative to identify sets of quality measures that payers have committed to using. The guiding principle of the Collaborative was to develop core measure sets that are meaningful to patients, consumers, and physicians, while reducing variability in measure selection, collection burden, and cost.[50]

In 2014, CMS began the implementation of Cross Setting Measures as mandated by the Impact Act.[51] The Impact Act requires the submission of standardized data by Long-Term Care Hospitals (LTCHs), SNFs, Home Health Agencies (HHAs), and Inpatient Rehabilitation Facilities

(IRFs). Examples of measures include the skin integrity and changes in skin integrity; functional status, cognitive function, and changes in function; transfer of health information and care preferences for transitions between levels of care; and, all-condition risk-adjusted potentially preventable hospital readmissions rates.

AHRQ is instrumental in advancing the study of measures, especially outcomes and the effectiveness of specific treatments. Criteria have been developed for the selection of measures based on attributes[52] that include the following:

- Standardization: Report the same kind of data in the same way.
- Comparability: If appropriate, results are risk adjusted for factors (e.g., age, gender, health status).
- Availability: Data will be available.
- Timeliness: Results will be available when most needed.
- Relevance: Results measure concerns of stakeholders and users.
- Validity: Measures have been tested so they consistently and accurately reflect the measure.
- Experience: Organizations have experience with the measure so it reflects actual performance.
- Stability: The measure is not likely to be removed from use.
- Evaluability: The measure can be evaluated as better or worse.
- Distinguishability: The measure denotes differences between organizations.
- Credibility: The measures can be audited.

Other sources of measures are shown in **TABLE 4-7**.

When measures are developed, or selected for use, there must be a context in which to determine whether the performance of a specific measure is good. To determine the goodness, there are several factors to consider. Does the evidence pre-establish the desired or expected performance level? If not, does any regulatory, accreditation, or payer agencies identify a desired or expected performance level? The use of comparative data helps set desired targets or goals and provides a method by which to determine how well the organization is performing compared with similar organizations, competitors, best in the industry, and best in class.

To support quality, safety, and performance improvement and other administrative functions, many organizations have moved in the direction of building large data warehouses that include information from all systems in the organization. For example, these data warehouses contain clinical, operational, financial, and human resources data. The data warehouses are supported by hardware (e.g., servers) and database software that combines the information into integrated data tables. The ability to integrate these data allows for robust reporting and analyses.

Data collection can be both expensive and time-consuming for any organization. Just enough data are collected; avoid

Table 4-7 Sources of Measures

Type	Examples of Measure Sources
Administrative data	Volume, admissions Discharges Length of stay (LOS) Billing data Uniform Hospital Discharge Data Set (UHDDS)
Medical records	Clinical care Medication use Surgery and procedural data
Patient surveys	Consumer Assessment of Healthcare Providers and Systems (CAHPS)
Standardized clinical data sets	Performance Measurement Reporting [The Joint Commission] (ORYX®) Outcome and Assessment Information Set (OASIS) National Surgical Quality Improvement Program (NSQIP) Healthcare Effectiveness Data and Information Set (HEDIS) AHRQ (Inpatient Quality Indicators, Patient Safety Indicators, Pediatric Quality Indicators) National Hospital Quality Measures National Database of Nursing Quality Indicators (NDNQI)
Other	Culture of safety surveys Feedback from patients and families Grievance and complaints Employee engagement surveys Leapfrog survey National Quality Forum

over-measurement in terms of both number of measures and frequency of measurement and analysis. Healthcare quality professionals can prevent duplicate data collection efforts among different groups and departments. It is preferable to pilot a new data collection process, even if it is new only to the organization. The development of a comprehensive data collection plan for improvement activities can leverage the warehouse and conserve resources. Planning includes the following steps:

- Determine the who, what, when, where, why, and how.
- Structure the design.
- Choose and develop the sampling method.
- Determine and conduct the necessary training.
- Delegate responsibilities and communicate timelines.

- Facilitate interdepartmental/cross-functional coordination.
- Forecast the budget requirements.
- Conduct pilot procedures for the forms and the data collection process.

Connected to the data warehouse is usually at least one business intelligence (BI) tool that allows end users, including quality, safety, and performance improvement staff, to create their own reports. The BI tools have the capability to filter data by diagnosis, location, or provider and produce sophisticated tables, graphs, and analyses. These tools also allow for trending over time and comparisons of different groups. Utilizing the BI tool enables the capability to analyze baseline information before a QI project starts, look at trends over time, and measure the impact of improve efforts. Further, analytical tools, such as R, SAS, or SPSS can be used on the data available in the warehouse to test for significant changes, control for varying patient characteristics, and build predictive models.

See *Performance and Process Improvement* and *Patient Safety* for more information on evaluation and measures.

Data Types

There are two general types of data: measurement/continuous and count/categorical. Ordinal data are a form of categorical data. Methods of sampling, data collection, and analysis are different for each type or level of data. This distinction is critical because quality, safety, and performance improvement work involves both types of data and their associated statistics. It is one of the most significant sources of confusion for people new to performance improvement and data analysis. Data levels are *categorical* (nominal and ordinal) and *continuous* (interval and ratio).

Categorical

Nominal. Nominal data are also called *count*, *discrete*, or *qualitative data*. In statistical process control (SPC) these are known as *attributes data*. Binary data are categorical data with only two possibilities (e.g., gender). Numerical values can be assigned to each category as a label to facilitate data analysis, but this is purely arbitrary with no quantitative value. There is no order to these data. Examples of nominal scale data are shown in **TABLE 4-8**.

Ordinal. For this type of data, characteristics are put into categories and are rank-ordered. Assignment to categories is not arbitrary. Examples of ordinal scale data are shown in **TABLE 4-9**.

Continuous. Continuous or "measured" data are assigned scales that theoretically have no gaps. The SPC term for this

Table 4-8 Examples of Nominal Variables

Nominal Variable	Values
Surgical patients	Preoperative
	Postoperative
Gender	Male
	Female
Patient education	Attended video session
	Did not attend video session

is *variables data*. There are two subtypes of continuous data: interval and ratio.

- *Interval.* For interval-level data, the distance between each point is equal and there is no true zero (e.g., the values on a Fahrenheit thermometer).
- *Ratio.* For ratio-level data, the distance between each point is equal and there is a true zero (e.g., height and weight).

Measurement/continuous data often can be converted to count/categorical data. For example, the number of pounds lost by a patient undergoing hemodialysis during treatment in relationship to his or her desired or "dry weight" is measurement data. If Mr. Jones was admitted at 170 lb and was discharged at his dry weight of 165 lb, then he measured a 5-lb weight loss. If the nurse manager wanted to know the number of patients finishing their treatments at their "dry weight" for the entire day, then this information would be an example of count data and would be converted into "yes/no" format.

Table 4-9 Examples of Ordinal Variables

Ordinal Variable	Values
Nursing staff rank	1. Nurse Level 1 2. Nurse Level II 3. Nurse Level III
Education	1. Diploma/Associate Degree 2. BS 3. MS 4. PhD/DNSc/DNP
Attitude toward research (Likert scale)	1. Strongly agree 2. Agree 3. Neutral 4. Disagree 5. Strongly disagree

A critical issue is whether the right data are measured or counted. A common criticism of quality, safety, and performance improvement activities is that readily available data, such as patient visits, deaths, infections, falls, cost, and laboratory tests, are analyzed for improvement specifically because the data are easy to retrieve.

Statistical Power

Categorical data are the least powerful statistically, and continuous data have the most power. The practical meaning of this when comparing patient outcomes after process change is that fewer data points (and fewer subjects) are needed if data in continuous form are collected, if the researcher has a choice. For example, when dealing with blood pressure, a healthcare quality manager might collect the data by categorizing subjects as either hypertensive or non-hypertensive, or by recording the measured levels of systolic and diastolic pressure. The latter form is more powerful and allows more flexibility in data analysis.

When a quality, safety, and performance improvement project is designed, each step must be planned and accountability assigned. Each organization can adopt an improvement model that facilitates performance improvement and is in alignment with its mission, vision, core values, goals, and strategic plan (for more information, see *Organizational Leadership* and *Performance and Process Improvement*).

Sampling Design

A *population* (*N*) is the total aggregate or group (e.g., all cases that meet a designated set of criteria for practitioners, all patients who died at a particular hospital, or all registered nurses with a tenure of 10 years or longer).

Sampling makes research more feasible because it allows researchers to sample a portion of the population to represent the entire population (*n*). A sample usually is selected from the accessible population; that is, the population that is available.

Sampling has several primary purposes, including providing a logical way of making statements about a larger group based on a smaller group and allowing researchers to make inferences or generalize from the sample to the population if the selection process was random and systematic (i.e., unbiased).

Types of Sampling

There are different methods that might be used to create a sample. Generally, they are grouped into one of two categories described below: probability sampling and nonprobability sampling.

Probability. Probability sampling requires every element in the population to have an equal or random chance of being selected for inclusion in the sample. The following are subsets of probability sampling:

- **Simple random sampling.** Everyone in the sampling frame (all subjects in the population) has an equal chance of being chosen (e.g., pulling a name out of a hat containing all possible names).
- **Systematic sampling.** After randomly selecting the first case, this method involves drawing every nth element from a population. For example, picking every third name from a list of possible names.
- **Stratified random sampling.** A subpopulation is a *stratum*, and *strata* are two or more homogeneous subpopulations. After the population is divided into strata, each member of a stratum has an equal probability of being selected. Examples of strata include sex, ethnicity, patients with certain diseases, or patients living in certain parts of the country.
- **Cluster sampling.** This method requires that the population be divided into groups, or clusters. For example, if a researcher is studying medical students, they may not have individual names but may have a list of medical schools in the area. The sample may be randomly derived from this list of medical schools.

Nonprobability. Nonprobability sampling provides no way of estimating the probability that each element will be included in the sample. When this approach is used, the results will be representative of the sample only and cannot be generalized to the available population. The following are subsets of nonprobability sampling:

- **Convenience sampling.** This approach allows the use of any available group of subjects. Because of the lack of randomization in this sampling method, subjects may be atypical in some way. Sending a survey to a list of members of an elder organization may not reflect the opinions of all elders, for example. Convenience sampling may include all patients at an organization who are undergoing a certain procedure over a 12-month period. Selection bias may be present in all convenience sampling because the selected subjects may not accurately reflect the population of interest.
- **Snowball sampling.** This is a subtype of convenience sampling. This method involves subjects suggesting other subjects for inclusion in the study so the sampling process gains momentum. With this type of sampling, subjects are recruited who are difficult to identify but are known to others because of an informal network.
- **Purposive or judgment sampling.** This method selects a group or groups based on certain criteria. This method is subjective, and the researcher uses their judgment to decide who is representative of the population. Using a group of nurses, because the researcher believes the group represents a cross-section of women, is an example of this type of sampling.
- **Expert sampling.** This is a type of purposive sampling that involves selecting experts in each area because of their access to the information relevant to the study. Expert sampling is used in the Delphi technique, in which several rounds of questionnaires are distributed on a selected topic and sent to experts to elicit their responses and then sent out again after the initial data analysis. The goal is to achieve rapid group consensus. A conference planning team serves as an example if it uses the Delphi method to identify potential program content that may be of interest to those in the same professions for an upcoming conference.
- **Quota sampling.** In this type of sampling, the researcher makes a judgment decision about the best type of sample for the investigation. That is, the researcher pre-specifies characteristics of the sample to increase its representativeness. The researcher identifies strata of the population and determines the proportions of elements needed from various segments of the population. Stratification may be based on any demographic, such as age or ethnicity.

Sample Size

Many factors may influence the determination of sample size, such as research purpose, design, level of confidence desired, anticipated degree of difference between study groups, and size of the population. Depending on these factors, a small or large sample size may be appropriate. However, except for case studies, the larger the sample, the more valid and accurate the study because a larger sample size is more likely to represent the population. The larger the sample, the smaller the sample error of the mean, which is a measure of fluctuation of a statistic from one sample to another drawn from the same population. Also, as the actual difference between study groups gets smaller, the size of the sample required to detect the difference gets larger. Outcomes that are measured on a continuous scale or using repeated measures require fewer subjects than do categorical outcomes. Using too large a sample to answer a research question is a waste of time and resources.

Variation

Use of an SPC chart clarifies and interprets a function or process. The performance of functions or processes varies over time. This variation is expected and predictable and is referred to as *random* or *common-cause variation*. A process is said to be "in control" if the variation is within the computed upper and lower limits and no trends are evident. There is no need to act if a process is in control. *Special-cause variation* occurs when activity falls outside the control limits or there is an obvious nonrandom pattern around the central line. This type of variation is interpreted as a trend and investigated.

Trends

When a trend is identified for a measure in an unanticipated direction, an investigation is initiated to determine the cause (e.g., RCA). For example, if the 30-day readmission rate is climbing 1% every month for a 6-month period there might be change in practice that needs to be addressed. In this case, an inter-professional team may be convened to further analyze and improve the process that is causing the increase. The team uses performance improvement principles and tools (e.g., histograms, flowcharts, Pareto charts, cause-and-effect diagrams, run charts; for more information, see *Performance and Process Improvement*). After thorough analysis of the process, the team selects and implements appropriate corrective measures.

Comparison Groups

One of the biggest challenges in making conclusions in the evaluation of QI interventions is the lack on "true" comparison group. While looking for changes over time is useful, there is more value in comparing to a group that did not get the intervention (e.g., change in process). Since random assignment to different groups is usually not possible, selecting a comparison group is based on convenience. For example, it might be possible to test a new standard of practice (i.e., intervention) to reduce pressure ulcers on several nursing units while maintaining the current practice on other nursing units (i.e., control). The problem is the patients on the units might not be the same. One approach to dealing with this problem is to use propensity score matching.[53] *Propensity score matching* is a multivariate approach to pairing up people with the same characteristics in the intervention and control groups to eliminate potential impact of variation between the groups that are not equal. Propensity score matching is an effective approach to equating groups and a tool that quality, safety, and performance improvement teams consider when analyzing data.

Measurement Tools

Instruments are the devices that healthcare quality professionals and researchers use to obtain and record data received from the subjects. These instruments can include questionnaires, surveys, rating scales, interview transcripts, and the like. It is critical to use the most credible tools possible (those with proven reliability and validity).

Reliability

Reliability is the extent to which an experiment, test, or measuring procedure yields the same results on repeated trials. For example, a scale that measures a person's weight as 110 lb one minute and then yields a reading of 160 lb a minute later would be considered unreliable and not capable of meeting the standards for accuracy or consistency.

- **Reliability coefficient.** The stability of an instrument is derived through procedures referred to as *test–retest reliability*. This is done by administering the test to a sample of people on two occasions and then comparing the scores obtained. The comparison results in a reliability coefficient, which is the numerical index of the test's reliability. The closer the coefficient is to 1.0, the more reliable the tool. In general, reliability coefficients of ≥0.70 are considered acceptable, although ≥0.80 is desired. The reliability coefficient can be determined by evaluating the internal consistency of a measure. This refers to the degree to which the subparts of an instrument are all measuring the same attribute or dimension. The "split-half" technique is one of the oldest methods for assessing internal consistency of an instrument and can be done by hand. It correlates scores on half of the measure with scores on the other half. The concept of *reliability by equivalence* is established by comparing scores from the various versions of the instrument that have been developed (e.g., parallel forms or alternate forms of a test). This concept is used to compare different translations of a measurement tool or different forms of the Certified Professional in Healthcare Quality (CPHQ) examination, for example.
- **Interrater reliability.** This concept refers to the degree to which two raters, operating independently, assign the same ratings in the context of observational research or in coding qualitative materials. The monitoring of the accuracy of a patient acuity system entails interrater reliability. The staff that monitors the system must be able to assign the same classification to the same patient to ensure reliability of their monitoring. Interrater reliability frequently is reported as a degree of concordance, or Cohen's kappa.

Validity

Validity is the degree to which an instrument measures what it is intended to measure. Validity usually is more difficult to establish than reliability. The validity and reliability of an instrument are not wholly independent of each other. An instrument that is not reliable cannot possibly be valid. However, an instrument that is reliable does not have to have validity. For example, a thermometer is a reliable instrument, but it is not valid for measuring height.

- **Content (face) validity.** This is the degree to which the instrument adequately represents the universe of content. Content validity, although necessary, is not a sufficient indication that the instrument measures what it is intended to measure. For example, a panel of rehabilitation specialists evaluated the functional independence measure (FIM™) tool and identified that it measured the key aspects of functional independence. On the other hand, a survey designed to measure patient satisfaction with their primary care provider would be considered inadequate in terms of content validity if it failed to cover the major dimensions of access, waiting time, practitioner–patient interaction, or engagement. Content validity includes judgments by experts or respondents about the degree to which a test appears to measure the relevant construct.
- **Construct validity.** This concept refers to the degree to which an instrument measures the theoretical construct or trait that it was designed to measure. For example, severity-adjustment scales are tools for measuring staffing needs. Risk-adjustment scales are tools for predicting the probability of outcomes such as morbidity and mortality. If a previously used satisfaction tool had demonstrated validity, a new, abbreviated tool can be compared to the "old" tool to determine whether the new tool has construct validity. Similarly, two functional status health outcome measures could be compared, such as the SF-36 and SF-12 instruments.
- **Criterion-related validity.** This concept refers to the extent that the score on an instrument can be related to a criterion (the behavior that the instrument is supposed to predict). Criterion-related validity can be either predictive or concurrent, depending on when the criterion variable is measured. If the criterion variable is obtained at the same time as the measurement under study, *concurrent validity* is assessed. If the criterion measure is obtained at some future time (after the predictor instrument was used), *predictive validity* is assessed. A patient acuity system has criterion-related validity because it predicts staffing needs (skill mix and number of staff required).

Statistical Techniques

The discussion of statistical techniques that follows is in no way a complete account of each topic. Other sources for more information on the various statistical techniques, including Hansen's CAN'T MISS series, are included in Suggested Reading & Online Resources at the end of this section.

Measures of Central Tendency

Measures of central tendency are statistical indexes that describe where a set of scores or values of a distribution cluster. *Central* refers to the middle value, and *tendency* refers to the general trend of the numbers. A healthcare quality manager or researcher might ask questions relating to central tendency when answering queries such as, "What is the average LOS for patients with chronic obstructive pulmonary disease?" or "What is the Apgar score of most infants born in the new birthing suites?" The three most common measures of central tendency are the mean, the median, and the mode. The type and distribution of the data determine which measures of central tendency (and spread) are most appropriate.

Mean. The *mean* (M) of a set of measurements is the sum of all scores or values divided by the total number of scores. The mean is also known as the average.

Example: If five infants had Apgar scores of 7, 8, 8, 9, and 8, the sum of the values is calculated, and then divided by the total number of infants: $7 + 8 + 8 + 9 + 8 = 40$; $40 \div 5 = 8$; therefore, 8 is the mean.

The mean is the most commonly used of all the measures of central tendency, but it is the most sensitive to extreme scores. In the example given above, if one infant was severely depressed at the time of Apgar scoring and was given a value of 1 instead of 9, the mean then would be 6.4 rather than 8. In this case, the mean is no longer representative of the entire group because it was substantially lowered by just *one* score. The median, described below would be a better statistic to use.

It is appropriate to compute the mean for interval or ratio data when variables can be added and the values show a bell-shaped or normal distribution. The mean also can be used with ordinal variables that have an approximately normal distribution.

Median. The *median* is the measure of central tendency that corresponds to the middle score; that is, the point on a numerical scale above which and below which 50% of the cases fall. To determine the median of data, first arrange the values in rank order. If the total of values is odd, count up (or down) to the middle value. If there are several identical values clustered at the middle, the median is that value. If the total number of values is even, compute the mean of the two middle values.

Example: Consider the following set of values: 2 2 2 3 4 5 6 6 8 9. The median for this set of numbers is 4.5, which is the value that divides the set exactly in half. Note that an important characteristic of the median is that the calculation does not consider the quantitative values of the individual scores. An example of this notion can be demonstrated in the sample above. If the last value of 9 were increased to the value 84, the median would remain the same because it does not enter the computation of the median; only the number of values and the values near the midpoint of the distribution enter the computation. The median, consequently, is not sensitive to extreme scores or statistical outliers. It is appropriate to compute the median for ordinal, interval, or ratio data, but not for nominal data.

Mode. The *mode* is the score or value that occurs most frequently in a distribution of scores. Of the three measures of central tendency, the mode is the easiest to determine; simply determine which value occurs most often in the data set.

Example: Look at the following distribution of numbers: 30 31 31 32 33 33 33 33 33 34 35 36. It is easy to determine that the mode is 33; the value of 33 appears five times, a higher frequency than for any other number. An easy way to determine the mode is by using a statistical package to run descriptive data frequencies and/or a stem-and-leaf plot. In research studies, the mode is seldom the only measure of central tendency reported. Modes are viewed as a quick and easy method to determine an "average," but they tend to be unstable. This instability means that the modes tend to fluctuate widely from sample to sample, even when drawn from the same population. Thus, the mode is reported infrequently, except when used as a descriptor for "typical" values on nominal data. For example, a research report may describe the sample population demographic data as follows: "The typical respondent was a Hispanic man who was married."

Measures of Variability

In the preceding section the purpose of measuring the central tendencies of data was to describe the ways subjects or cases group together. In contrast, *variability* looks at the dispersion, or how the measures are spread out. Variability further may be defined as the degree to which values on a set of scores differ. For example, it is expected that there is greater variability of age within a hospital than within a nursing home or pediatric intensive care unit. Measures of variability are interpreted as distances on a scale of values, which are unlike averages that are points representing a central value.

The three measures of variability that are presented in this review are the range, SD, and interpercentile measures.

Range. The *range* is the difference between the highest and lowest values in a distribution of scores. Although it indicates the distance on the score scale between the lowest and highest values, the range is best reported as the values themselves and not as the distance between the values. Range offers advantages: It is a quick estimate of variability and it provides information about the two endpoints of a distribution. Disadvantages of range include its instability because it is based on only two scores: its tendency to increase with sample size, and its sensitivity to extreme values.

Example: Test scores for students range from 98 to 60. The range is 98 minus 60, or 38. When the range is reported in research findings, it normally would be written as a maximum and a minimum, without the subtracted value.

Standard Deviation. The *SD*, an average of the deviations from the mean, is the most frequently used statistic for measuring the degree of variability in a set of scores. Standard refers to the fact that the deviation indicates a group's average spread of scores or values around their mean; deviation indicates how much each score is scattered from the mean. The larger the spread of a distribution, the greater the dispersion or variability from the mean; consequently, the SD will be a larger value and is said to be heterogeneous. The more the values cluster around the mean, the smaller the amount of variability or deviation and the more homogeneous the group is said to be and it will have a smaller SD. The standard bell curve illustrates this measure of variability (FIG. 4-2). A histogram can be used to display data distribution and to determine if data are normally distributed. When computing the SD, as with the mean, all the scores or values in a distribution are taken into consideration. Use of the SD is most appropriate with normally distributed interval or ratio scale data. SDs (and means) also may be calculated for normally distributed values from a broad ordinal scale. SDs can be calculated by hand or with statistical software.

Example: The researcher may compare coping-scale scores for two groups of patients, with each group having a different

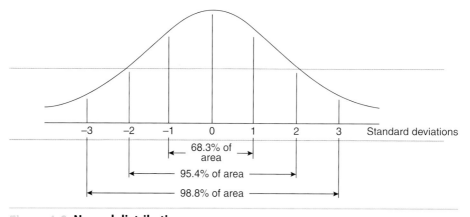

Figure 4-2 **Normal distribution.**

ethnic background. Although each distribution demonstrated a mean score of 30, the SDs were computed at 3 and 8, respectively. The investigator could conclude that although the means were alike, one sample was more homogeneous (or had less variance) in its coping skills.

Interpercentile Measures. Although there are several interpercentile measures of variability, the most common is the *interquartile range*, a stable measure of variability based on excluding extreme scores and using only middle cases. The interquartile range is more stable than the range and is determined by lining up the measures in order of size and then dividing the array into quarters. The range of scores that includes the middle 50% of the scores is the interquartile range; that is, the range between scores comprising the lowest quartile, or quarter, and the highest quartile. The interquartile range demonstrates how the middle 50% of the distribution is scattered. The first quartile ends at the 25th percentile. Interquartile range values often are presented in "box plots."

Example: Growth charts are one of the most commonly used interpercentile measures. Normal growth is represented by measurements between the 25th and 75th percentiles on the National Center for Health Statistics growth charts.

Example: Clinical pathways are developed based on the interquartile range of the designated population. Paths can be designed around the average patient or those in the middle quartiles.

Statistical Tests

Significance tests are categorized as either *parametric* or *nonparametric*. Parametric tests are used with data measured on a continuous scale (i.e., interval or ratio data, which also are known as variables data). Nonparametric tests are used with categorical (attributes) data and used with ordinal data, especially if the ordinal categories have a small range of possible values or a non-normal distribution. **TABLE 4-10** summarizes statistical options for each type of data and the best types of statistical tests for healthcare studies.

Table 4-10 Statistical Options for Different Data Types

	Categorical	Ordinal	Continuous
	Statistical process control (SPC): "attribute," nominal, discrete, binary (0/1)	*Ordinal categorical*	*SPC: "variables" measured*
Examples	Gender, vital status, ethnicity	Age in categories, functional independence measure (FIM) items, patient satisfaction	Age, FIM total, charges, LOS
Usually reported as	Percentage in each category	Percentage in each category (but not always)	Mean, median, min, max, percentiles
Usual statistical test of differences between groups	Chi square (χ^2)	χ^2 for most scales; *t*-tests may be appropriate (>6 levels) if there is a broad scale between groups and data are normally distributed	*t*-Tests
Control chart[a]	p if rate > 1/100 u if 1,000 < rate <1/100 c if rate < 1/1,000	Depends on scale, data distribution, and whether regrouped	p charts, c charts, x bar and R charts
Rules of thumb for sample sizes per plotted point	For p charts; ± 40 common events; up to 200 for rarer events	(see p chart rules)	Calculate mean based on 2–10 randomly selected values (3–4 optimal)
Usual regression technique[b]	Logistic	Logistic (if regrouped as 0/1 outcome)	"Ordinary least squares"

[a]Most commonly used type; lists not exhaustive
[b]Regression is the preferred method for simultaneous control of numerous "demographic" variables (e.g., gender, age, ethnicity, severity) and is most commonly used in research settings. To control for the influence of a single demographic variable, consider stratifying the analysis by levels of that demographic variable.

Parametric Tests. *Parametric tests are based on assumptions about the distribution of the underlying population from which the sample was taken. The most common parametric assumption is that data are approximately normally distributed.*[54]

t-Test. The *t*-test assesses whether the means of two groups are statistically different from each other. When determining whether the difference between two group means is significant, a distinction must be made regarding the two groups. The two groups may be independent; that is, a control group and an experimental group, or they can be dependent, wherein a single group yields pretreatment and posttreatment scores.

Example: A healthcare quality manager wants to test the effect of a special educational program on departmental heads' attitudes toward using graphical or visual displays of data in their performance improvement team meeting. Ten of the 20 department heads are randomly assigned to an experiment group, which will be exposed to videos, discussion groups, and lectures on the use of the basic quality control tools and management and planning tools. The remaining 10 department heads comprise the control group, which will not receive special instruction on using the tools. At the end of the experiment, both groups are administered a scale measuring attitudes toward using these tools. The two-sample independent *t*-test helps the researcher determine if there was a significant statistical difference between the two groups (i.e., whether any difference was due to chance).

Alternatively, if all 20 department heads received the training with pre- and post-training testing scores, the statistical significance of any changes in average scores would be measured using a "paired sample" *t*-test.

Regression Analysis. Regression analysis is based on statistical correlations, or associations among variables. A correlation between two variables is used to evaluate the usefulness of a prediction equation. If this correlation were perfect (i.e., $r = 1$ or $r = -1$), it would be possible to make a perfect prediction about the score on one variable given the score on the other variable. Unfortunately, this is never the case because there never are perfect correlations; consequently, it never is possible to make perfect predictions. The higher the correlation between variables, the more accurate the degree of prediction. If there were no correlation between two variables (i.e., $r = 0$), knowing the score of one would not help to estimate the score on the other. In simple linear regression, one variable (x) is used to predict a second variable (y). For example, simple regression can be used to predict weight based on height or to predict response to a diabetes management program. Regression analysis is performed with the intent to make predictions about phenomena. The ability to make accurate predictions has substantial implications in the healthcare industry.

Multiple Regression Analysis. Multiple regression analysis estimates the effects of two or more independent variables (x) on a dependent measure (y). For example, the objective may be to predict intravenous (IV) site infiltration (y) based on predictors (x), which may include osmolarity of the IV solution and addition of an irritating medication, such as potassium, to the IV.

Nonparametric Tests. *One might define nonparametric statistical procedures as a class of statistical procedures that do not rely on assumptions about the shape or form of the probability distribution from which the data were drawn.*[54]

Chi-Square (χ^2) Tests and Categorical (Attributes) Data. Much of the data collected by healthcare quality professionals is counted, not measured. Being counted (e.g., 15 male and 30 female patients in the clinic today) means that many arithmetic operations do not apply (it is not possible to calculate the average gender of patients). But it certainly is possible to describe the ratio of the counts (e.g., there were twice as many woman as men in the clinic today) or to compare proportions with counted data (50% of male vs. 75% of female patients, came for their appointments today). The chi-square test (χ^2) measures the statistical significance of a difference in proportions and is the most commonly reported statistical test in the medical literature. It is the easiest statistical test to calculate manually (see the CAN'T MISS series). It is a statistical test commonly used to compare observed data with data that one would expect to obtain per a specific hypothesis.

Example: Using the previously furnished appointment data, 15 of 30 men (50%) with appointments failed to keep them, while only 10 of 40 women (25%) failed to appear. The referent rate of missed appointments in men would be 0.5/0.25 = 2 (i.e., men are twice as likely to not show up as women). While that may or may not fit the hypothesis about men's behavior in this situation, the statistical question is whether this 25% difference in the proportion of no-shows might have happened by chance sampling (in this case, scheduling might be causing the difference). The null hypothesis is that men and women fail to show up for appointments at about the same rate (i.e., rate = 1). Thus, χ^2 tests indicate the likelihood of noting a twofold difference in no-shows between the groups if in fact men and women fail to keep their appointments at the same rate. The actual χ^2 value (test statistic) for these data is 5.84, which corresponds to a statistical significance (p) value of less than 0.02, meaning fewer than 2 out of every 100 days would result in a schedule with which men were twice as likely to not show up. In other words, there is a 2% probability that the difference in no-shows by gender is due to chance, but there is a 98% probability the difference is due to some other factor or factors.

Tests of Significance. Tests for statistical significance are used to determine the probability that a relationship between two variables is just a chance occurrence. Discussed here are confidence interval (CI) and level of significance.

Confidence Interval. A *CI* provides a range of possible values around a sample estimate (a mean, proportion, or ratio) that is calculated from data. CIs commonly are used when comparing groups, but they also have other applications. They reflect the uncertainty that always is present when working with samples of subjects. The sample estimate(s) are a best guess about the true value of interest. For example, continuing the missed appointment example above, it is estimated that 50% of men miss their appointments, but the true value may be higher or lower. There is similar uncertainty about the true proportion of women who miss their appointments and about the ratio of the men's and women's proportions. Using the measure of variation from a sample, it is possible to construct a CI that, with a stated level of probability, holds the true value of interest.

Example*:* It was observed (hypothetically) that men are twice as likely to miss their appointments as women. The 95% CI around the referent rate of 2 is (1.27 to 3.13), meaning there is 95% certainty that men are between 1.27 and 3.13 times more likely to miss their appointment. A lower level of confidence would include a narrower range of values. For example, the 90% CI around the referent rate for the appointment data would be (1.44 to 2.77).

Level of Significance. The level of significance (p) gives the probability of observing a difference as large as the one found in a study when, in fact, there is no true difference between the groups (i.e., when the null hypothesis is true). A small p value indicates a small chance that the null hypothesis is true and favors the alternative hypothesis that there is a significance between the two groups. Historically, when the p value is less than 0.05, healthcare quality managers and researchers declared their results statistically significant and "rejected the null hypothesis."

Example*:* The p value for the ratio of missed appointment rates above was 0.02, so it was concluded that there was little evidence that men and women had the same rate of missed appointments ("the null") and determined that men probably had a higher rate of missed appointments. How much higher? There is 95% confidence that the odds ratio lies between 1.27 and 3.13 times more likely to miss their appointments (see the CI example above). Note that if the p value had been >0.05, the 95% CI would have included 1.0, determining that there was no difference in the proportions of men and women who miss their appointments.

Described next are decision-making methods and tools, SPC, and types of variation, and examples of these tools.

Methods and Tools

The management of data, analysis of information, and management through knowledge are necessary to change and improve healthcare organizations. For the tools to be successful, a strong team facilitator is necessary. Many tools are useful in the analysis of current processes and the design of new processes; this discussion is not meant to be all-inclusive. Various charts and diagrams can be used by healthcare professionals when considering the data collected to make sense of them. These tools typically represent the data in a visual way to assist stakeholders in making decisions about improvement.

Activity Network Diagram

This tool also is known as an *arrow diagram* (FIG. 4-3) (in industry it also is called the program evaluation and review technique or a critical path method chart). In the arrow diagram, arrows connect articles (nodes) that represent a start and finish of activities. The arrows themselves represent the activities to be completed. Using the arrow diagram, a sequence of events is depicted. It is useful when several simultaneous paths must be coordinated.

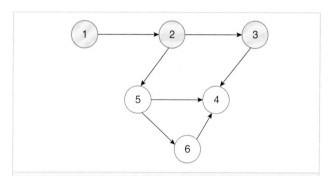

How to construct

1. List all the necessary tasks, one per card, to complete a project from start to finish.
2. Use the cards to sequence the activities for each path.
3. Identify the places in the paths where there are connections with other paths. These places identify parts of one path that cannot be initiated until a point in another path is reached.
4. Determine the time duration for each task.
5. Calculate the shortest possible time to complete the project.
6. Review and revise the diagram as needed.

When to use

- When a task is complex or crucial to an organization
- When simultaneous implementation of several paths must be coordinated

Figure 4-3 Activity network diagram.

Stratification Chart

Stratification charts (FIG. 4-4) are designed to show where a problem does and does not occur or to demonstrate underlying patterns. One such chart is called the is/is-not matrix.

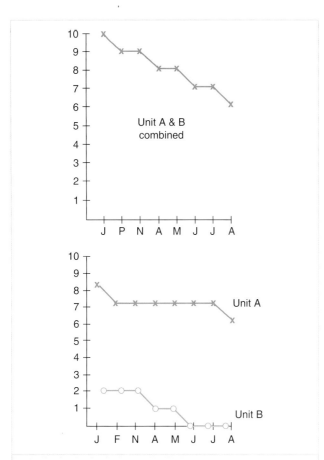

How to construct

1. Examine the process to identify characteristics that could lead to biases and systematic differences in your results.
2. Enter data onto data collection forms (such as day of week or month, shifts or workers).
3. Look for patterns related to time and sequence.

Alternate tool: Is/is-not matrix

1. Enter data (such as where, when, what kind or how much, and who) onto a matrix in the column on the left.
2. Across the top of the matrix list three columns: Is (when does something occur); Is Not (when does something not occur); and Therefore (what might explain the pattern of occurrence).
3. Fill in the boxes.

When to use

- Before data collection to know what difference or patterns to look for
- After data collection to determine which factors affected the results

Figure 4-4 Stratification charts.

This matrix is used to organize knowledge and information so that patterns can be identified.

Histogram or Bar Chart

Before further analyzing a data set, the distribution of values for each of the variables is reviewed (FIG. 4-5). The optimal tool for reviewing a distribution depends on the amount of information. A bar chart with a separate bar for each value may be used when data are sparse (e.g., fewer than 12 values), but, as the data increase, it becomes

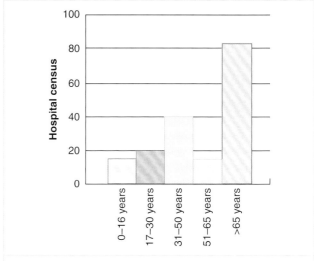

How to construct

1. Accumulate at least 25 data points (to give them at least five bars).
2. Rank the data points from the smallest to the largest.
3. Calculate the range of the data by subtracting the smallest value from the largest.
4. Estimate the number of bars to be displayed (equals the square root of the number of data points).
5. Determine the width of the bars by dividing the range by the calculated number of bars, rounding the numbers as necessary.
6. Draw the vertical axis to show the number of times a value of the data falls with each bar.
7. Draw the horizontal axis to show the number of times a value of the data falls with each bar.
8. At the left side, draw bars with heights equal to the number of times the data fall within the bounds of each bar.
9. Label the histogram and describe the source, data, and author.

When to use

- Show the data distribution or spread
- Show whether the data are symmetric shape (approximately the same on both sides) or skewed (right or left)
- Show whether there are extreme data values (outliers)

Figure 4-5 Histogram or bar chart.

necessary to organize and summarize them. *Histograms* are a specialized type of bar graph used to summarize groups of data. It is the most commonly used frequency distribution tool that presents the measurement scale of values along the *x* axis (each bar is equal-sized interval) and the frequency scale along the *y* axis (counts or percentages). Plotting the frequency of each interval reveals the pattern of the data, showing their center and spread (including outliers) and whether there is symmetry or skew. This is important information because it may reveal problems in the data and may influence the choice of measure of central tendency and spread.

An important distinction must be made regarding bar charts and histograms. With a bar chart, the *x* axis consists of discrete categories (each bar is a separate group). An example of this would be plotting systolic blood pressure >140 by ethnic group. The height of the bar represents the frequency of elevated blood pressure for each 1 mm Hg change in each ethnic group. A histogram's *x* axis is divided into categories using equally sized ranges of values along the axis. The variable is measured on a continuous scale, and the bars are not separated by gaps. To continue with the systolic blood pressure example, the groupings of the *x* axis could be equal-sized, with ranges defined, for example, as 90 to 99, 100 to 119, or 120 to 129 mmHg. Histograms can be constructed manually or automatically with various statistical software programs.

Pie Chart

Pie charts (FIG. 4-6) are useful for understanding all the responses on a measure, usually expressed as percentages. For example, if a home care agency wanted to visualize the discharge disposition of patients when they leave care the agency would count the number staying home with no care, referred to an SNF, readmitted to the hospital or any other category. The slices of the pie would then represent percentage in each group. Bigger slices represent a greater proportion of patients.

Pareto Diagram/Pareto Chart

A *Pareto diagram or chart* (FIG. 4-7) displays a series of bars with which the priority for problem solving can easily be seen by the varying height of the bars. The tallest bar is the most frequently occurring issue. The bars always are arranged in descending height. This tool is related to the Pareto principle (named after the 19th-century economist Vilfredo Pareto), which states that 80% of the problems or effects come from 20% of the causes. Therefore, by tackling 20% of the most frequent causes, an 80% improvement can be achieved.

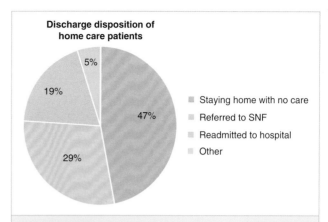

How to construct

1. Values on the pie chart should equal 100%.
2. Draw sectors that are equal in size to the quantity represented.
3. Color code sectors of pie.
4. Label units of measurement.
5. Provide a legend for sector categories.
6. Insert Title.

When to use

- Graphical display to show the distribution or spread of comparative data
- During any stage of PDSA to communicate data distribution. This is a visual representation of data, but not an analysis
- Answer questions
  - Where do more of the incidents occur?
  - Which location experiences the least incidents?

Figure 4-6 Pie chart. (Adapted from National Association for Healthcare Quality. *Data Analysis and Reporting: Quick Reference Guide.* Chicago, IL: NAHQ; 2016; Centers for Disease Control and Prevention. *Evaluation briefs: Using graphs and charts to illustrate quantitative data;* 2008. https://www.cdc.gov/healthyyouth/evaluation/pdf/brief12.pdf.)

Cause-and-Effect, Ishikawa, or Fishbone Diagram

A *cause-and-effect diagram* (FIG. 4-8) is used to analyze and display the potential causes of a problem or the source of variation. There generally are at least four categories in the diagram. Some of the common categories include the four Ms: manpower, methods, machines, and materials; or the five Ps: patrons (users of the system), people (workers), provisions (supplies), places to work (work environment), and procedures (methods and rules).

Scatter Diagram or Plot

A *scatter diagram* (FIG. 4-9) is used to determine the extent to which two variables (quality effects or process causes) relate to one another. These diagrams often are used in

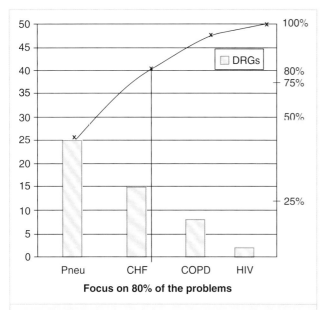

Focus on 80% of the problems

How to construct

1. Identify the independent categories and the way to compare, either by frequency (count), time, cost, or other unity of analysis.

   Note: For four to six categories, have at least 30 data points. For 7–10 categories, have at least 60 data points. For 11 or more categories, have at least 100 data points.

2. Rank order the data in descending categories.
3. Calculate the percentage of the total each category depicts.

The steps can be put into a data table.

1. Draw the left, or vertical, axis with the unit of comparison.
2. Draw the horizontal axis with the categories, the largest to the smallest.
3. Draw a bar for each category.
4. Draw the right vertical axis from 0 to 100.
5. Draw a line graph of the cumulative percentage.
6. Label the axes and the diagram, noting the data source, date, and author.

When to use

- Use when there is a need to identify the most frequent or most important factors contributing to cost, problems, etc.

Figure 4-7 **Pareto diagram or chart.**

combination with fishbone or Pareto diagrams/charts. The extent to which the variables relate is called *correlation*. Scatter plots can be created manually or with statistical or spreadsheet software.

Run or Trend Chart

Run or *trend charts* (FIG. 4-10) are graphic displays of data points over time. Run charts are control charts without

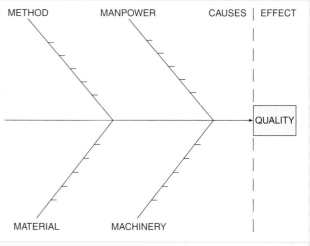

How to construct

1. Determine the effect or the label for the diagram and put it on the far right side of the diagram.
2. Draw a horizontal line to the left of the effect.
3. Determine the categories (the four Ms or the five Ps).
4. Draw a diagonal line for half of the categories above the line and half below the line.
5. Brainstorm the list for each of the categories.
6. Organize each of the causes on each bone.
7. Draw branch bones to show the relationships.

When to use

- Identify and organize possible causes of problems
- Identify factors that will lead to success
- Conducting a root cause analysis

Figure 4-8 **Cause-and-effect, Ishikawa, or fishbone diagram.**

the control limits. Their name comes from the fact that the user is looking for trends in the data or a significant number of data points going in one direction or on one side of the average.

Trends generally indicate a statistically important event that needs further analysis. Resist the tendency to see every variation in the data as significant; wait to interpret the results until at least 10 (or even better, 20) data points are plotted. As indicated in this example, it is best to not analyze data too frequently. For example, looking at quarterly data may more accurately reflect trends over time than reviewing data monthly.

Statistical Process Control

SPC is an approach to monitoring quality by looking at whether a process or outcome is within the bounds of what is expected. Control charts are typically used to visualize data to detect

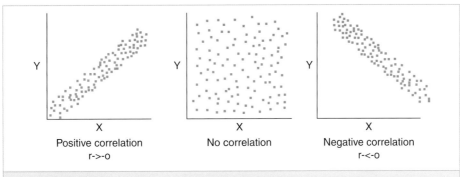

How to construct

1. Collect at least 25 pairs of data for the two variables.
2. Draw and label the data over the equal distance on the graph.
3. Spread the data over equal distances on the graph.
4. Plot the paired sets of data by marking the intersection of their values.
5. Label the scatter diagram and describe the source, date, and author.

When to use

- Determining whether there is a relationship between two variables
- Determining the strength of the relationship—tight, loose, or outliers

  Tight. The factors appear to be responsible for most of the variation

  Loose. Other factors probably affect the data

  Outliers. Special causes probably are present
- Determining the type of relationship with variables—positive, negative, or no relationship

  Positive. As one variable increases, the other increases

  Negative. As one variable increases, the other decreases

Figure 4-9 **Scatter diagram or scatter plot.**

and prevent problems. There are two basic types of control charts—univariate control chart that is a graphical display (chart) of one quality characteristic and multivariate control chart that is a graphical display of a statistic that summarizes or represents more than one quality characteristic. *Control charts* are run charts to which control limits have been added above and below the center line (mean). These lines are calculated from the data and show the range of variation in the output of a process. In general, upper control limits (UCLs) and lower control limits (LCLs) are determined by adding and subtracting three SDs to or from the mean. Assuming a normal distribution and no special-cause variation 99% of data points would be expected to fall between the UCL and LCL.

There are many types of control charts for both variable and attributes data.

- Variables data: 1 Range Bar chart, median and range chart, x and s chart, XmR chart, moving average chart;
- Attributes data: P chart, NP chart, U chart, C chart.

One common chart presents individual values (X) and calculates limits based on the moving range (mR); this is the XmR chart. The XmR chart is used when data are obtained on

a periodic basis, such as once a day or once a week, which is common in quality and performance improvement activities. See FIGURE 4-11 for example of control chart.

Types of Variation

By design, control charts are very useful in identifying variation in quality measures. The challenge for the healthcare quality professional is determining whether what they are seeing is common or special-cause variation so that appropriate action can be taken.

- **Common-cause variation.** Variation is inherent in any process. On a control chart this type of variation is exhibited as points between the control limits in no particular pattern. This is variation that normally would be expected from a process. If this type of variation is treated as being unpredictable, it could tamper with the process and, in fact, make things worse. The root cause of the variation must be identified before trying to "fix" the problem.
- **Special-cause variation.** Variation that arises from sources that are not inherent in the process are unpredictable.

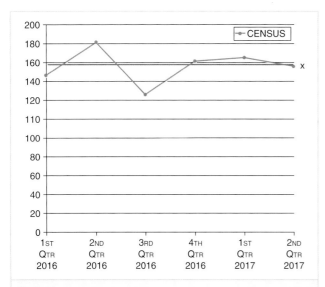

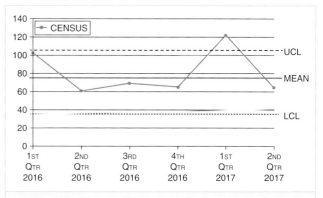

How to construct

1. Draw vertical and horizontal axes.
2. Label the vertical axis with the indicator or the variable and determine the scale.
3. Label the horizontal axis with the unit of time or sequence for which the data were collected.
4. Plot the data points.
5. Connect the data points.
6. Determine the mean of the plotted numbers and draw a mean line on the graph.
7. Label the chart and name the source of the data, the date, and the author.

When to use

- Use to display variation
- Use to detect variation (presence or absence of special causes)
- Use when observing the effects of process improvement (observe the effects of interventions on change)

Figure 4-10   Run chart or trend chart.

On a control chart this type of variation is exhibited as points that fall outside the control limits, or, when inside the control limits, exhibits certain patterns. These special-cause variations are addressed any time they occur with interventions appropriate to eliminate the special cause, if possible.

Force Field Analysis. *Force field analysis* (FIG. 4-12) is a method to systematically identify the various forces that facilitate or increase the likelihood of success, and the opposite factors that decrease or restrain the likelihood of success or improvement in the process. This chart is like listing the pros and cons of an action.

Frequency Distribution. Bell curves, histograms, and 2×2 tables are all types of *frequency distributions* (FIG. 4-13). When

How to construct

1. Construct the chart as you would a run or trend chart.
2. Calculate control limits using the appropriate statistical formula or via a computer program.
3. Plot the control limits on the chart and examine the data for variation as described below.

When to use

- Distinguish variation from common and special causes
- Assist with eliminating special-cause variation
- Observe effects of a process improvement

Figure 4-11   Control chart.

people describe a normal distribution, they are referring to a bell curve. Displaying the frequency distribution can help determine if one or more processes are occurring. For example, a frequency distribution can be a bimodal distribution of the ages of patients undergoing a total hip replacement. In other words, the data essentially have two different bell curves present and possibly two different processes. Conceivably, the demographics and risk factors may be different, and each age distribution may need a separate quality, safety or performance improvement focus.

See *Performance and Process Improvement* for more discussion of tools and methods to better understand how to use data, how to translate data to information, and using information to drive improvement efforts.

Data-Driven Decision-Making

The analysis, ultimate interpretation of data, and reporting are meaningful to various audiences. Good presentation of data creates interest and enhances understanding. Data are reported and analyzed on a regular basis. In this process, it is important to validate that the data were collected accurately. Data can be displayed in a format that is easily understood, and a summary provided. Those involved in the process being monitored are asked to help with the analysis. There is an analysis of variances and identification of unexpected

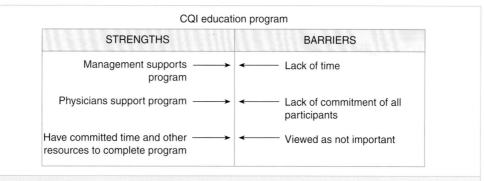

How to construct

1. Identify the issue.
2. Create two columns on a piece of paper. Label one "strengths" and one "barriers."
3. Brainstorm and list potential strengths and barriers on the chart.
4. Determine actions to be taken to increase the strengths and to decrease or eliminate the barriers.

When to use

Identify the strengths of barriers for the success of the project

Figure 4-12 **Force field analysis.**

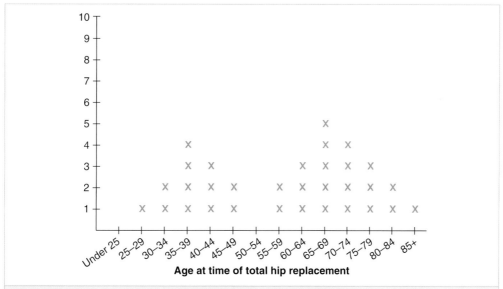

How to construct

1. Develop a scale based on the range of data to be collected.
2. Count the data and mark the appropriate spot on the scale.

When to use

- When the spread or distribution of the data is important
- When the occurrence of more than one process is suspected

Figure 4-13 **Frequency distribution.**

patterns among caregivers, services, and patients. If there are trends, ask people to identify possible causes and solutions.

Displaying Data

A challenge for performance improvement or quality analytics staff is to display data in a meaningful way to be used by the involved departments or interprofessional teams. Graphic display of the data enhances the understanding and use of results. Bader and Bohr[23] describe the use of tables, graphics, infographics and visuals. Tables are the most common format to present information. By highlighting the most pertinent information, readers can quickly and efficiently hone in on key information. For tables to be most effective they are understandable and use minimal abbreviations or jargon. They have columns clearly identified, with specific findings highlighted with boldface type, underlining, or other distinguishing marks. Graphics and visuals provide a snapshot of an organization's status; where the variations lie; the relative importance of identified problems; and the impact, if any, of changes that have been instituted.[55]

There are books and other publications available on the visual display of data and information. The emphasis is telling stories through graphic representation of data.[56] Common presentations of data discussed in the previous sections include the following:

- Pareto diagram/chart: prioritizes a series of problems or possible causes of problems;
- Histogram: illustrates the variability or distribution of data;
- Scatter diagram: displays possible cause and effect, illustrates whether one variable might have an impact upon another variable, and can illustrate the strength of that impact;
- Run chart: used to monitor processes over time;
- Control chart: used to statistically illustrate upper and lower limits of a process and the variation of an organization's process within those limits; and
- Stratification: breaks down single values into meaningful categories or classifications to focus on improvement opportunities or corrective action.[55]

To effectively present data for interpretation and discussion, it is essential to provide a contextual background. Because most people are visually oriented, a graph is used to display data. A table of values can accompany the graph. There is an explanation of specifics regarding the data collection (how, when, and where the data were collected, and from whom they were obtained). There is a report summarizing the meaning of the values and how they were computed. If outliers were removed from the sample, that is stated. The time-order of the data collection can be included in the presentation to determine whether a pattern exists.

Balanced Scorecards

In 1992, Kaplan and Norton[57] described a framework for performance improvement that relies on reporting key metrics representing all aspects of the business. The concept of the balanced scorecard is the presentation of a mixture of measures each compared to a target value. The target values can be set by the organization or be based on external benchmarks. In reporting on quality, balanced scorecards can be developed that focus on multiple dimensions that underlie care delivery. For example, the key quality metrics typically can be grouped into the following domains: process, outcomes, utilization, and patient experience. A balanced scorecard would then have several measures in each of these domains with appropriate targets. One of the biggest benefits is that balanced scorecards can be used for easy communication of the quality measures to executives in the organization (e.g., Chief Executive Officer [CEO], Chief Medical Officer [CMO], Chief Nursing Officer [CNO], etc.). Examples of measures used in balanced scorecards can be found in FIGURE 4-14.

Dashboards

Organizations often develop "Dashboards" to represent key management and performance indicators.[58] As a decision support tool, the Dashboard can provide insights that are seldom seen with mere gut and intuition using a combination of the right metrics with visualization that will help "provide context and meaning that go beyond the buzzwords and technologies."[59(p1)] Dashboards can be used to analyze and forecast various organizational systems. These dashboards frequently incorporate external benchmarks, which allow organizations to compare performance to national, state, or regional norms. Benchmarks are available from CMS, state health department websites, medical specialty groups, published literature, and organizations such as The Leapfrog Group. An example is shown as FIGURE 4-15.

Benchmarking

No matter what data display or reporting tool is used, benchmarking offers the organization to establish performance goals for administrative, financial, and clinical outcomes. The performance improvement team can determine whether it wants to be "average" (the industry standard) or raise the bar to a much higher level of performance. When comparison reveals differences, the healthcare organization's management staff can begin to ask questions to determine the factors contributing to variances. Benchmarking includes routinely comparing indicators (structure, process, and outcomes) against best performance and seeking out ways to make improvements with the greatest impact on outcomes. It offers another approach to compare an organization's or individual

People and Workforce	Service and Care Management	Quality and Patient Safety	Growth and Strategic Goals	Financial and Operational Excellence
Labor cost per adjusted day	Overall patient satisfaction	Patients receiving known allergen	Admissions	Readmissions
FTEs per adjusted occupied bed	Patients seen by admission coordinators within 24 h	% of patients receiving asthma home management plan of care	Patient days	Operating margin
Total operating revenue per FTE	Pre-registered accounts fast tracked	Employee perception of top management commitment to patient safety	Adjusted patient days	Hospital FTEs per acuity adjusted occupied bed
Total average compensation per FTE	ED patients waiting >3 h to see MD	Total number of health deficiencies on health last nursing home inspection	Operating Room minutes	Cost per acuity adjusted inpatient day no greater than 3% over budget
Employee injury/illness rate	ED decision to admit room assignment	Return to OR within 24 h	Ambulatory visits	Days in accounts receivables
Employee turnover rate	Call answer rate by customer service	Employee likely to report medical errors	Primary Care Physician referrals	YTD days cash on hand
RN vacancy rate	ED arrival to triage	HIM record completion	Ancillary outpatient tests/treatments	Supply chain cost/adjusted patient day
Education and training investment per FTE	Short-stay residents successfully discharged to the community	Employee perception of department commitment to patient safety	Operating room visits	Net collection rate
Total temp/registry	Recommend organization to others	National Patient Safety Goals • Universal protocol	Average daily census	YTD obligated group days cash on hand
Total productive support staff cost per clinic	Leaving emergency department without being seen	• HAIs • Patient identification	Ambulatory behavioral health center admits	Total expense/adjusted patient day
Number of successors on key posts	Complaints from community MDs	• Medication management	New ACO partner contracts	Administration costs

Figure 4-14 **Balanced scorecard measures for hospitals and other healthcare organizations.** (Created by Christy L. Beaudin, PhD LCSW CPHQ for general education purposes. ©2011, 2012.)

practitioner's results against a reference point. Ideally, the reference point is a demonstrated best practice.

Internal or external benchmarks can be used depending on the measure and what the organization is trying to accomplish. In their discussion about the use of benchmarking and continuous QI, Ettorchi-Tardy et al.,[60(pe110)] advantages of internal benchmarking are it is rapid, less expensive, and offers a learning method. For external benchmarking for clinical practices, some of the challenges might be specificity of the indicators to be used and how these practices might be compared against other healthcare organizations. External sources help develop best practices by implementing the same or similar processes to achieve better results. For example, an organization is focusing on improving vaccination rates among healthcare workers using the "timely and effective care: healthcare worker influenza vaccination" measure. Using

Hospital Compare, the organization can assess progress in its vaccination rates with data provided by the Centers for Disease Control and Prevention (CDC) via the National Healthcare Safety Network (NHSN) tool. Another example is using Medical Office User Comparative Database Reports to identify key indicators for benchmarking from the Culture of Safety Survey.

One of the most critical decisions an organization makes when launching a benchmarking initiative is selecting the source of comparative data. Organizations like Milliman have developed benchmarks for different aspects of operations such as efficiency benchmarks (the level of resource required for the completion of a defined number of transactions) and quality benchmarks (the level of consistency applied to similar transactions against recognized standards and the relative level of value of those services). According to

Core metrics dashboard for risk-adjusted measures

This dashboard allows exploration of the progress of selected core measures over time and in relation to the 2016 targets, when available.

Summary view

Select a data period and measurement population to view from the drop down menus.

Click on a measure description to see trends in the time series view. Hover on any mark for more details.

Choose data period*
201503-201602

Choose group to view
All groups (Maine care, Comm., & Medicare)

■ Progress made
░ Distance remaining
▓ Target not established

Maine Commercial Payers did not endorse a target.

Medicare targets were developed in collaboration with the Maine State Innovation Model program staff and Center for Medicare and Medicaid Innovation staff with the intent to drive Maine's healthcare reform improvements. The measures are specific to Maine and the measures and targets are not endorsed by Medicare.

MaineCare targets ⓘ   Medicare targets ⓘ

Data and trend information available for all populations by clicking below on the measure or on the target circle itself.

Measure		MaineCare targets	Medicare targets
Developmental screenings in the first 3 years of life		100.00% complete	N/A for Population
Results	Higher is better Out of 100%	2015Q3-2016Q2: 36.70	2015:
Well-child visits (ages 3–6)		99.80% complete	N/A for Population
Results	Higher is better Out of 100%	2015Q3-2016Q2: 68.86	2015:
Children 7–11 access to primary care practitioners		95.52% complete	N/A for Population
Results	Higher is better Out of 100%	2015Q3-2016Q2: 81.19	2015:
All-cause readmissions	Lower is better	86.32% complete	94.76% complete
Results	Out of 100%	2015Q3-2016Q2: 15.06	2015: 12.98
Diabetic care HbA1c (ages 18–75)	Higher is better	84.11% complete	96.18% complete
Results	Out of 100%	2015Q3-2016Q2: 76.54	2015: 86.61
Follow-up after hospitalization for mental illness	Higher is better	86.76% complete	83.23% complete
Results	Out of 100%	2015Q3-2016Q2: 71.14	2015: 58.26
Median fragmented care index	Lower is better Median FCI	71.17% complete	Target not established
Results	Index	2015Q3-2016Q2: 0.58	2015: 0.00
Non-emergent ED use	Lower is better Out of 1,000 Member	98.40% complete	100.00% complete
Results	Months	2015Q3-2016Q2: 112.80	2015: 48.32
Use of imaging studies for low back pain	Higher is better	100.00% complete	93.01% complete
Results	Out of 100%	2015Q3-2016Q2: 86.77	2015: 79.06

*MaineCare metrics look at the most updated data we have and is reported from Q3 of a given calendar year through Q2 of the following year. Commercial and Medicare metrics are reported on a calendar year Q1 through Q4 basis.
Data for 2016 are available only for MaineCare at this time.

**Well-child visits (ages 3–6), children 7–11 access to primary care practitioners, and follow-up after hospitalization for mental illness data for Commercial are forthcoming.

Figure 4-15 Sample Core Metrics Dashboard.

Source: Evaluation Dashboards. (nd). Maine State Innovation Model, Maine Department of Health and Human Services. http://www.maine.gov/dhhs/sim/evaluation/dashboard.shtml

Zolelzer,[61] these performance benchmarks define the vision for what is possible in "Best Practice" operations and can identify strengths and weaknesses in operations and support operational improvement initiatives. Using Milliman's administrative performance benchmarking, a health plan can analyze the efficiency of operational areas including claims, medical management, customer service, and administration and look at resource allocations in comparison to peers and competitors.[61] FIGURE 4-16 illustrates benchmarks for administrative costs by functional area.

Activity-Level PM PM Cost		Benchmarks PM PM				Client Results	
		Median				$	%ile
Functions	Activities	High	Comp	Peer	Low	PM PM	
Claims	Mallroom and Claims Preparation	$0.25	$0.13	$0.14	$0.07	$0.14	44%
	Data Capture	$0.20	$0.10	$0.11	$0.06	$0.18	10%
	Adjudication	$0.75	$0.38	$0.41	$0.21	$0.68	9%
	COB/TPL/Subrogation	$0.25	$0.13	$0.14	$0.07	$0.14	44%
	Adjustments and Rework	$0.25	$0.13	$0.14	$0.07	$0.14	44%
	Audit, Training and Setup	$0.13	$0.06	$0.07	$0.03	$0.05	72%
Provider Management	Provider Services	$0.75	$0.38	$0.41	$0.21	$0.25	87%
	Provider Contracting	$1.00	$0.50	$0.55	$0.28	$0.87	13%
Member Services	Customer Service	$2.50	$1.25	$1.38	$0.69	$1.25	50%
	Membership	$1.25	$0.63	$0.69	$0.34	$0.55	63%
Medical Management	Utilization and Quality Review	$2.00	$1.00	$1.10	$0.55	$0.78	75%
	Care Management	$1.25	$0.63	$0.69	$0.34	$0.35	99%
	Medical Director	$0.50	$0.25	$0.28	$0.14	$0.20	72%
	Other Healthcare Services	$1.25	$0.63	$0.69	$0.34	$1.00	20%
Business Development	Marketing	$2.00	$1.00	$1.10	$0.55	$1.23	39%
	Sales	$7.00	$3.50	$3.85	$1.93	$6.00	14%
	External Brokers	$12.00	$6.00	$6.60	$3.30	$6.00	50%
Finance	Finance and Accounting	$1.00	$0.50	$0.55	$0.28	$0.37	79%
	Actuarial and Underwriting	$0.75	$0.38	$0.41	$0.21	$0.55	27%
Information Systems	Operations and Support	$2.50	$1.25	$1.38	$0.69	$1.00	72%
	Development and Integration	$6.00	$3.00	$3.30	$1.65	$4.50	25%
Corporate Services and Administration	Executive Office	$4.00	$2.00	$2.20	$1.10	$2.50	38%
	Taxes	$4.00	$2.00	$2.20	$1.10	$3.00	25%
	TOTAL	$51.58	$25.79	$28.37	$14.18	$31.73	39%

Figure 4-16 **Example of Milliman operational benchmarks—administrative costs (sample data for illustrative purposes only).** (Reprinted from Zolelzer, N. *Managing Administrative Expenses with Operational Benchmarking. Milliman Healthcare Analytics Blog*. https://info.medinsight. milliman.com/2013/07/managing-administrative-expenses-with-operational-benchmarking/, with permission. Sample data for illustrative purposes only. Copyright © 2013 Milliman, Inc. All rights reserved.)

Healthcare quality professionals often coordinate an organization's benchmarking efforts. Most healthcare regulatory agencies require benchmarking as part of a comprehensive quality, safety, and performance improvement program. Potential data sources for benchmarking include the following:

- Government data available from CMS, the CDC, and state government agencies;
- Alliances such as large healthcare systems (partnership organizations often provide data extrapolation for their members, frequently providing databases for internal and external benchmarking);
- State peer review organizations and state hospital associations that offer free benchmarking opportunities for hospitals within their state; and
- For-profit database companies that offer software that helps hospitals or organizations extrapolate and compile their own benchmark data or provide benchmarking data through a centralized database compiled by the company.

These data are reported to regulatory and accreditation agencies as part of routine reporting (e.g., ORYX, Outcome and Assessment Information Set [OASIS], and HEDIS). **TABLE 4-11** illustrates examples of benchmarking projects.

Reporting

The final product of every quality, safety, or performance improvement project is reporting. For example, reporting can include three documents shared across the organization and be used with different audiences.

- First: a high-level presentation used in meetings to discuss the overall findings and outline suggestions for improvements.
- Second: a one-page executive summary or infographic shared broadly and summarizes the project, findings, and improvement recommendations.
- Third: a detailed report describing what was done; features all the analyses, tables, and figures; interprets the findings; and offers the specific details about next steps. The detailed report is sent to chairs of departments, quality leaders, and senior administrators.

Another avenue of communication to consider is quarterly or semiannual events/forums that include presentations and posters on recent quality, safety, or performance improvement projects. These events can be offered to a broad audience and widely publicized. Other options for disseminating quality, safety, and performance improvement findings to staff include monthly newsletters, e-mails, blogs, and other social media distribution networks.

Myriad data analysis and graphic display tools are available to assist with understanding a process at a point in time and

Table 4-11 Benchmarking Examples

Type of Benchmarking	Example Topic	Measure
Internal	Cesarean section rate	Physician A versus B versus C; physician group Practice A versus B versus C; physicians versus midwives
Internal	Time to antibiotic for XYZ Infection	Emergency department versus unit A versus unit B Emergency department versus urgent care setting
Internal	Resident satisfaction	Overall satisfaction with nursing care by unit Unit supervisor pays attention to resident safety problems
External	Use of ACE inhibitors with acute myocardial infarction	Health system or proprietary database Performance of all hospitals versus region versus similar-size hospital versus own hospital
External	Central-line-associated blood stream infection rates	Hospital unit versus National Healthcare Safety Network data for similar units; can compare by quartile or median rates (industry standard)
External	Wrong site/wrong procedure/wrong person surgery	Facility's incidence versus zero incidence

over time. Although no single tool can support an entire process improvement team, tools can be used in combination to facilitate making data-based decisions. However, the use of tools alone does not guarantee accurate and effective decision-making. Quality, safety, and performance improvement teams must be configured to include frontline caregivers, key stakeholders across disciplines, and healthcare quality professionals with expertise in quality, safety, and performance improvement design, implementation, and evaluation (including the tools and statistics described in this section).

See *Performance and Process Improvement, Organizational Leadership*, and *Patient Safety* for more discussion about data-driven decision-making and tools to support performance excellence.

Section Summary

A historical perspective and new developments in health data analytics puts into context the importance of information management in the work of the healthcare quality professional. The analysis of data and translation to meaningful information are critical given national quality and safety priorities and initiatives. Healthcare reform includes an emphasis on data and information related to individuals, populations, and organizations. Strategies are proposed to foster the use of data in decision-making. The public reporting of quality data promotes value-based purchasing—accountability for is part of the equation. Factoring into the equation are evidence-based quality management, measurement and decision support, systematic healthcare QI, and MISs. Finally, sound study design and analysis support the healthcare quality professional's efforts to achieve performance excellence and sustain a culture of safety and quality.

References

1. Juran JM. Quality and its assurance: an overview. Presented at the Second NATO Symposium on Quality and Its Assurance, London; 1977.
2. Deming WE. *The New Economics for Industry, Government, Education*. Cambridge, MA: MIT Press; 2000.
3. Juran JM. Product quality: a prescription for the west. The Management Review; 1981, June and July. (First presented at the 25th Conference of the European Organization for Quality Control, Paris.)
4. Juran JM. The QC circle phenomenon. *Ind Control*. 1967 January;23:329–336.
5. Grandia L. Healthcare information systems: a look at the past, present, and future. https://www.healthcatalyst.com/healthcare-information-systems-past-present-future. Accessed May 25, 2017.
6. Davenport TH. Competing on analytics. *Harvard Bus Rev*. 2006;84(1):98–107, 134.
7. The Advisory Board. *Big Data in Health Care: Educational Briefing for Non-IT Executives*. Washington, DC: Author; 2017.
8. Walker M. Data veracity. *Data Sci Central*; 2012. www.datasciencecentral.com/profiles/blogs/data-veracity. Accessed May 18, 2017.
9. Kayyali B, Knott D, Van Kuiken S. The big-data revolution in US health care: accelerating value and innovation; 2013. http://www.mckinsey.com/industries/healthcare-systems-and-services/our-insights/the-big-data-revolution-in-us-health-care. Accessed July 16, 2017.
10. National Institutes of Health. What is big data? 2015. https://datascience.nih.gov/bd2k/about/what. Accessed May 16, 2017.
11. National Institutes of Health. About BD2K; 2016. https://datascience.nih.gov/bd2k/about. Accessed May 16, 2017.
12. President's Information Technology Advisory Committee. Health care delivery and information technology subcommittee: draft recommendations; April 13, 2004. www.itrd.gov/pitac/meetings/2004/20040413/20040413_draft_hit.pdf. Accessed May 16, 2017.
13. Bates DW, Gawande AA. Improving safety with information technology. *New Eng J Med*. 2003;348(25):2526–2534. doi:10.1056/NEJMsa020847
14. Weiner M, Callahan CM, Tierney WM, et al. Using information technology to improve health care of older adults. *Ann Int Med*. 2003;139:430–436.
15. Jamoom E, Yang N. *Table of Electronic Health Record Adoption and Use Among Office-Based Physicians in the US, by State: 2015 National Electronic Health Records Survey*. Atlanta, GA: Centers for Disease Control and Prevention, National Center for Health Statistics; 2016.
16. National Committee on Vital and Health Statistics. Letter to the secretary: recommendations for the first set of PMRI standards. Washington, DC: Author; 2002, February 27. https://www.ncvhs.hhs.gov/subcommittees-work-groups/subcommittee-on-standards/020227lt.htm. Accessed May 16, 2017.
17. Healthcare Information and Management Systems Society (HIMSS). Evaluating HIT standards: key principles to support healthcare IT interoperability in the United States; 2013. http://www.himss.org/sites/himssorg/files/FileDownloads/2013-09-23-EvaluatingHIT Standards-FINAL.pdf. Accessed May 16, 2017.
18. Institute of Medicine, Committee on Patient Safety and Health Information Technology. *Health IT and Patient Safety: Building Safer Systems for Better Care*. Washington, DC: National Academies Press; 2012.
19. HealthIT.gov. Meaningful use definition & objectives; 2017. www.healthit.gov/providers-professionals/meaningful-use-definition-objectives. Accessed May 16, 2017.
20. Nutley T, Reynolds HW. Improving the use of health data for health system strengthening. *Global Health Action*. 2013;6:1–10. doi:10.3402/gha.v6i0.20001
21. Gudea S. Data, information, knowledge: a healthcare enterprise case. *Perspect Health Inf Manag*. 2005;2:8. doi: 10.1.1.104.6709
22. Quality Measurement and Management Project. *Hospital Quality-Related Data: Recommendations for Appropriate Data Requests, Analysis, and Utilization*. Chicago: American Hospital Association; 1991.
23. Bader BS, Bohr D. *Guide to the Interpretation and Use of Quality of Care Data*. Chicago: American Hospital Association, The Hospital Research and Education Trust; 1991.
24. Byers JF, Beaudin CL. Critical appraisal tools facilitate the work of the quality professional. *J Healthcare Qual*. 2001;23(5):35–38, 40–43. doi:10.1111/j.1945-1474.2001.tb00374.x
25. Chassin MR, Loeb JM, Schmaltz SP, Wachter RM. Accountability measures—using measurement to promote quality improvement. *New Engl J Med*. 2010;363(7):683–688. doi:10.1056/NEJMsb1002320
26. Sackett D, Rosenberg WMC, Muir-Gray JA, Haynes RB, Richardson WS. Evidence-based medicine: what it is and what it isn't. *Br Med J*. 1996;312(13):71–72. doi:10.1136/bmj.312.7023.71
27. Greenhalgh T. Narrative based medicine: narrative based medicine in an evidence based world. *Br Med J*. 1999;318(7179):323–325. doi:10.1136/bmj.318.7179.323
28. Tonelli M. The limits of evidence-based medicine. *Respir Care*. 2001;46(12):1435–1440.

29. Institute of Medicine, Committee on Quality of Health Care in America. *Crossing the Quality Chasm: A New Health System for the 21st Century*. Washington, DC: National Academies Press; 2001.

30. Deaton C. Outcomes measurement and evidence-based nursing practice. *J Cardiovasc Nurs*. 2001;15(2):83–86.

31. Weiss NS. The new world of data linkages in clinical epidemiology: are we being brave or foolhardy? *Epidemiology*. 2011;22(3):292–294. doi:10.1097/EDE.0b013e318210aca5

32. Kindig DA, Stoddart G. What is population health? *Am J Public Health*. 2003;93:380–383.

33. Lewis N. Populations, population health, and the evolution of population management: making sense of the terminology in US health care today; 2014. http://www.ihi.org/communities/blogs/_layouts/15/ihi/community/blog/itemview.aspx?List=81ca4a47-4ccd-4e9e-89d9-14d88ec59e8d&ID=50. Accessed May 24, 2017.

34. Boult C, Wieland, GD. Comprehensive primary care for older patients with multiple chronic conditions. *J Am Med Assoc*. 2010;304(17):1936–1943.

35. Tweed-Weber, Inc. *Total Quality Management in Home Health Care*. Reading, PA: Author; 1992.

36. Higgins TC, Crosson J, Peikes D, et al. Using health information technology to support quality improvement in primary care; AHRQ Publication No. 15-0031-EF. Rockville, MD: Agency for Healthcare Research and Quality; 2015.

37. O'Rourke LM, Bader BS. An illustrative quality and performance report for the governing board. *Qual Lett Healthcare Leaders*. 1993;5(2):15–28.

38. U.S. Department of Health & Human Services, Office of the National Coordinator for Health Information Technology (ONC). Adoption of electronic health record systems among U.S. non-federal acute care hospitals: 2008-2014; 2015. https://www.healthit.gov/sites/default/files/data-brief/2014HospitalAdoptionDataBrief.pdf. Accessed May 16, 2017.

39. Rontal R. Information and decision support in managed care. *Manag Care Q*. 1993;1(3):3–14.

40. Bright TJ, Wong A, Dhurjati R, et al. Effect of clinical decision-support systems: a systematic review. *Ann Int Med*. 2012; 157(1):29–43.

41. U.S. Code of Federal Regulations Parts 160 and 164. Standards for privacy of individually identifiable health information: final rule. Federal Register; 2002. www.gpo.gov/fdsys/pkg/CFR-2002-title45-vol1/xml/CFR-2002-title45-vol1-sec164-514.xml. Accessed May 16, 2017.

42. White SV. Interview with a quality leader: David Brailer on information technology and advancing healthcare quality. *J Healthcare Qual*. 2004;26(6):20–25. doi:10.1111/j.1945-1474.2004.tb00531.x

43. Rosati RJ. Creating quality improvement projects. In: Siegler EL, Mirafzali S, Foust JB, eds. *A Guide to Hospitals and Inpatient care*. New York: Springer; 2003:326–338.

44. Berwick DM, Nolan TW, Whittington J. The triple aim: care, health and cost. *Health Affairs*. 2008;27(3):759–769. doi:10.1377/hlthaff.27.3.759

45. Sikka R, Morath JM, Leape L. The quadruple aim: care, health, cost, and meaning in work. *BMJ Qual Saf Online*. 2015;1–3. doi:10.1136/bmjqs-2015-004160

46. Oleske DM. *Epidemiology and the Delivery of Health Care Services: Methods and Applications*. New York: Springer; 2009.

47. McGlynn EA. Identifying, categorizing, and evaluating health care efficiency measures. Final Report (prepared by the Southern California Evidence-based Practice Center—RAND Corporation, under Contract No. 282-00-0005-21). AHRQ Publication No. 08-0030. Rockville, MD: Agency for Healthcare Research and Quality; April 2008.

48. Centers for Medicare & Medicaid Services. eCQM library; 2017. https://www.cms.gov/Regulations-and-Guidance/Legislation/EHRIncentivePrograms/eCQM_Library.html. Accessed May 22, 2017.

49. Agency for Healthcare Research and Quality. AHRQ quality indicators; n.d. https://www.qualityindicators.ahrq.gov/. Accessed May 24, 2017.

50. Centers for Medicare & Medicaid Services. Core measures; 2016. https://www.cms.gov/Medicare/Quality-Initiatives-Patient-Assessment-Instruments/QualityMeasures/Core-Measures.html.

51. Centers for Medicare & Medicaid Services. IMPACT Act of 2014 & cross setting measures; 2015. https://www.cms.gov/Medicare/Quality-Initiatives-Patient-Assessment-Instruments/Post-Acute-Care-Quality-Initiatives/IMPACT-Act-of-2014-and-Cross-Setting-Measures.html. Accessed May 22, 2017.

52. Agency for Healthcare Research and Quality. Enabling health care decision-making through health information technology; 2012. https://healthit.ahrq.gov/ahrq-funded-projects/enabling-health-care-decisionmaking-through-use-health-information-technology. Accessed May 16, 2017.

53. Iezzoni L. *Risk Adjustment for Measuring Healthcare Outcomes*. 4th ed. Chicago, IL: Health Administration Press; 2012.

54. Hoskin T. Parametric and nonparametric: demystifying the terms. BERD at Mayo Clinic; 2012. https://www.mayo.edu/mayo-edu-docs/center-for-translational-science-activities-documents/berd-5-6.pdf. Accessed May 28, 2017.

55. Brassard M, Ritter D. *The Memory Jogger II*. Methuen, MA: Goal/QPC; 1994.

56. Tufte E. *Beautiful Evidence*. Columbia, MD: Graphics Press; 2006.

57. Kaplan RS, Norton DP. The balanced scorecard—measures that drive performance. *Harvard Bus Rev*. 1992;70(1):71–79.

58. Russell D, Rosenfeld P, Ames S, Rosati RJ. Using technology to enhance the quality of home health care: three case studies of health information technology initiatives at the visiting nurse service of New York. *J Healthcare Qual*. 2010;32(5):22–28.

59. Nelson GS. The healthcare performance dashboard: linking strategy to metrics; 2010. Paper 167-2010 from SAS Global Forum. http://support.sas.com/resources/papers/proceedings10/167-2010.pdf. Accessed May 28, 2017.

60. Ettorchi-Tardy A, Levif M, Michel P. Benchmarking: a method for continuous quality improvement in health. *Healthcare Policy*. 2012;7(4):e101–e119.

61. Zolelzer N. Managing administrative expenses with operational benchmarking; 2013. Milliman Healthcare Analytics Blog. https://info.medinsight.milliman.com/2013/07/managing-administrative-expenses-with-operational-benchmarking/. Accessed May 28, 2017.

Suggested Readings

Amland RC, Dean BB, Yu H, et al. Computerized clinical decision support to prevent venous thromboembolism among hospitalized patients: proximal outcomes from a multiyear quality improvement project. *J Healthcare Qual*. 2015;37(4):221–231.

Lyden JR, Zickmund SL, Bhargava TD, et al. Implementing health information technology in a patient-centered manner: patient experiences with an online evidence-based lifestyle intervention. *J Healthcare Qual*. 2013;35(5):47–57.

Hansen JP. CAN'T MISS—conquer any number task by making important statistics simple. Part 1. Types of variables, mean, median, variance, and standard deviation. *J Healthcare Qual*. 2003;25(4):19–24. doi:10.1111/j.1945-1474.2003.tb01070.x

Hansen JP. CAN'T MISS—conquer any number task by making important statistics simple. Part 2. Probability, populations, samples, and normal distributions. *J Healthcare Qual.* 2003;25(4):25–33. doi:10.1111/j.1945-1474.2003.tb01071.x

Hansen JP. CAN'T MISS—conquer any number task by making important statistics simple. Part 3. Standard error, estimation, and confidence intervals. *J Healthcare Qual.* 2003;25(4):34–39. doi:10.1111/j.1945-1474.2003.tb01072.x

Hansen JP. CAN'T MISS—conquer any number task by making important statistics simple. Part 4. Confidence intervals with t distributions, standard error, and confidence intervals for proportions. *J Healthcare Qual.* 2004;26(4):26–32. doi:10.1111/j.1945-1474.2004.tb00504.x

Hansen JP. CAN'T MISS—conquer any number task by making important statistics simple. Part 5. Comparing two confidence intervals, standard error of the difference between two means and between two proportions. *J Healthcare Qual.* 2004;26(4):33–42. doi:10.1111/j.1945-1474.2004.tb00506.x

Hansen JP. CAN'T MISS—conquer any number task by making important statistics simple. Part 6. Tests of statistical significance (z test statistic, rejecting the null hypothesis, p value), t test, z test for proportions, statistical significance versus meaningful difference. *J Healthcare Qual.* 2004;26(4):43–53. doi:10.1111/j.1945-1474.2004.tb00507.x

Hansen JP. CAN'T MISS: conquer any number task by making important statistics simple. Part 7. Statistical process control: x–s control charts. *J Healthcare Qual.* 2005;27(4), 32–43. doi:10.1111/j.1945-1474.2005.tb00566.x

Hansen JP. CAN'T MISS: conquer any number task by making important statistics simple. Part 8. Statistical process control: n, np, c, u control charts. *J Healthcare Qual.* 2005;27(4):45–52. doi:10.1111/j.1945-1474.2005.tb00567.x

Mandavia R, Yassin G, Dhar V, Jacob T. Completing the audit cycle: the impact of an electronic reporting system on the feedback loop in surgical specialties. *J Healthcare Qual.* 2013;35(6):16–23.

Mitchell JP. Electronic healthcare's relationship with patient satisfaction and communication. *J Healthcare Qual.* 2016;38(5):296–303.

O'Leary KJ, Balabanova A, Patyk M, et al. Medical inpatients' use of information technology: characterizing the potential to share information electronically. *J Healthcare Qual.*; 2015:37(4):207–220.

Pellegrin KL, Miyamura JB, Ma C, Taniguchi R. Improving accuracy and relevance of race/ethnicity data: results of a statewide collaboration in Hawaii. *J Healthcare Qual.* 2016;38(5):314–321.

Raglan GB, Margolis B, Paulus RA, Schulkin J. Electronic health record adoption among obstetrician/gynecologists in the United States: physician practices and satisfaction. *J Healthcare Qual.* Post Author Corrections: May 23, 2015.

Reddy CK, Aggarwal CC. *Healthcare Data Analytics.* UK, London: Chapman and Hall/CRC; 2015.

Rico F, Liu Y, Martinez DA, et al. Preventable readmission risk factors for patients with chronic conditions. *J Healthcare Qual.* 2016;38(3):127–142.

Spiva L, Hand M, VanBrackle L, McVay F. Validation of a predictive model to identify patients at high risk for hospital readmission. *J Healthcare Qual.* 2016;38(1):34–41.

Strome TL. *Healthcare Analytics for Quality and Performance Improvement.* Hoboken, NJ: John Wiley and Sons; 2013.

Westover C, Arredondo PH, Chapa G, Cole E, Campbell CR. Quality of care in a low-income consumer-driven health plan: assessment of Healthcare Effectiveness Data Information Set (HEDIS) scores for secondary prevention. *J Healthcare Qual.* 2014;36(3):28–34.

Online Resources

Advisory Board
- **Disease Registries**
  https://www.advisory.com/international/topics/doctor-relations/disease-registries

Agency for Healthcare Research and Quality
  www.ahrq.gov
- **Module 7. Measuring and Benchmarking Clinical Performance**
  https://www.ahrq.gov/professionals/prevention-chronic-care/improve/system/pfhandbook/mod7.html
- **Computerized Registries**
  https://healthit.ahrq.gov/key-topics/computerized-disease-registries
- **Healthcare Cost and Utilization Project**
  https://hcup-us.ahrq.gov/databases.jsp
- **Medical Expenditure Panel Survey**
  https://meps.ahrq.gov/data_stats/onsite_datacenter.jsp
- **National Quality Measures Clearinghouse**
  www.qualitymeasures.ahrq.gov
- **Quality and Patient Safety**
  www.ahrq.gov/qual/kt
- **Surveys on Patient Safety Culture**
  https://www.ahrq.gov/professionals/quality-patient-safety/patientsafetyculture/index.html
- **State Snapshots**
  https://www.ahrq.gov/research/data/state-snapshots/index.html

American Society for Quality
  www.asq.org

American Health Information Management Association
  http://www.ahima.org/

Australian Commission on Safety and Quality in Health Care
  www.safetyandquality.gov.au

Best Practice Guidelines Clearinghouses
- **Centre for Effective Practice**
  https://effectivepractice.org/

Centers for Disease Control and Prevention
- **Behavioral Risk Factor Surveillance System: Annual Survey Data**
  https://www.cdc.gov/brfss/annual_data/annual_data.htm
- **National Vital Statistics System**
  https://www.cdc.gov/nchs/nvss/
- **National Center for Health Statistics**
  https://www.cdc.gov/nchs/

Centers for Medicare & Medicaid Services Program Statistics
  https://www.cms.gov/Research-Statistics-Data-and-Systems/Statistics-Trends-and-Reports/CMSProgramStatistics/index.html

The Dartmouth Atlas of Healthcare
  http://www.dartmouthatlas.org/tools/benchmarking.aspx

DARTNet Institute
  http://www.dartnet.info/

eCQI Resource Center
  http://ecqi.healthit.gov/

Health and Medicine Division of National Academies of Sciences, Engineering, and Medicine (previously Institute of Medicine)

- **Population Health Metrics That Matter for Population Health Action: Workshop Summary (2016)**
  https://www.nap.edu/catalog/21899/metrics-that-matter-for-population-health-action-workshop-summary
- **Refining the Concept of Scientific Inference When Working with Big Data: Proceedings of a Workshop**
  https://www.nap.edu/catalog/24654/refining-the-concept-of-scientific-inference-when-working-with-big-data

HealthData.gov
https://www.healthdata.gov/

Health Information Management and Systems Society
http://www.himss.org/

Health Quality Ontario
http://www.hqontario.ca/Quality-Improvement/Our-Programs/Quality-Improvement-in-Long-Term-Care

Health Resources & Services Administration
- **Data Warehouse**
  https://datawarehouse.hrsa.gov/
- **Health Workforce Data**
  https://bhw.hrsa.gov/health-workforce-analysis/data

Institute for Healthcare Improvement
www.ihi.org
- **IHI Open School**
  http://www.ihi.org/education/ihiopenschool/Pages/default.aspx
- **The Improvement Project**
  http://www.ihi.org/education/InPersonTraining/ImprovementProject/Pages/default.aspx

The International Society for Quality in Health Care
www.isqua.org

The Joint Commission
www.jointcommission.org

The Leapfrog Group
www.leapfroggroup.org

National Association for Healthcare Quality
www.nahq.org

National Committee for Quality Assurance
http://www.ncqa.org/org

National Guideline Clearinghouse
www.guideline.gov

National Health Service, UK
www.nhs.uk/Pages/HomePage.aspx

National Institutes of Health
- **BD2K Initiative**
  https://datascience.nih.gov/bd2k/aboutNational
- **List of Registries**
  https://www.nih.gov/health-information/nih-clinical-research-trials-you/list-registries

National Patient Safety Foundation
www.npsf.org

National Quality Forum
www.qualityforum.org

NHS National Patient Safety Agency
www.npsa.nhs.uk

RAND Corporation
www.rand.org

SAFTINet
http://www.aafp.org/patient-care/nrn/studies/all/SAFTINet.html

Society for Human Resource Management
www.shrm.org

Substance Abuse and Mental Health Services Administration
- **National Survey on Drug Use and Health (NSDUH; Population Data)**
  https://www.samhsa.gov/data/population-data-nsduh
- **Treatment Episode Data Set (TEDS; Client Level Data)**
  https://www.samhsa.gov/data/client-level-data-teds
- **National Survey of Substance Abuse Treatment Services (NSSATS; Substance Use Facility Data)**
  https://www.samhsa.gov/data/substance-abuse-facilities-data-nssats
- **National Mental Health Services Survey (NMHSS; Mental Health Facility Data)**
  https://www.samhsa.gov/data/mental-health-facilities-data-nmhss
- **Drug Abuse Warning Network (DAWN; Emergency Department Data)**
  https://www.samhsa.gov/data/emergency-department-data-dawn

Acronyms

A

AAAHC	Accreditation Association for Ambulatory Health Care
ACA	Affordable Care Act
ACF	Administration for Children & Families
ACGME	Accreditation Council for Graduate Medical Education
ACHC	Accreditation Commission for Health Care
ACL	Administration for Community Living
ACO	Accountable Care Organization
ACR	American College of Radiology
ACS	American College of Surgeons
ACUG	Accreditation and Certification Users Group
AHA	American Hospital Association
AHIMA	American Health Information Management Association
AHRQ	Agency for Healthcare Research and Quality
AIDET	Acknowledge, Introduce, Duration, Explanation, Thank You
AIDS	Acquired Immune Deficiency Syndrome
ALOS	Average Length of Stay
AMA	American Medical Association
AMI	Acute Myocardial Infarction
ANCC	American Nurses Credentialing Center
APA	American Psychological Association
APIC	Association for Professionals in Infection Control and Epidemiology
APIE	Assess, Plan, Implement, Evaluate
APM	Alternate Payment Model
ARRA	American Recovery and Reinvestment Act
ASA	American Society of Anesthesiologists
ASC	Ambulatory Surgery Center
ASHRM	American Society of Healthcare Risk Management
ASP	Antibiotic Stewardship Program
ASQ	American Society for Quality
ATSDR	Agency for Toxic Substances and Disease Registry

B

BAA	Business Associate Agreement
BD2K	Big Data to Knowledge
BI	Business Intelligence
BSC	Balanced Scorecard

C

CAH	Critical Access Hospital
CAHPS	Consumer Assessment of Health Care Providers and Systems
CAP	Corrective Action Plan
CAP	College of American Pathologists
CARF	CARF International
CAS	Complex Adaptive Systems
CAUTI	Catheter-Associated Urinary Tract Infections
CBA	Cost–Benefit Analysis
CDC	Centers for Disease Control and Prevention
CDSS	Clinical Decision Support Systems
CEC	Content Expert Certification
CEO	Chief Executive Officer
CER	Comparative Effectiveness Research
CfC	Conditions for Coverage
CFR	Code of Federal Regulations
CHAP	Community Health Accreditation Partner
CI	Confidence Interval
CLABSI	Central Line-Associated Blood Stream Infection
CLAS	Culturally and Linguistically Appropriate Services in Health and Health Care (the National CLAS Standards)
CLIA	Clinical Laboratory Improvement Amendments
CM	Case Management
CMO	Chief Medical Officer
CMS	Centers for Medicare & Medicaid Services
CNO	Chief Nursing Officer; Also Chief Nurse Executive (CNE)
COLA	Commission of Office Laboratory Accreditation
CoP	Conditions of Participation
COPIS	Customer-Output-Process-Input-Supplier
CORF	Comprehensive Outpatient Rehabilitation Facility
CPG	Clinical Practice Guideline
CPHQ	Certified Professional in Healthcare Quality
CPM	Critical Path Method
CPOE	Computerized Prescriber Order Entry
CPR	Cardiopulmonary Resuscitation
CPRC	Cancer Prevention Research Center
CQHCA	Committee on Quality of Health Care in America
CQI	Continuous Quality Improvement
CRM	Crew Resource Management
CSR	Continuous Survey Readiness
CVO	Credentials Verification Organization

D

DHHS	Department of Health and Human Services
DM	Disease Management
DMAIC	Define, Measure, Analyze, Improve, Control
DMEPOS	Durable Medical Equipment, Prosthetics, Orthotics, and Supplies

DNP	Doctor of Nursing Practice
DNSc	Doctor of Nursing Science
DNV GL	DNV GL National Integrated Accreditation for Healthcare Organizations (NIAHO)
DoD	Department of Defense
DOJ	Department of Justice
DPH	Department of Public Health
DPMO	Defects Per Million Opportunities
DRG	Diagnosis-Related Groups

E

EBP	Evidence-Based Practice
eCQMs	Electronic Clinical Quality Measures
EHR	Electronic Health Record
EMC	Emergency Medical Condition
EMR	Electronic Medical Record
EMTALA	Emergency Medical Treatment & Active Labor Act
EP	Eligible Professional
ERISA	Employee Retirement Income Security Act of 1974
ERM	Enterprise Risk Management
ESC	Evidence of Standard Compliance
ESRD	End-Stage Renal Disease

F

FAIR	Findable, Accessible, Interoperable, and Reusable
FDA	Food & Drug Administration
FMEA	Failure Mode and Effects Analysis
FPPE	Focused Professional Practice Evaluation

H

HAI	Healthcare-Associated Infection
HBIPS	Hospital-Based Inpatient Psychiatric Services
HCAHPS	Hospital Consumer Assessment of Healthcare Providers and Systems
HCDIT	Health Care Delivery and Information Technology
HCFAC	Health Care Fraud and Abuse Control Program
HCP	Healthcare Personnel
HCW	Healthcare Worker
HEDIS	Healthcare Effectiveness Data and Information Set
HFAP	Healthcare Facilities Accreditation Program
HFMEA	Healthcare Failure Mode and Effects Analysis
HHA	Home Health Agency
HHS	U.S. Department of Health & Human Services
HIE	Health Information Exchange
HIIN	Hospital Improvement Innovation Network
HIM	Health Information Management
HIMSS	Healthcare Information and Management Systems Society
HIP	Health Information Products
HIPAA	Health Insurance Portability and Accountability Act
HIPDB	Healthcare Integrity and Protection Data Bank

HIT	Health Information Technology
HITECH	Health Information Technology for Economic and Clinical Health Act
HIV	Human Immunodeficiency Virus
HMD	Health and Medicine Division of the National Academy of Sciences (formerly IOM)
HMO	Health Maintenance Organization
HPA	Health Plan Accreditation
HQCC	Healthcare Quality Certification Commission
HRET	Health Research & Education Trust
HRM	Healthcare Risk Management
HRO	High Reliability Organization
HRSA	Health Resources & Services Administration

I

ICF/MR	Intermediate Care Facilities for Persons with Mental Retardation
ICU	Intensive Care Unit
IHI	Institute for Healthcare Improvement
IHS	Indian Health Service
IJ	Immediate Jeopardy
IMPACT	Improving Medicare Post-Acute Care Transformation Act of 2014 (the IMPACT Act)
IOM	Institute of Medicine (now Health and Medicine Division of the National Academy of Sciences)
IPC	Infection Prevention and Control
IPFCC	Institute for Patient and Family-Centered Care
IRF	Inpatient Rehabilitation Facility
ISMP	Institute for Safe Medication Practices
IT	Information Technology
ITL	Immediate Threat to Life
IV	Intravenous

J

JCAH	Joint Commission on Accreditation of Hospitals (now The Joint Commission)
JCAHO	Joint Commission on Accreditation of Healthcare Organizations (now The Joint Commission)
JHQ	Journal for Healthcare Quality

K

KPI	Key Performance Indicator
KRI	Key Risk Indicator

L

LCL	Lower Control Limit
LEP	Limited English Proficiency
LIP	Licensed Independent Practitioner
LOS	Length of Stay
LTC	Long-Term Care
LTCH	Long-Term Care Hospital

M

M & M	Morbidity and Mortality
MACRA	Medicare Access and CHIP Reauthorization Act

MBHO	Managed Behavioral Healthcare Organization
MCO	Managed Care Organization
MD	Medical Doctor
MDS	Minimum Data Set
MIPS	Merit-Based Incentive Payment System
MIS	Management Information System
MQSA	Mammography Quality Standards Act
MRSA	Methicillin-Resistant *Staphylococcus aureus*
MS	Master of Science
MSDS	Material Safety Data Sheet
MSE	Medical Screening Examination

N

NAHQ	National Association for Healthcare Quality
NAIC	National Association of Insurance Commissioners
NCVHS	National Committee on Vital and Health Statistics
NCQA	National Committee for Quality Assurance
NEJM	New England Journal of Medicine
NGC	National Guideline Clearinghouse
NHIN	Nationwide Health Information Network
NHSN	National Healthcare Safety Network
NIAHO	National Integrated Accreditation for Healthcare Organizations
NIH	National Institutes of Health
NIOSH	National Institute for Occupational Safety and Health
NPDB	National Practitioner Data Bank
NPP	National Priorities Partnership
NPSF	National Patient Safety Foundation
NPSG	National Patient Safety Goal
NQF	National Quality Forum
NQS	National Quality Strategy
NSQIP	National Surgical Quality Improvement Program

O

OASIS	Outcome and Assessment Information Set
OCR	Office of Civil Rights
OIG	Office of Inspector General
OMH	Office of Minority Health
ONC	Office of the National Coordinator
OPO	Organ Procurement Organization
OPPE	Ongoing Professional Practice Evaluation
OPSC	Oregon Patient Safety Commission
ORYX	Performance Measurement Reporting (The Joint Commission)
OSHA	Occupational Safety and Health Administration

P

PACE	Programs of All-Inclusive Care for the Elderly
PCMH	Patient-Centered Medical Home
PCP	Primary Care Physician or Primary Care Provider
PDCA	Plan Do Check Act

PDSA	Plan Do Study Act
PERT	Program Evaluation and Review Technique
PFCC	Patient- and Family-Centered Care
PhD	Doctor of Philosophy
PHI	Protected Health Information
PHQ	Physician and Hospital Quality
PHR	Personnel Health Record
PI	Performance Improvement
PICU	Pediatric Intensive Care Unit
PoC	Plan of Correction
PPACA	Patient Protection and Affordable Care Act
PPE	Personal Protective Equipment
PPPSA	Physician Practice Patient Safety Assessment
PPS	Prospective Payment System
PSCHO	Patient Safety Climate in Healthcare Organizations
PSNet	AHRQ Patient Safety Network
PSO	Patient Safety Organization
PSWP	Patient Safety Work Product

Q

QA	Quality Assurance
QC	Quality Circle
QFD	Quality Function Deployment
QI	Quality Improvement
QPI	Quality and Performance Improvement
QPP	Quality Payment Program

R

RCA	Root Cause Analysis
RCA2	Root Cause Analysis and Action
RHC	Rural Health Clinic
RM	Risk Management
RN	Registered Nurse
ROI	Return on Investment
RPIW	Rapid Process Improvement Workshop

S

6S	Sort (Seiri), Straighten (Seiton), Scrub/Shine (Seiso), Standardize (Seiketsu), Systematize/Sustain (Shitsuke), Safety
SAFER	Survey Analysis for Evaluating Risk
SAMHSA	Substance Abuse and Mental Health Services Administration
SAQ	Safety Attitudes Questionnaire
SBAR	Situation Background Assessment Recommendation
SIPOC	Supplier-Input-Process-Output-Customer
SMART	Specific, Measurable, Achievable, Relevant, and Time-Bound
SNF	Skilled Nursing Facility
SNOMED	Systemized Nomenclature of Medicine
SOM	State Operations Manual
SPC	Statistical Process Control
SRE	Serious Reportable Event
SSI	Surgical Site Infection

T

Team STEPPS	Team Strategies and Tools to Enhance Performance and Patient Safety
TJC	The Joint Commission
TPO	Treatment, Payment, or Business Operations
TQM	Total Quality Management

U

UCL	Upper Control Limit
UHDDS	Uniform Hospital Discharge Data Set
UM	Utilization Management
US	United States
USB	Universal Serial Bus
USPSTF	U.S. Preventive Services Task Force

V

VA	Veterans Affairs
VHA	Voluntary Hospital Association
VLER	Virtual Lifetime Electronic Record
VOC	Voice of the Customer
VTE	Venous Thromboembolism

W

WHO	World Health Organization
WHP	Wellness and Health Promotion
XML	Extensible Markup Language

Glossary

This *Glossary* has been developed and structured to reflect the nature of healthcare quality—concepts, thinking, applications, and practices. Although comprehensive, the *Glossary* is not exhaustive. Terms relate to the content of *HQ Solutions*. Many definitions come from authoritative sources and may also be cited in a section. See the *Bibliography* at the end of the section.

6S: Method used to create and maintain a clean, orderly, and safe work environment. 6S is based on the five pillars (5S) of the visual workplace in the Toyota Production System, plus another pillar for safety. 6S is often the first method companies implement in their Lean journey, because it serves as the foundation of future continual improvement efforts.

85/15 Theory: Deming claimed that about 85% of organizational failures are because of system breakdowns involving factors such as management, machinery, or work rules; 85% of the problems detected are process or system-related, whereas only 15% are traceable to workers.

A

A3: Lean/Six Sigma tool used to capture an improvement opportunity. A standard format is used to address an improvement process (i.e., seven or nine blocks). This usually includes the background, current condition, goal, analysis, proposal/recommendation/countermeasure, plan, and follow-up.

Access: Ability to obtain needed healthcare services in a timely manner including the perceptions and experiences of people regarding their ease of reaching health services or health facilities in terms of proximity, location, time, and ease of approach (e.g., timeliness of response or services, time until next available appointment, and availability of services within a community).

Accountability: An obligation or willingness to accept responsibility for performance.

Accountable Care Organization (ACO): Network of healthcare providers that band together to provide the full continuum of healthcare services for patients. Receives a payment for all care provided to a patient and held accountable for the quality and cost of care. Goal is to improve quality and reduce costs by allowing them to share in any savings achieved because of these efforts.

Accreditation: Process in which a local, national, or internationally recognized agency assesses operations and performance to determine whether a set of recognized and accepted standards are met. Official authorization or approval, or recognition for conforming to standards, or to recognize as outstanding.

Activity Network Diagram: Using an arrow diagram, a sequence of events is depicted. It is useful when several simultaneous paths must be coordinated. Also known as arrow diagram, program evaluation and review technique (PERT), or critical path method (CPM) chart.

Affinity Diagram: Tool that organizes numerous ideas or issues into groupings based on their natural relationships within the groupings. Typically used by teams to analyze or chart a process and to structure and organize issues to provide a new perspective to help solve a problem.

B

Balanced Scorecard (BSC): Approach to performance management where performance measures provide a comprehensive view of organizational performance and not be overly dependent on a few choice indicators. The BSC helps organizations better link long-term strategy with short-term activities.

Baldrige Award: Competitive award that is given to organizations demonstrating a commitment to quality excellence based on successfully meeting the Baldrige National Health Care Criteria for Performance Excellence.

Bar Chart: Tool to visually demonstrate comparisons among various categories. Bar charts can be organized horizontally or vertically, to demonstrate the relationship between one or more categorical variables relative to a single continuous variable. A bar chart is a visual tool only and improvement decisions should not be made using this tool.

Benchmark: Sustained superior performance, which can be used as a reference to raise the mainstream of care by other providers, organizations, and delivery systems. The relative definition of superior will vary situation to situation.

Benchmarking: Comparison of an organization's or an individual practitioner's results against a reference point. Ideally, the reference point is a demonstrated best practice.

Best Practice: Procedure shown by research and experience to produce optimal results and that is established or proposed as a standard suitable for widespread adoption.

Biomedical Big Data: The complexity, challenges, and new opportunities presented by the combined analysis of data. In biomedical research, these data sources include the diverse, complex, disorganized, massive, and multimodal data being generated by researchers, hospitals, and mobile devices around the world.

Black Belt: Practitioner of Six Sigma methods with significant theoretical and practical experience and mentors others newer to this problem-solving framework (e.g., yellow belts, white belts, green belts).

Brainstorming: To institute a shared method for a team to rapidly and creatively generate many ideas in an efficient way for any topic. The use of this methodology fosters freedom of criticism and judgment while encouraging openness in thinking. Brainwriting is brainstorming in the written format.

Budgeting: Formal annual or periodic process through which financial performance goals and actual results are evaluated for the current and previous fiscal years, allowing for the development of formal goals for the next fiscal year.

Bundle: Small set of evidence-based interventions for a defined patient segment.

C

Capital Budgeting: Process by which an organization evaluates and selects which long-term investments (or capital expenditures) it will make. Typically, this is an annual activity, but it also may be triggered by events such as requests for new programs or equipment.

Care Bundle: Population and care setting that, when implemented together, result in significantly better outcomes than when implemented individually.

Case Management: Process of coordinating medical care provided to patients with specific diagnoses or those with high healthcare needs. These functions are performed by case managers who can be physicians, nurses, or social workers. Case management varies depending on the practice setting. Also called *care management*.

Cause-and-Effect Diagram: Used to display, explore, and analyze all the potential causes related to a problem or condition and to discover the root causes of variation. Also known as *Ishikawa* or *Fishbone diagram*.

Central Tendency: *Central* refers to the middle value, and *tendency* refers to the general trend of the numbers. The three most common measures of central tendency are the mean, the median, and the mode.

Certification: Formal, focused process that an organization, program, individual, or technology undergoes with an assessment by a neutral party or local, national,

internationally recognized, or regulatory agency to demonstrate compliance and competency with developed standards. Recognition for meeting special qualifications within a field. Being certified is not the same as being accredited.

Certified Professional in Healthcare Quality® (CPHQ): Individual who passed the certification examination, demonstrating competent knowledge, skill, and understanding of program development and management, quality improvement concepts, coordination of survey processes, communication and education techniques, and departmental management.

Champion: Person who translates the company's vision, mission, goals and metrics to create an organizational deployment plan; identifies individual projects and resources; and removes roadblocks.

Checklist: Allow complex pathways of care to function with high reliability by giving users the opportunity to pause and take stock of their actions before proceeding to the next step. Also, a standard way to ensure completion of critical tasks for a process or activity. The checklist ensures accuracy, accountability, completeness, and efficiency.

Chi-Square (χ^2): Test of statistical significance that assesses the difference in proportions among two or more variables.

Chronic Disease Management: Integrated care approach to managing illness, which includes screenings, check-ups, monitoring and coordinating treatment, and patient education. It can improve quality of life while reducing healthcare costs by preventing or minimizing the effects of a disease.

Clinical Decision Support System (CDSS): Health information technology functionality that builds upon the foundation of an electronic health record (EHR) to provide persons involved in care processes with general and person-specific information, intelligently filtered and organized, at appropriate times, to enhance health and healthcare.

Clinical Information System: Designed to support direct patient care processes; automated clinical information systems have great potential for analyzing and improving the quality of patient care.

Clinical Pathway: Document-based tools that provide a link between the best available evidence and clinical practice. Clinical pathways, also known as care pathways, critical pathways, integrated care pathways, or care maps, are one tool used to manage the quality in healthcare concerning the standardization of care processes.

Clinical Pertinence: Assessment of the documentation in the electronic medical record (EMR)/electronic health record (EHR) in terms of the patient's condition, diagnostic results, intervention procedures, vital signs, and other information. This review may determine that documentation was appropriate or not appropriate to the standard of care, key elements of the assessment, treatment plan, interventions, and medication management.

Clinical Practice Guideline (CPG): Statement that includes recommendations that intend to optimize patient care. CPGs are informed by a systematic review of evidence and an assessment of the benefits and harms of alternative care options.

Clinical Quality Measure (CQM): Mechanism used for assessing the degree to which a provider competently and safely delivers clinical services that are appropriate for the patient in an optimal time frame. CQMs are a subset of the broader category of performance measures that conform to practice guidelines, medical review criteria, or standards of quality.

Clinical Risk Management: Process of assessing potentially preventable defects in care and acting to mitigate those risks in a comprehensive and multi-stakeholder way that emphasizes systems thinking.

Cluster Sampling: Cluster sampling is a sampling technique used when "natural" but relatively heterogeneous groupings are evident in a statistical population. It is often used in marketing research. In this technique, the total population is divided into these groups (or clusters) and a simple random sample of the groups is selected.

Common Cause Variation: Fluctuation caused by unknown factors resulting in a steady but random distribution of output around the average of the data. It is a measure of the process potential, or how well the process can perform when special-cause variation is removed.

Complex Adaptive Systems (CAS): *Complex* implies the inclusion of a significant number of elements. *Adaptive* refers to the capacity to change and the ability to learn from experience. A *system* is a set of interdependent or connected items that are referred to in CAS as independent agents.

Complexity Science: Study of complex adaptive systems (CAS) is a field applied to healthcare to understand complex human organizations.

Compliance: Deliberate and good-faith adherence to regulatory or statutory requirements. Often demonstrated through a compliance program, which formalizes processes and procedures to ensure this adherence. Conformity in fulfilling official requirements.

Composite Performance Measure: Combination of two or more component measures, each of which individually reflects quality of care, into a single performance measure with a single score. Also called *composite measures.*

Confidence Interval (CI): Type of estimate of a population parameter based on sampled data. CIs offer an estimated range of values likely to include this population parameter. The CI offers a range wherein the true value is likely to fall based on those samples.

Construct Validity: Degree to which a measurement instrument correctly assesses the theoretical construct or trait that it was designed to measure (e.g., severity adjustment scales are tools for measuring staffing needs).

Content Validity: Degree to which a measurement instrument adequately represents the universe of content; includes judgments by experts or respondents about the degree to which the test appears to measure the relevant construct. Also known as *face validity.*

Continuous Data: Set of data where the values can assume any value within a defined range.

Continuous Quality Improvement (CQI): Process that continually monitors program performance. When a quality problem is identified, CQI develops a revised approach to that problem and monitors implementation and success of the revised approach. The process includes involvement at all stages by all organizations, which are affected by the problem and/or involved in implementing the revised approach.

Continuous Survey Readiness (CSR): Attitude and value demonstrated throughout the organization in goals and practices that yield an uninterrupted state of mental preparedness by demonstrating that staff throughout the organization are immediately physically ready or available to demonstrate compliance.

Continuous Variable: Measure score in which each individual value for the measure can fall anywhere along a continuous scale, and can be aggregated using a variety of methods such as the calculation of a mean or median (e.g., mean number of minutes between presentation to the emergency department to the time of admission).

Control Chart: Focuses attention on detecting and monitoring process variation over time; distinguishes special from common causes of variation; provides guidance for ongoing control of a process.

Convenience Sampling: Method of sampling a population that relies on a sample frame consisting of subjects easily available to the researcher, instead of a randomized sample from the whole population.

Corrective Action Plan (CAP): Collection of documents that organize improvements needed for organizations to be in full compliance with standards or regulations. The CAP is written in response to a survey, inspection, or gap analyses from assessments that define observations as well as recommendations for actions to achieve compliance for a given standard. Known as a plan of correction, improvement plan, and action plan.

Correlation: Extent to which variables relate.

Cost: An amount, usually specified in dollars, related to receiving, providing, or paying for medical care. Things that contribute to cost include visits to healthcare providers, healthcare services, equipment and supplies, and insurance premiums. The cost of care is a measure of total healthcare spending, which includes total resource use and unit price(s), by payer or consumer, for a healthcare service or group of healthcare services, associated with a specified patient population, time period, and unit(s) of clinical accountability.

Cost–Benefit Analysis (CBA): Analysis performed to determine the viability and broader benefits of proposed capital expenditures. The CBA helps organizations better use financial and human resources and includes a time frame to demonstrate the costs and benefits of the project over specific periods of time.

Credentialing: Process of appointing or hiring physicians and other health professionals and granting privileges to licensed independent practitioners utilizing standard, empirically based criteria. These criteria may include peer review information, education and/or board certifications to ensure the practitioner is well-qualified and able to deliver the highest quality care.

Criterion-Related Validity: Assessment of the relationship between a measure and an outcome. *Concurrent validity* refers to the outcome at the point a measure is assessed (i.e., a snapshot in time). *Predictive validity* refers to the positive predictive power of a measure relative to some future event (e.g., the assessment of blood pressure as a predictor of later heart failure).

Critical Path Method (CPM): Deterministic project management tool used to plan, monitor, and update the project as it progresses. It follows steps, uses network diagrams, schedules individual activities, and determines earliest to latest start and finish times for each activity. CPM focuses on time/cost tradeoffs.

Cultural Screen: A change management tool focusing on the cultural aspect of change and identifying those factors associated with the culture of the organization that should be assessed to achieve successful change.

Culture of Safety: A culture that encompasses acknowledgment of the high-risk nature of an organization's activities and the determination to achieve consistently safe operations, a blame free environment where individuals can report errors or near misses without fear of reprimand or punishment, encouragement of collaboration across ranks and disciplines to seek solutions to patient safety problems and organizational commitment of resources to address safety concerns.

Culture: The set of shared attitudes, values, goals, and practices that characterizes a company or corporation. A system of beliefs and actions that characterize a group. Culture also refers to norms of behavior and shared values among a group of people. The social "glue" that holds people together. At the heart of culture is the notion of shared values (what is important) and behavioral "norms" (the way things are done). Cultures are described as strong when the core values are intensely held and widely shared.

Customer: Actual and potential users of an organization's products, programs, or services. Customers include the end users of services as well as others who might be their immediate purchasers or users. These others might include distributors, agents, or organizations that further use services.

D

Dashboard: Collection of various individual metrics used to assess the performance of a product, service, or project. Often used to monitor standardized business processes.

Data: Set of discrete values, either qualitative or quantitative. The abstract representation of things, facts, concepts, and instructions that are stored in a defined format and structure on a passive medium (e.g., paper, computer, microfilm).

Deeming Authority: Granted by Centers for Medicare & Medicaid Services (CMS) to accrediting organizations to determine, on CMS's behalf, whether an organization evaluated by the accrediting organization is following corresponding Medicare regulations.

Delphi Method: Combination of brainstorming, multivoting, and nominal group techniques. This technique is used when group members are not in one location; it is frequently conducted by mail and/or email when a meeting is not feasible.

Denominator: Lower part of a fraction used to calculate a rate, proportion, or ratio. It can be the same as the initial population or a subset of the initial population to further constrain the population for measurement. Continuous variable measures do not have a denominator, but instead define a measure population.

Departmentation: How jobs are grouped together. Jobs can be grouped by function, product or service, geography, and process or customer.

Deployment Chart: Used to project schedules for complex tasks and their associated subtasks. It usually is used with a task for which the time for completion is known. The tool is also used to determine who has responsibility for the parts of a plan or project. This tool is also called *planning grid*.

The grid helps the group organize key steps in the project to reach milestones and the desired goal.

Diagnosis-Related Group (DRG): Classification system that groups patients by diagnosis, type of treatment, age, and other relevant criteria. Under the prospective payment system, hospitals are paid a set fee for treating patients in a single DRG category, regardless of the actual cost of care for the individual.

Disruptive Innovation: Phenomenon by which an innovation transforms an existing market or sector by introducing simplicity, convenience, accessibility, and affordability where complication and high cost are considered the norm. Initially, a disruptive innovation is formed in a specialized market that may appear unattractive or inconsequential to industry insiders, but eventually the new product or idea completely redefines the industry.

E

eCQM: Measure that uses data from electronic health records (EHR) and/or health information technology systems to measure healthcare quality. The Centers for Medicare & Medicaid Services use eCQMs in a variety of quality reporting and incentive programs.

Effective: Producing expected results. Based on scientific knowledge of who will likely benefit and with a philosophy of restraint from providing care unlikely to benefit the patient.

Efficient: Activities performed effectively with minimum of waste or unnecessary effort, or producing a high ratio of results to resources (e.g., equipment, supplies, ideas, and energy). Efficiency of care can be measured by the cost of care associated with a specific level of performance.

Electronic Health Record (EHR): Electronic clinical documentation, results reporting and management, electronic prescribing, clinical decision support, barcoding, and patient engagement tools.

Empowerment: Sharing of effective power between formal leaders and lower ranked colleagues. Typically includes higher level of information sharing, participation in decision-making and delegation of problem-solving authority at the level closest to a situation.

Enterprise-Wide Risk Management: Comprehensive business decision-making process instituted and supported by the healthcare organization's board, executive management, and medical staff leadership. A comprehensive framework for making risk management decisions, which maximize value protection and creation by managing risk and uncertainty and their connection to total value.

Episode of Care: Treatment of many health conditions crosses time and place. An episode of care includes all care related to a patient's condition over time, including prevention of disease, screening and assessment, appropriate treatment in any setting, and ongoing management.

Equitable Care: All individuals have access to affordable, high-quality, culturally and linguistically appropriate care in a timely manner. This includes regular preventive care, in addition to emergency care, as well as mental health support. Does not vary based on a patient's individual characteristics like sex, gender identity, ethnicity, geographic location, or socioeconomic status.

Evidence-Based Practice (EBP): The conscientious, explicit, and judicious use of current best evidence in making decisions about the care of patients.

Expert Sampling: Type of purposive sampling that involves selecting experts in each area because of their access to the information relevant to the study.

External Quality Review Organization (EQRO): Federal law and regulations require States to use an EQRO to review the care provided by capitated managed care entities. EQROs may be Peer Review Organizations (PROs), another entity that meets PRO requirements, or a private accreditation body.

F

Failure Mode and Effects Analysis (FMEA): Preventive approach to identify failures and opportunities for error; can be used for processes as well as equipment. An FMEA is a systematic method of identifying and preventing failures before they occur. The Veterans Affairs National Center for Patient Safety created the Healthcare FMEA (HFMEA).

Feasibility: This principle makes sure that the information needed to calculate a measure is readily available so that the effort of measurement is worth it. The most feasible measures use electronic data that are routinely collected during the delivery of care.

First-Order Change: Adjustment of variables (people, processes, technologies) within a system but without altering the structure of the system in which those variables occur.

Flowchart or Process Flowchart: Graphical display of a process outlining the sequence and relationship of the pieces of the process.

Focused Professional Practice Evaluation (FPPE): Privilege-specific competency evaluation of a practitioner that is undertaken for all newly requested privileges and/or whenever a question arises regarding a practitioner's ability to provide safe, high-quality patient care.

Focused Review: Processes or outcomes are reviewed using pre-established criteria or indicators. Also known as *intensive review*.

Force Field Analysis: Performance improvement technique to map the nature and relative strength of individual factors leading to, and opposing, the success of an improvement process.

Frequency Distribution: When people describe a normal distribution, they are referring to a bell curve. Displaying the frequency distribution can help determine if one or more processes are occurring. Bell curves, histograms, and 2×2 tables are all types of frequency distributions.

G

Goal: Broad, general statement specifying a purpose or desired outcome; may be more abstract than an objective (one goal can have several objectives). Establishing a goal is an early step in the strategic planning process and sets the direction for the activities to follow.

Goal Congruence: Integration of multiple goals, either within an organization or between multiple groups. Congruence is a result of the alignment of goals to achieve an overarching mission.

Green Belt: Member of a project team who assists with data collection and helps carry out Six Sigma projects under the direction of a Black Belt.

Guideline: Guidelines are systematically developed by appropriate groups to assist practitioners and patient decisions about appropriate healthcare for specific clinical circumstances.

H

Health Data Analytics: Approach to quality that converts data into information that is presented through compelling visualizations and journalist-style narratives so that any audience, at any level, can clearly understand the stakes and the path.

Health Information Technology: Hardware, software, integrated technologies or related licenses, intellectual property, upgrades, or packaged solutions provided as services that are designed for or support the use by healthcare entities or patients for the electronic creation, maintenance, access, or exchange of health information.

Healthcare Effectiveness Data and Information Set (HEDIS): One of the most widely used performance measure data sets, targeted toward health plans, wellness and health promotion, and disease management programs.

Healthcare Quality: Degree to which health services for individuals and populations increase the likelihood of desired health outcomes and are consistent with current professional knowledge. Quality of care is a measure of performance on specified aims (e.g., safety, timeliness, effectiveness, efficiency, equity, and patient centeredness).

Healthcare Quality Professional: Personnel who work in every healthcare setting to enhance care delivery, optimize value, and improve outcomes by leading activities in one or more of the following core quality functions: Patient Safety, Regulatory and Accreditation, Quality Review and Accountability, Performance and Process Improvement, Health Data Analytics, and Population Health and Care Transitions.

High Reliability: Operating in complex, high-risk environments for extended periods without significant failures, accidents, or avoidable errors. Focus is on standard workflows for more predictable outcomes and level of performance.

High Reliability Organization (HRO): An organization operating in an industry that is complex and has high risk for harm that consistently performs at high levels of safety over long periods of time.

Histogram: Tool used to illustrate the variability or distribution of data. It presents the measurement scale of values along its x-axis (broken into equal-sized intervals) and the frequency scale (as count or percent) along the y-axis. Also called *bar chart*.

Hoshin Planning: Japanese term for policy deployment; a component of the total quality management/quality improvement system used to ensure that the vision set forth by top management is being translated into planning objectives. Also includes the actions that both management and employees will take to accomplish long-term organizational strategic goals.

Human Factors: Knowledge of human capabilities and limitations in the design of products, processes, systems, and work environments, which affect health and safety. For example, employee attitudes, motivation, health (physical and psychological), education, training, and cognitive functioning can influence the likelihood of a medical error.

I

Immediate Jeopardy: Mechanism to escalate crisis survey issues immediately within both State and Federal agencies and with the healthcare provider. It is determined when a crisis is identified in which the health and safety of individual(s) are at immediate risk.

Incentive and Penalty Programs: Series of programs created by healthcare payers that are comprised of incentives and reductions for payment (referred to as "adjustments" by the Centers for Medicare & Medicaid Services). At their inception, most programs offer an incentive to participate, currently however, most of the Federal and State programs associated with Medicare and Medicaid, are entering the penalty phase of such programs.

Information: Obtained when data are translated into results and statements that are useful for decision-making. For information to be meaningful, data must be considered within the context of how they were obtained and how they are to be used.

Innovation: Making meaningful change to improve an organization's services, processes, and organizational effectiveness and create new value for stakeholders.

Instruments: Devices that quality professionals and researchers use to obtain and record data received from the subjects. These instruments can include questionnaires, surveys, rating scales, interview transcripts, and the like. It is critical to use the most credible tools possible (those with proven reliability and validity).

Interoperability: Ensures that health-related information flows seamlessly; refers to the architecture and standards that make it possible for diverse EHR systems to work compatibly in a true information network.

Interpercentile Measures: Although there are several interpercentile measures of variability, the most common is the *interquartile range*, a stable measure of variability based on excluding extreme scores and using only middle cases. Growth charts are one of the most commonly used interpercentile measures. Clinical pathways are developed based on the interquartile range of the designated population.

Inter-rater Reliability: Degree to which two raters, operating independently, assign the same ratings in the context of observational research or in coding qualitative materials.

Interrelationship Diagram: Drawing that organizes a complex problem by sorting and displaying the cause-and-effect relationships among its various aspects.

Interval Data: The distance between each data point is equal (e.g., the values on a Fahrenheit thermometer).

J

Journey to Zero: Innovative strategies to eradicate hospital-associated infections through a process of laying the foundation (sizing the burden), crafting a multipronged strategy (establishing frontline awareness and minimizing pathogen opportunity), and ensuring sustainable success and promoting long-term gains.

Just Culture: Awareness by everyone throughout the organization about the inevitability of medical errors; but all errors and unintended events are reported, even when the events may not cause patient injury. A culture of safety balances learning and accountability for behavioral choices with organizational and individual values, and fosters transparency, trust, and open communication: all that promote the delivery of highly reliable, safe, and quality care.

K

Kaizen: A long-term approach to work that systematically seeks to achieve incremental changes to improve efficiency and quality. It focuses on removing process waste and maximizing value to the customer (e.g., patient, family).

Knowledge Management: Process of recording, storing, categorizing, and socializing information within an organization.

L

Leadership: Ability to influence an individual or group toward achievement of goals; determining the correct direction or path.

Lean Enterprise: System that uses value stream analysis (a tool for exposing waste), root cause analysis (RCA, a method for pursuing perfection), and new technologies to facilitate more efficient practices. The major focus in a lean enterprise is to eliminate waste in the following areas: production, waiting time, inappropriate processing, inventory, transporting, and defects.

Learning Healthcare System: Designed to generate and apply the best evidence for the collaborative healthcare choices of each patient and provider; to drive the process of discovery as a natural outgrowth of patient care; and to ensure innovation, quality, safety, and value in healthcare.

Learning Organization: Where people continually expand their capacity to create the results they truly desire, where new and expansive patterns of thinking are nurtured, where collective aspiration is set free, and where people are continually learning to see the whole together.

Level of Significance: Gives the probability of observing a difference (p) as large as the one found in a study when, in fact, there is no true difference between the groups (i.e., when the null hypothesis is true).

M

Managed Care: Integrates the financing and delivery of appropriate healthcare services to covered individuals by means of arrangements with selected providers to furnish a comprehensive set of healthcare services to members, explicit criteria for the selection of healthcare providers, and significant financial incentives for members to use providers and procedures associated with the plan. Managed care plans typically are labeled as Health Maintenance Organizations (HMOs) (staff, group, Independent Practice Association, and mixed models), Preferred Provider Organizations, or Point of Service plans. Managed care services are reimbursed via a variety of methods including capitation, fee for service, and a combination of the two.

Management Information System (MIS): Contains both the manual and the automated methods that provide information for decision-making. The term, as it commonly is used, refers to an automated or computerized system. Other names for an MIS, which are used interchangeably, include data-processing structure, medical information system, hospital information system, or decision support system

Matrix Diagram: Permits a team to methodically discover and analyze the relationships between two or more sets of information. A rating system is used, which helps to identify patterns of responsibilities. This visual provides clarity and helps a team reach consensus. Provides structure for decision-making.

Mean: Sum of all scores or values divided by the total number of scores. Also known as *average.*

Measure: Mechanism to assign a quantity to an attribute by comparison to a criterion. A measure may stand alone or belong to a composite, subset, set, and/or collection of measures. A healthcare performance measure is a way to calculate whether and how often the healthcare system does what it should. Measures are based on scientific evidence about processes, outcomes, perceptions, or systems that relate to high-quality care.

Measurement: Systematic process of data collection, repeated over time or at a single point in time.

Median: Number that divides a set of numerically ordered data into a lower and an upper half; also considered the 50th percentile.

Medical Error: An event that caused, or could have caused, harm to a patient and which could have been prevented given the current state of medical knowledge and processes in place to prevent the error.

Mission: Organization's purpose or reason for existing. A mission statement answers such questions as "Why are we here?" "Whom do we serve?" and "What do we do?"

Mistake Proofing: Use of process or design features to prevent errors or the negative impact of errors; also known as Poka Yoke.

Misuse: Occurs when patients received appropriate medical services provided poorly, adding to the risk for preventable complications.

Mode: Value that occurs most frequently within a defined set of numbers.

Morbidity: In common clinical usage, any disease state, including diagnosis and complications, is referred to as morbidity.

Morbidity Rate: Disease rate or proportion of diseased people in a population. The number of people ill during a time period divided by the number of people in the total population.

Mortality Rate: Death rate often made explicit for a characteristic (e.g., gender, sex, or specific cause of death). Mortality rate contains three essential elements: the number of people in a population exposed to the risk of death (denominator), a time factor, and the number of deaths occurring in the exposed population during a certain time period (the numerator).

Multiple Regression Analysis: Exercise that estimates the effects of two or more independent variables (x) on a dependent measure (y).

Multi-voting: Easy method for prioritizing items on a list in a team setting. This method builds consensus using a series of votes to reduce the list to a more manageable size.

N

Never Event: Medical error that should never occur (e.g., wrong-site surgery); this informal term is often used in place of serious reportable event. Eliminating harm completely is important but difficult to do.

Nominal Data: A set of data distinguished by a name that has no intrinsic relational meaning. For example, ethnicity is nominal whereas temperatures are not.

Nominal Group Technique: Group decision-making process for generating many ideas in which each member initially works by himself or herself. Also known as *brainwriting.*

Nonparametric Tests: Type of statistical test that does not require the population's distribution to be characterized by certain parameters. Nonparametric tests are used when there is no assumption that the population is normally distributed, for example.

Nonprobability Sampling: Method that provides no way of estimating the probability that each element will be included in the sample. When this approach is used, the results will be representative of the sample only and cannot be generalized to the available population. The following are subsets of nonprobability sampling: convenience, snowball, purposive or judgment, expert, and quota.

Numerator: Upper portion of a fraction used to calculate a rate, proportion, or ratio. Also called *measure focus,* it is the target process, condition, event, or outcome. Numerator criteria are the processes or outcomes expected for each patient, procedure, or other unit of measurement defined in the denominator. A numerator statement describes the clinical action that satisfies the conditions of the performance measure.

O

Objectives: Specific statements that detail how goals will be achieved and are relatively narrow and concrete. Objectives represent the organization's commitment to achieving specific outcomes.

Ongoing Professional Practice Evaluation (OPPE): Documented summary of ongoing data collected for assessing a practitioner's clinical competence and professional behavior. The OPPE information gathered during this process factors into decisions to maintain, revise, or revoke existing privileges.

Ordinal Data: In statistics ordinal data have an order, such as nursing staff rank (nurse level 1, nurse level 2), educational level (BS, MS, MD), or attitude toward research scale (strongly agree, agree, neutral, disagree, strongly disagree). No assumption is made that the distances between the points are the same.

Organizational Learning: Pattern of learning carried out in organizations skilled at creating, acquiring, and transferring knowledge and at modifying behavior to reflect new knowledge and insights.

Outcome Measure: Assesses the results of healthcare that are experienced by patients: clinical events, recovery and health status, experiences in the health system, and efficiency/cost.

Outcome: Result of performance (or nonperformance) of a function or process. The results of care (e.g., increased satisfaction, decreased morbidity, improved quality of life or wellbeing) or the change in a patient's current and future health status that can be attributed to antecedent healthcare. A measure that assesses the results of healthcare that are experienced by patients: clinical events, recovery and health status, experiences in the health system, and efficiency/cost.

Overuse: Repeated use of therapy when additional applications have not been proven to be medically necessary or therapeutically beneficial.

P

Parametric Tests: Statistical tests that assume an underlying data set is normally distributed (i.e., follows the bell curve).

Pareto Diagram/Chart: Tool used to prioritize a series of problems or possible causes of problems. Displays a series of bars in which the varying height of the bars clearly displays the priority for problem solving.

Patient: Represents any label for someone who is registered for and/or uses healthcare services such as client, resident, consumer, customer, stakeholder, recipient, or partner.

Patient- and Family-Centered Care: Meaningful interpersonal relationships between the patient and the provider(s) and honoring the whole person and family; respecting individual values, preferences, and choices; and ensuring continuity of care with the goal of ensuring a positive patient experience; also may be referred to as *patient and family-engaged care*.

Patient Safety: Any improvement effort focused on preventing medical errors; prevention and mitigation from harm; the degree to which the healthcare environment is free from hazards or dangers.

Patient Safety Organization: An organization that collects and analyzes data, reports, educates, and advocates for the reduction of medical errors; privilege, and confidentiality protections are conferred to providers who work with PSOs.

Patient Safety Practice: Type of process or structure whose application reduces the probability of adverse events resulting from exposure to the healthcare system across the range of diseases and procedures.

Patient Safety Solution: Any system design or intervention that has demonstrated the ability to prevent or mitigate patient harm stemming from the processes of healthcare.

Pay for Performance: A healthcare payment system in which providers receive incentives for meeting or exceeding quality, and sometimes cost, benchmarks. Some systems also penalize providers who do not meet established benchmarks. The goal of pay for performance programs is to improve the quality of care over time.

Payment Models: Healthcare payment models consist of formulas for reimbursing healthcare providers (e.g., hospitals, physicians).

Peer Review: An episode of care review is conducted to improve the quality of patient care or the use of healthcare resources. It is a process protected by statute in most states, although this varies, and by federal statute for federal healthcare facilities. A peer is generally defined as a healthcare professional with comparable education, training, experience, licensure, or similar clinical privileges or scope of practice.

Peer Review Organization (PRO): Organization funded by the U.S. Department of Health & Human Services to determine the appropriateness and quality of medical care provided to Medicare beneficiaries.

Percentile: A number that corresponds to one of the equal divisions of the range of a variable in a sample and that characterizes a value of the variable as not exceeded by a specified percentage of all the values in the sample (e.g., a score higher that 95% of those attained is said to be in the 95th percentile).

Performance: The way in which an individual, group, or organization carries out or accomplishes its important functions or processes.

Performance and Process Improvement: Performance and process involves setting goals, implementing changes, measuring outcomes and results, and spreading and/or sustaining improvements. This approach of continuous improvement applies to any healthcare services.

Performance Assessment: Involves the analysis and interpretation of performance measurement data to transform it into useful information for purposes of continuous performance improvement.

Performance Improvement Projects: Examine and seek to achieve improvement in major areas of clinical and non-clinical services. These projects are usually based on information such as enrollee characteristics, standardized measures, utilization, diagnosis and outcome information, data from surveys, grievances, appeals, and other processes. A project measures performance at two periods of time to ascertain if improvement has occurred.

Performance Management: Strategy to promote change in organizational culture, systems, and processes by helping to set agreed upon performance goals, allocating and prioritizing resources, informing managers to either confirm or change current policy or program direction to meet those goals, and sharing results of performance in pursuing those goals.

Performance Measures: A gauge used to assess the performance of a process or function of any organization. Quantitative or qualitative measures of the care and services delivered to patients (process) or the result of that care and services (outcomes). Performance measures can be used to assess other aspects of an individual or organization's performance such as access and availability of care, utilization of care, health plan stability, patient characteristics, and other structural and operational aspect of healthcare services.

Performance Monitoring: The impact and effectiveness of a quality improvement action is monitored, which involves the collection and analysis of qualitative or quantitative data.

Person- and Family-Centered Care: Respectful care that is responsive to patient preferences, needs, and values and ensures that patient values guide all clinical decisions; meaningful interpersonal relationships between the patient and the provider(s) and honoring the whole person and family, respecting individual values, preferences and choices, and ensuring continuity of care with the goal of ensuring a positive patient experience. Also referred to as *patient- and family-centered care.*

Pilot testing: Measurement testing that is divided into two main types: alpha testing (also called *formative testing*) and beta testing (also called *field testing*).

Plan-Do-Check-Act: Four-step process designed to continuously improve quality, originally conceived by Shewhart.

Plan-Do-Study-Act: Later adaptation by Deming of the Plan–Do–Check–Act cycle; also referred to as the Deming Cycle or the Deming Wheel.

Population: Any complete group (e.g., all residents of a community, all cases that meet a designated set of criteria for practitioners, all registered nurses).

Population Health Management: Design, delivery, coordination, and payment of high-quality healthcare services for a population using the best resources available within the healthcare system; may also be referred to as *population medicine.*

Population Health: Outcomes for a group of individuals including outcomes within a group. Maintaining the health and wellness of populations depends on determinants of health, including medical care, public health, genetics, personal behaviors and lifestyle, and a broad range of social, environmental, and economic factors.

Preventive Care: Healthcare that emphasizes the early detection and treatment of diseases. The focus on prevention is intended to keep people healthier for longer, thus reducing healthcare costs over the long term.

Prioritization Matrix: Tool that organizes tasks, issues, or actions and prioritizes them based on agreed-upon criteria. The tool combines the tree diagram and the L-shaped matrix diagram, displaying the best possible effect.

Private Reporting: Sharing quality measurement results with internal stakeholders only, such as within a single health system.

Probability Sampling: Method of sampling in which every item in the population has an equal chance of being selected for inclusion in the sample.

Process Analysis: An industrial quality improvement technique to improve clinical or administrative outcomes by analyzing its processes. For example, process analysis occurs whenever a group of individuals diagrams a healthcare process.

Process Decision Program Chart: Maps the identified events and contingencies that can occur between the time a problem is stated and solved. It attempts to identify potential deviations from the desired process, allowing the team to anticipate and prevent the deviation.

Process Improvement: Methodology utilized to make improvements to a process using continuous quality improvement methods.

Process: Involves the set of activities that go on within and between practitioners and patients.

Process Measure: Focuses on a sequence of actions or steps that should be followed to provide high-quality, evidence-based care. There should be a scientific basis for believing that the process, when executed well, will increase the probability of achieving a desired outcome.

Process: The goal-directed, interrelated series of actions, events, mechanisms, or steps.

Program Evaluation and Review Technique (PERT): A probabilistic project management tool used to plan, monitor, and update the project as it progresses. It follows steps, uses network diagrams, schedules individual activities, and determines earliest to latest start and finish times for each activity.

Project: Endeavor involving a connected sequence of activities and a range of resources designed to achieve specific outcomes considering the constraints of time, costs, and quality used to introduce change.

Project Management: Application of a collection of tools and techniques to direct the use of resources to accomplish a unique, complex, one-time task within time, cost, and quality constraints.

Project Selection Matrix: A tool that ranks and compares potential project areas for implementation. Ranking criteria may include organizational and strategic goals, potential financial impact to the organization, effect on patient and employee satisfaction, likelihood of success, and completion within a specified time frame.

Propensity Score Matching: Multivariate approach to pairing up people with the same characteristics in the intervention and control groups to eliminate potential impact of variation between the groups due to there not being equal.

Proportion: Score derived by dividing the number of cases that meet a criterion for quality (the numerator) by the number of eligible cases within a given time frame (the denominator) where the numerator cases are a subset of the denominator cases (e.g., percentage of eligible women with a mammogram performed in the last year).

Public Reporting: Sharing quality measurement results with the general public, such as through a website or printed report.

Purposive Sampling: Method in which a group or groups are selected based on certain criteria. It is subjective, because the researcher uses his or her judgment to decide who is representative of the population. Also known as *judgment sampling*.

Q

Quality Assurance: Process of looking at how well a healthcare service is provided. The process may include formally reviewing healthcare given to a person, or group of persons, locating the problem, correcting the problem, and then checking to see what worked.

Quality Function Deployment (QFD): Focused methodology for carefully listening to the voice of the customer (VOC) and then effectively responding to those needs and expectations. Also called matrix product planning, decision matrices, and customer-driven engineering.

Quality Improvement (QI): A means by which quality performance is achieved at unprecedented levels by establishing the infrastructure needed to secure annual QI; identifying the specific areas for improvement; establishing clear accountability for bringing QI projects to a successful conclusion; and providing the resources, motivation, and training needed by the teams (e.g., to diagnose the causes, stimulate establishment of a remedy, and establish controls to hold the gains).

Quality Measure: Numeric quantification of healthcare quality for a designated accountable healthcare entity, such as hospital, health plan, nursing home, clinician, etc. A healthcare performance measure is a way to calculate whether and how often the healthcare system does what it should. Measures are based on scientific evidence about processes, outcomes, perceptions, or systems that relate to high-quality care. Also known as *performance measure*.

Quality: Product performance that results in customer satisfaction; freedom from product deficiencies, which avoid customer dissatisfaction.

Quota Sampling: Method where the researcher makes a judgment about the best type of sample for the investigation and specifies characteristics of the sample to increase its representativeness.

R

Random Sample: Group selected for study, which is drawn at random from the universe of cases by a statistically valid method.

Range: Difference between the highest and lowest values in a distribution of scores; usually expressed as a maximum and minimum.

Rapid Cycle Improvement: Strategy whereby organizations collaborate to identify and prioritize aims for improvement and gain access to methods, tools, and materials that will enable them to conduct sophisticated, evidence-based quality improvement activities that they could not conduct individually.

Ratio Data: Where the distance between each point is equal and there is a true zero (e.g., weight and height).

Ratio: Score derived by dividing a count of one type of data by a count of another type of data (e.g., the number of patients with central lines who develop infection divided by the number of central line days).

Red Rules: These are rules that must be followed to the letter; if there is a condition or situation that poses risk, red rules "stop the line."

Reengineering: Efforts focused on work force redesign or on the restructuring of systems and departments into more efficient processes.

Regression Analysis: Statistical procedure to predict outcomes based on the identification of individual variables and how they interact (jointly and individually) with the process being measured.

Regulations: Requirements issued by various governmental agencies to carry out the intent of legislation enacted by Congress, state legislatures, and local authorities. Compliance with regulations is mandatory by law.

Reliability Coefficient: Numerical index of the test's reliability. The closer the coefficient is to 1.0, the more reliable the tool. In general, reliability coefficients of ≥ 0.70 are considered acceptable, although ≥ 0.80 is desired. The reliability coefficient can be determined by evaluating the internal consistency of a measure.

Reliability: Extent to which an experiment, test, or measuring procedure yields the same results on repeated trials.

Resilience: Process of adapting well in the face of adversity, trauma, tragedy, threats, or even significant sources of stress—such as family and relationship problems, serious health problems, or workplace and financial stressors. It means "bouncing back" from difficult experiences.

Resource Use: Resources are the goods or services that are combined to produce medical care. They are inputs that have a price assigned to them. When a procedure is done many times, resource use can be measured and predicted (e.g., people and things needed to perform cataract surgery are a set of resources).

Reversibility: Ability to stop the adoption or use of the innovation and return to a normal or "safe" position if the innovation is not effective.

Risk Adjustment: Technique used to adjust payments to providers in a manner that adjusts for the fact that different patients with the same diagnosis have conditions or characteristics that affect how well they respond to treatment.

Risk Management: Strategies deployed to protect the organization from unintended negative consequences including financial losses; organized effort to identify, assess, and reduce, where appropriate, risk to patients, visitors, staff, and organizational assets. See also *Enterprise-Wide Risk Management*.

Robust Process Improvement: Combination of Lean, Six Sigma, and change management as a new set of tools to achieve high reliability and maintain patient safety.

Root Cause Analysis and Assessment (RCA²): To improve the effectiveness and to prevent future harm, necessary actions coupled with the root cause analysis (RCA), need to be put in place. To emphasize the importance of "action" coupled with RCA, the National Patient Safety Foundation coined Root Cause Analysis and Action (RCA² or RCA "squared").

Root Cause Analysis (RCA): Collective term that describes a range of approaches, tools, and techniques used to uncover the true or root causes of problems.

Run Chart: Graphic display of data points over time; also called *trend chart*. Run charts are control charts without the control limits.

S

Safe Care: Reduces harm and avoids patient injury during the process of care or treatment intended to help them.

Sample: Small number of cases or events that is used to make statements about a population. Researchers use samples to make statistical inferences about the population when the population is too large to study in its entirety.

Sanctions: Administrative remedies and actions (e.g., exclusion, Civil Monetary Penalties) available to the Office of the Inspector General to deal with questionable, improper, or abusive behaviors of providers under the Medicare, Medicaid, or any State health programs.

SBAR: Acronym for Situation, Background, Assessment, Recommendation, which is an evidence-based standardized communication tool used in healthcare settings to facilitate communication.

Scatter Diagram: Tool used to display possible causes and effects. Can determine the extent to which two variables (quality effects or process causes) relate to one another. Often used in combination with fishbone or Pareto diagrams or charts.

Scatter Plot: Method of graphing two related continuous variables by showing a dot on the intersection of values on an XY axis. For example, a patient's temperature may be displayed with a scatter plot by putting the date or time on one axis and the temperature on the other.

Second-Order Change: A complex change that requires a significant alteration in thinking and behavior. Also known as an "out of the box" change.

Sensitivity: As a statistical term, sensitivity refers to the proportion of actual positives that are correctly identified as such (e.g., the percentage of people with diabetes who are correctly identified as having diabetes). See *Specificity*.

Sentinel Event: Any patient safety event that reaches the patient and causes death, permanent harm, or severe temporary harm and intervention required to sustain life.

Sentinel Event: Any patient safety event that reaches the patient and causes death, permanent harm, or severe temporary harm and intervention required to sustain life.

Serious reportable adverse events: Also known as *never events*. The Centers for Medicare & Medicaid Services withholds payment to hospitals if any of these events occur in an acute care facility.

Severity Factors: Frequently, the presence of additional diagnoses helps to define the severity of a group of patients within a Diagnosis-Related Group (DRG), on an individual patient level, or both. A component of risk adjustment.

Severity of Harm: In an FMEA, an estimation of how serious the effects or harm would be if a given failure did occur.

Simple Random Sampling: A method in which everyone in the sampling frame (all subjects in the population) has an equal chance of being chosen (e.g., pulling a name out of a hat containing all possible names).

Six Sigma: Established improvement methodology that uses statistical analysis and other methods to eliminate defects in business processes. Six Sigma is named after six standard deviations from the mean of a normal curve. At this point on a curve of defects, there are only 3.4 defects per million opportunities (dpmo).

Snowball Sampling: Subtype of convenience sampling that allows subjects to suggest other subjects for inclusion in the study, so that the sample size increases. Snowball sampling is often used when subjects are difficult to identify but are known to others through an informal network.

Spaghetti Diagram: Graphic representation of the flow of traffic or movement. Also called *layout diagram*.

Special-Cause Variation: In statistical process control (SPC), a variation in performance that falls outside the control limits or when an obvious nonrandom pattern occurs in a process. This type of variation requires investigation.

Specification: Measure specifications are the technical instructions for how to build and calculate a measure. They describe a measure's building blocks: numerator, denominator, exclusions, target population, how results might be split to show differences across groups (stratification scheme), risk adjustment methodology, how results are calculated (calculation algorithm), sampling methodology, data source, level of analysis, how data are attributed to providers and/or hospitals (attribution model), and care setting.

Specificity: As a statistical term, specificity refers to the proportion of negatives that are correctly identified (e.g., the percentage of healthy people who are correctly identified as not having the condition). Perfect specificity would mean that the measure recognizes all actual negatives (e.g., all healthy people will be recognized as healthy). See *Sensitivity*.

Spread: The intentional and methodical expansion of the number and type of people, units, or organizations using the improvements; based on theory and application on Diffusion of Innovation (Knowledge, Persuasion, Decision, Implementation, and Confirmation).

Stakeholder: All groups that are or might be affected by an organization's actions and success. Examples of key stakeholders might include customers, the workforce, partners, collaborators, governing boards, stockholders, donors, suppliers, taxpayers, regulatory bodies, policy makers, funders, and local and professional communities.

Standard Deviation (SD): Describes the dispersion of a data set around the mean. The SD, represented by sigma (e.g., in Six Sigma approaches), suggests variability in normally distributed data; lower SDs suggest more of the data points cluster around the mean whereas higher SDs suggest broader dispersion of values around the mean.

Standards: Evidence-based guidelines developed and established by consensus or research of an authoritative body. They are used as a guide for optimum achievement and outcomes. Compliance with standards is voluntary, though standards may be named in regulations thereby granting them legal status.

Statistical Process Control (SPC): Measurement of randomly selected outputs of a process to determine whether the process is affected by special-cause variation. SPC is applied to monitor and control a process per customer expectations and business science, ensuring that the process operates at its full potential.

Steward: Person responsible for the fitness and management of data elements within an organization. Also called *measure owner*, this is an individual or organization that owns a measure and is responsible for maintaining the measure. Measure stewards are often the same as measure developers, but not always. Measure stewards are also the ongoing point of contact for people interested in each measure.

Strategic Goal: Broadly stated or long-term outcome written as an overall statement that relates to a philosophy, a purpose, or a desired outcome.

Strategic Objective: Specific statement written in measurable and observable terms using quantitative and qualitative measurement criteria. Written as an action-oriented statement, it indicates the minimum acceptable level of performance and specific time limit or degree of accuracy.

Strategic Planning: Development and codification of a major direction for an organization's future.

Strategy: Plans and activities developed by an organization in pursuit of its goals and objectives, particularly about positioning itself to meet external demands relative to its competition.

Stratification Chart: Tool designed to show where a problem does and does not occur or to demonstrate underlying patterns.

Stratification: Divides a population or resource services into distinct, independent groups of similar data, enabling analysis of the specific subgroups. This type of adjustment can show where disparities exist or where there is a need to expose differences in results.

Stratified Random Sampling: Method in which a population is divided into categories (e.g., patients with particular diseases) and each member of every category has an equal probability of being selected.

Structural Measure: Assesses features of a healthcare organization or clinician relevant to its capacity for healthcare delivery.

Structure: Represents the resources available for care delivery and system design.

Supplier-Input-Process-Output-Customer (SIPOC): Tool in process management to identify key drivers of a process.

System: Regularly interacting or interdependent group of items forming a unified whole.

Systematic Sampling: Method in which, after the first case is randomly selected, every nth element from a population is selected (e.g., picking every third name from a list of possible names).

T

Target Population: The numerator (cases) and denominator (population sample meeting specified criteria) of the measure.

Team: Group of people who are interdependent with respect to information, resources, and skills and who seek to combine their efforts to achieve a common goal.

Teamwork: Dynamic process involving two or more health professionals with complimentary backgrounds and skills, sharing common health goals and exercising concerted physical and mental effort in assessing, planning, or evaluating patient care.

Test-Retest Reliability: Test is administered to a sample on two occasions and then the scores obtained are compared.

Timely Care: Wait times and harmful delays for those who receive and provide care are eliminated.

Total Quality: Attitude or an orientation that permeates an entire organization, and the way that an organization performs its internal and external business. Total quality integrates fundamental management techniques, existing improvement efforts, and the use of technical tools utilizing a disciplined statistical quality control (SQC).

Total Quality Management (TQM): An approach to organizational development and change that ensures that the organization meets or exceeds customer expectations. TQM is a strategic, integrated management system that involves all managers and employees and uses quantitative methods to continuously improve an organization's processes to meet and exceed customer needs, wants, and expectations. The four principles of TQM are: do it right the first time to eliminate costly rework; listen to and learn from customers and employees; make continuous quality improvement an everyday matter; and build teamwork, trust, and mutual respect.

Tracer: A self-assessment methodology designed to "trace" the care experiences that a patient had while at an organization. It is a way to analyze the organization's system of providing care, treatment, or services using actual patients as the framework for assessing standards compliance. Can be individual, system or focused.

Transparency: Communicating and operating in such a way that it is easy for others to see what actions are performed; the full, accurate, and timely disclosure of information. For safe healthcare, such openness and accountability are needed among staff, between caregivers and patients, among institutions, and in public reporting.

Tree Diagram: Method that maps out the full range of paths and tasks that are involved in a process and must be accomplished to achieve a goal; resembles an organizational chart.

Trialability: Degree to which an innovation can be tested/piloted on a small scale.

Triple Aim: Includes better care, smarter spending, and healthier populations. Workforce engagement and workforce safety can be added as a fourth aim.

***t*-test:** Used to analyze the difference between two means to determine whether the difference between them is significant; a distinction must be made regarding the two groups.

U

Underuse: Situation in which patients do not receive beneficial health services (e.g., 65% of people with severe symptoms of depression who are not getting help from a mental health professional).

Usability: This principle checks that users of a measure—employers, patients, providers, hospitals, and health plans—will be able to understand the measure's results and find them useful for quality improvement and decision-making.

Utilization Management: An organized, comprehensive approach to analyze, direct, and conserve organizational resources, to provide care that is high-quality and cost-effective (e.g., medical necessity appropriateness review; discharge planning and monitoring; overutilization and underutilization surveillance; and identification of overutilization and underutilization).

V

Validation: Process by which the integrity and correctness of data are established. Validation processes can occur immediately after a data item is collected or after a complete set of data is collected.

Validity: Degree to which an instrument measures what it is intended to measure. Validity usually is more difficult to establish than reliability.

Value: The value of healthcare is subjective. It weighs costs against the health outcomes achieved, including patient satisfaction and quality of life. Value is the measure of a specified stakeholder's preference-weighted assessment of a particular combination of quality and cost of care performance (e.g., patients, consumer organizations, payers, providers, governments, or societies).

Value Stream Mapping: Map of the process in which only value-added steps for the customer are retained and waste removed. This Lean tool analyzes a process from a systems perspective and creates a visual depiction of the sequential steps in a process from beginning to end.

Values: Statement describes what the organization believes in and how it will behave. It defines the deeply held beliefs and principles of the organizational culture. These core values are an internalized framework that is shared and acted on by leadership.

Variability: Degree to which values on a set of scores differ.

Variation Analysis: Method to identify the contributors to a process that results in consistently inconsistent results. The contributors to variation include clinical factors, patient characteristics, data collection procedures, or organizational attributes like staffing levels.

Vision: An organization's statement of its goals for the future, described in measurable terms that clarify the direction for everyone in the organization. An organization's direction is built upon its mission and is guided, through leadership, by its vision.

Voice of the Customer (VOC): Tool used at the start (or "Fuzzy Front End") of any new product, process, or service design initiative to understand better the customer's wants and needs. The VOC can serve as key input for new product definition, Quality Function Deployment (QFD), or the setting of detailed design specifications.

W

Work Motivation: The psychological forces that determine the *direction* of a person's behavior in an organization, a person's level of *effort,* and a person's level of *persistence.*

BIBLIOGRAPHY

American Psychological Association. The road to resilience: what is resilience? www.apa.org/helpcenter/road-resilience.aspx. Accessed January 14, 2017.

American Society for Quality. Six sigma belts, executives and champions – what does it all mean? http://asq.org/learn-about-quality/six-sigma/overview/belts-executives-champions.html

Baldrige Performance Excellence Program. *2017–2018 Baldrige Excellence Framework: A Systems Approach to Improving Your Organization's Performance.* Gaithersburg, MD: U.S. Department of Commerce, National Institute of Standards and Technology, 2017:p. 43. https://www.nist.gov/baldrige

Becher EC, Chassin MR. Improving the quality of healthcare: who will lead? *Health Affairs.* 2001;20:164–179. doi:10.1377/hlthaff.20.5.164

Begun J, Zimmerman B, Dooley K. Health care organizations as complex adaptive systems. In: Mick S, Wyttenbach M, eds. *Advances in Health Care Organization Theory.* San Francisco, CA: Jossey-Bass; 2003:253–258.

Berwick DM, Nolan TW, Whittington J. The triple aim: care, health and cost. *Health Affairs.* 2008;27(3):759–769. doi:10.1377/hlthaff.27.3.759

Bodenheimer T, Sinsky C. From triple to quadruple aim: care of the patient requires care of the provider. *Ann Fam Med.* 2014;12(6):573–576.

Business Dictionary. *Goal congruence.* http://www.businessdictionary.com/definition/goal-congruence.html. Accessed January 14, 2017.

Centers for Medicare & Medicaid Services. Glossary; 2006. https://www.cms.gov/apps/glossary/

Centers for Medicare & Medicaid Services. State operations manual: Appendix Q: Guidelines for determining immediate jeopardy; 2004. cms.hhs.gov/Regulations-and-guidance/Guidance/Manuals/downloads//som107ap_q_immedjeopardy.pdf. Accessed January 14, 2017.

Chassin MR, Loeb JM. High-reliability health care: getting there from here. *Milbank Q.* 2013;91(3):459–490.

Christensen CM, Bohmer RMJ, Kenagy J. Will disruptive innovations cure health care? *Harvard Bus Rev.* 2000;78(5):102–112, 199.

CMS Office of the National Coordinator for Health Information Technology (ONC); U.S. Department of Health & Human Services. Glossary of eCQI Terms. https://ecqi.healthit.gov/content/glossary-ecqi-terms

Deming WE. *Out of the Crisis.* Cambridge, MA: MIT Press; 2000.

Donabedian A. *The Definition of Quality and Approaches to Its Assessment.* Ann Arbor, MI: Health Administration Press; 1980:79, 83.

Frampton SB, Guastello S, Hoy L, et al. *Harnessing Evidence and Experience to Change Culture: A Guiding Framework for Patient and Family Engaged Care.* Discussion paper. Washington, DC: National Academy of Medicine; 2017. https://nam.edu/wp-content/uploads/2017/01/Harnessing-Evidence-and-Experience-to-Change-Culture-A-Guiding-Framework-for-Patient-and-Family-Engaged-Care.pdf. Accessed April 17, 2017.

George JM, Jones GR. *Organizational Behavior.* 3rd ed. Upper Saddle River, NJ: Prentice Hall; 2002.

Grout JR. Mistake-proofing the design of health care processes (AHRQ Publication No. 07-P0020). Rockville, MD: Agency for Healthcare Research and Quality; 2007, May. www.ahrq.gov/qual/mistakeproof/mistakeproofing.pdf

Institute of Medicine, Committee on Quality of Health Care in America. *Crossing the Quality Chasm: A New Health System for the 21st Century.* Washington, DC: National Academies Press; 2001.

Institute of Medicine, Roundtable on Evidence-Based Medicine. *The Learning Healthcare System: Workshop Summary.* Washington, DC: National Academies Press; 2007.

Institute of Medicine. *Medicare: A Strategy for Quality Assurance* (Vol. 2). Washington, DC: National Academy Press; 2000:128–129.

Institute of Medicine. *Clinical Practice Guidelines We Can Trust.* Washington, DC: The National Academies Press; 2011. http://www.iom. edu/Reports/2011/Clinical-Practice-Guidelines-We-Can-Trust. aspx. Accessed May 2, 2017.

Juran JM. *Juran on Leadership for Quality: An Executive Handbook.* New York: Free Press; 1989.

Kaiser Family Foundation. Health Reform Glossary; 2017. http:// www.kff.org/glossary/health-reform-glossary/

Kaplan R, Norton D. Using the balanced scorecard as a strategic management system. *Harvard Bus Rev.* 1996;74:75–85.

Kavaler F, Spiegel A. *Risk Management in Health Care Institutions: A Strategic Approach.* Sudbury, MA: Jones & Bartlett; 1997.

Kindig DA, Stoddart G. What is population health? *Am J Public Health.* 2003;93:380–383.

Latino Health Coalition for a Healthy California. Social and economic opportunity. http://www.lchc.org/health-equity-resources-data/ social-economic-opportunity/equitable-health-care-access/

Lewis N. Populations, population health, and the evolution of population management: making sense of the terminology in US health care today; 2014. http://www.ihi.org/communities/ blogs/_layouts/15/ihi/community/blog/itemview.aspx?List=-81ca4a47-4ccd-4e9e-89d9-14d88ec59e8d&ID=50. Accessed May 24, 2017.

McGlynn EA. Identifying, categorizing, and evaluating health care efficiency measures. Final Report (prepared by the Southern California Evidence-based Practice Center—RAND Corporation, under Contract No. 282-00-0005-21). AHRQ Publication No. 08-0030. Rockville, MD: Agency for Healthcare Research and Quality; 2008.

Merrriam-Webster. Accredit. https://www.merriamwebster.com/ thesaurus/accreditation. Accessed January 15, 2017.

Merriam-Webster. Best practice. https://www.merriam-webster.com/ dictionary/best practice. Accessed January 22, 2017.

Merriam-Webster. Certify. https://www.merriam-webster.com/ dictionary/certify. Accessed January 15, 2017.

Merriam-Webster. Compliance. https://www.merriam-webster.com/ dictionary/compliance. Accessed January 15, 2017.

Merriam-Webster. Culture. https://www.merriam-webster.com/ dictionary/culture. Accessed January 15, 2017.

Merriam-Webster. System. https://www.merriam-webster.com/ dictionary/system. Accessed January 15, 2017.

National Institutes of Health. What is big data? 2015. https://data-science.nih.gov/bd2k/about/what. Accessed May 16, 2017.

National Patient Safety Foundation. RCA[2] Improving root cause analyses and actions to prevent harm (Version 2); 2016. http://www. npsf.org/?page=RCA2. Accessed April 17, 2017.

National Quality Forum. Phrase book: a plain language guide to NQF jargon. http://public.qualityforum.org/NQFDocuments/ Phrasebook.pdf

Pelletier LR, Stichler JE. Patient-centered care and engagement: nurse leaders' imperative for health reform. *J Nurs Admin.* 2014;44(9): 473–480. doi:10.1097/NNA.0000000000000102, p. 473.

Quality Measurement and Management Project. *Hospital Quality-Related Data: Recommendations for Appropriate Data Requests, Analysis, and Utilization.* Chicago: American Hospital Association; 1991.

Rao MV. Project Management - CPM/PERT. Guru Gobind Singh Educational Society's Technical Campus; 2016. https://www.slide-share.net/annaprasad/project-management-cpmpert-61847309. Accessed June 3, 2016.

Resar R, Griffin FA, Haraden C, Nolan TW. *Using Care Bundles to Improve Health Care Quality.* IHI Innovation Series white paper. Cambridge, MA: Institute for Healthcare Improvement; 2012. http:// www.ihi.org/resources/Pages/IHIWhitePapers/UsingCareBundles. aspx. Accessed May 2, 2017.

ReVelle JB. *Quality Essentials: A Reference Guide from A to Z.* Milwaukee, WI: ASQ Quality Press; 2004.

Robbins SP. *Organizational Behavior.* 8th ed. Upper Saddle River, NJ: Prentice Hall; 2001.

Rogers EM. *Diffusion of Innovations* (4th ed.). New York: The Free Press; 1995.

Rokeach M. *The Nature of Human Values.* New York: Free Press; 1973.

Sackett D, Rosenberg WMC, Muir-Gray JA, Haynes RB, Richardson WS. Evidence-based medicine: what it is and what it isn't. *Br Med J.* 1996;312(13):71–72. doi:10.1136/bmj.312.7023.71

Safer Healthcare. Checklists: a critical patient safety tool & guide. http://www.saferhealthcare.com/high-reliability-topics/checklists/. Accessed February 16, 2017.

Senge PM. *The Fifth Discipline: The Art and Practice of the Learning Organization.* New York: Doubleday; 1990.

Shook J. *A3 templates from Lean Enterprise Institute.* Cambridge, MA: Lean Enterprise Institute; 2010. http://www.lean.org/common/display/?o=1314

Shortell SM, Morrison E, Robbins S. Strategy-making in health care organizations: a framework and agenda for research. *Med Care Rev.* 1985;2:219–266. doi:10.1177/107755878504200203, p. 220.

Sikka R, Morath JM, Leape L. The quadruple aim: care, health, cost, and meaning in work. *BMJ Qual Saf Online;* 2015. http://quali-tysafety.bmj.com/content/qhc/24/10/608.full.pdf. Accessed April 17, 2017.

Society for Human Resource Management. Mission & Vision Statements: What is the difference between mission, vision and values statements? 2012. https://www.shrm.org/ResourcesAndTools/tools-and-samples/ hr-qa/Pages/Isthereadifferencebetweenacompany%E2%80%99 smission,visionandvaluestatements.aspx

Stamatis DH. *Total Quality Management in Healthcare: Implementation Strategies for Optimum Results.* Chicago: Irwin; 1996:58.

The Advisory Board Company. *The Journey to Zero: Innovative Strategies for Minimizing Hospital-Acquired Infections.* Washington, DC: Author; 2008.

The Joint Commission. Sentinel event policy and procedure. https://www.jointcommission.org/sentinel_event_policy_and_ procedures/. Accessed January 27, 2017.

The Joint Commission. Sentinel event policy and procedure. https:// www.jointcommission.org/sentinel_event_policy_and_procedures/. Accessed January 27, 2017.

The Joint Commission. The SAFER™ Matrix: A new scoring methodology. *Joint Comm Perspect.* 2016;36(5). https://www.jointcommis-sion.org/assets/1/6/SAFER_Matrix_New_Scoring_Methodology. pdf. Accessed January 13, 2017.

The Joint Commission. The SAFER™ Matrix and changes to the post-survey process; 2016. https://www.jointcommission.org/assets/1/18/The_Safer_Matirx_and_Changes_to_Post_Survey_Process.pdf. Accessed January 13, 2017.

The Joint Commission, Joint Commission International, World Health Organization. Patient safety solutions preamble; 2007. http://www.who.int/patientsafety/solutions/patientsafety/Preamble.pdf. Accessed April 17, 2017.

Thompson L. *Making the Team: A Guide for Managers.* Upper Saddle River, NJ: Prentice Hall; 2000.

U.S. Department of Health & Human Services, Office of the National Coordinator. Interoperability basics: defining interoperability; 2015. https://www.healthit.gov/providers-professionals/implementation-resources/interoperability-basics-training

U.S. Environmental Protection Agency. Lean Manufacturing and Environment, November 10, 2011. http://www.epa.gov/lean/environment/methods/fives.htm

Watkins MD. What is organizational culture? And why should we care? *Harvard Bus Rev.* May 15, 2013. https://hbr.org/2013/05/what-is-organizational-culture

World Health Organization. Patient safety checklists. http://www.who.int/patientsafety/implementation/checklists/en/. Accessed April 17, 2017.

Xyrichis A, Ream E. Teamwork: a concept analysis. *J Adv Nurs.* 2008;61:232–241. doi/10.1111/j.1365-2648.2007

Index

Note: Page numbers followed by "f" indicate figures; those followed by "t" indicate tables.